MEDICAL MANAGEMENT OF TYPE 1 DIABETES

SEVENTH EDITION

Cecilia C. Low Wang, MD, FACP

Avni C. Shah, MD

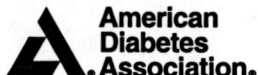

American Diabetes Association.

Director, Book Publishing, Abe Ogden; *Managing Editor,* Rebekah Renshaw; *Acquisitions Editor,* Victor Van Beuren; *Project Manager,* Lauren Wilson; *Production Manager and Composition,* Melissa Sprott; *Cover Design,* Jody Billert; *Printer,* LightningSource.

Printed in the United States of America
1 3 5 7 9 10 8 6 4 2

The suggestions and information contained in this publication are generally consistent with the *Standards of Medical Care in Diabetes* and other policies of the American Diabetes Association, but they do not represent the policy or position of the Association or any of its boards or committees. Reasonable steps have been taken to ensure the accuracy of the information presented. However, the American Diabetes Association cannot ensure the safety or efficacy of any product or service described in this publication. Individuals are advised to consult a physician or other appropriate health care professional before undertaking any diet or exercise program or taking any medication referred to in this publication. Professionals must use and apply their own professional judgment, experience, and training and should not rely solely on the information contained in this publication before prescribing any diet, exercise, or medication. The American Diabetes Association—its officers, directors, employees, volunteers, and members—assumes no responsibility or liability for personal or other injury, loss, or damage that may result from the suggestions or information in this publication.

♾ The paper in this publication meets the requirements of the ANSI Standard Z39.48-1992 (permanence of paper).

American Diabetes Association titles may be purchased for business or promotional use or for special sales. To purchase more than 50 copies of this book at a discount, or for custom editions of this book with your logo, contact the American Diabetes Association at the address below or at booksales@diabetes.org.

American Diabetes Association
2451 Crystal Drive, Suite 900
Arlington, VA 22202

DOI: 10.2337/9781580406307

Library of Congress Cataloging-in-Publication Data
Names: Low Wang, Cecilia C., editor. | Shah, Avni C., editor. | American Diabetes Association, publisher.
Title: Medical management of type 1 diabetes / [edited by] Cecilia C. Low Wang and Avni C. Shah.
Other titles: Medical management of type one diabetes
Description: 7th edition. | Alexandria : American Diabetes Association, [2016] | Includes bibliographical references and index.
Identifiers: LCCN 2016016080 | ISBN 9781580406307 (alk. paper)
Subjects: | MESH: Diabetes Mellitus, Type 1
Classification: LCC RC660 | NLM WK 810 | DDC 616.4/6206--dc23
LC record available at https://lccn.loc.gov/2016016080

Contents

Special Situations   163

A Word about This Guide

Type 1 diabetes is a life-changing diagnosis. The disease impacts every decision about food, activity, and medication that a patient makes, and though it may not be obvious to others, it is always lurking in the background for individuals with diabetes. This is the 7th edition of the American Diabetes Association's *Medical Management of Type 1 Diabetes*. What is known and what is being investigated in the field of diabetes management continues to expand rapidly. We have carefully reviewed the previous edition of this book, updated and overhauled every section, and added in a few new ones, while soliciting the expert input of our contributors who so generously volunteered their time and expertise. We present to you what we hope are practical and useful strategies for the management of all of the key aspects of type 1 diabetes throughout the continuum of human development—from childhood through old age. Interacting with patients who have taken on the challenge of diabetes management and have refused to allow a diagnosis of type 1 diabetes to limit their potential continues to inspire us. We wish you the best as you help your patients with type 1 diabetes successfully navigate their way through life with this often challenging disease.

Contributors to the Seventh Edition

EDITORS

Cecilia C. Low Wang, MD, FACP
University of Colorado School of
Medicine
  Division of Endocrinology,
  Metabolism, and Diabetes
Aurora, CO

Avni C. Shah, MD
Stanford University
  Division of Endocrinology and
  Diabetes
Stanford, CA

CONTRIBUTORS

Barry P. Conrad, MPH, RD, CDE
Stanford University
  Division of Endocrinology and
  Diabetes
Stanford, CA

Daniel DeSalvo, MD
Baylor College of Medicine/
Texas Children's Hospital
  Section of Pediatric Diabetes and
  Endocrinology
Houston, TX

Thomas J. Jensen, MD
University of Colorado School of
Medicine
  Division of Endocrinology,
  Metabolism, and Diabetes
Aurora, CO

Trang Ly, MBBS, FRACP, PhD
Stanford Univeristy
  Division of Endocrinology and
  Diabetes
Stanford, CA

Aaron W. Michels, MD
University of Colorado School of
Medicine
  Barbara Davis Center for Diabetes
Aurora, CO

Diana Naranjo, PhD
Stanford University Dept. of Medicine
  Division of Child and Adolescent
  Psychiatry and Child Development
Stanford, CA

Sarit Polsky, MD, MPH
University of Colorado School of
Medicine
  Barbara Davis Center for Diabetes
Aurora, CO

Irene E. Schauer, MD, PhD
University of Colorado School of
Medicine
  Division of Endocrinology,
  Metabolism, and Diabetes
Aurora, CO

Emily B. Schroeder, MD, PhD
Institute for Health Research, Kaiser
Permanente Colorado
Denver, CO

**Stacey A. Seggelke, RN, MS,
ACNS-BC, CB-ADM**
University of Colorado School of
Medicine
  Division of Endocrinology,
  Metabolism, and Diabetes
Aurora, CO

Acknowledgments

C ecilia C. Low Wang and Avni C. Shah would like to acknowledge the colleagues who contributed their time and expertise to this edition of *Medical Management of Type 1 Diabetes* and the peer reviewers and staff at the American Diabetes Association. Cecilia is grateful for her mentors, colleagues, and patients, and the unending support from Michael and Maia. Avni would also like to acknowledge her mentors, colleagues, patients, and family—Rajiv, Lila, and Diya.

Diagnosis and Classification/Pathogenesis

Highlights

Highlights
Diagnosis and
Classification/Pathogenesis

CLASSIFICATION AND DIAGNOSIS

- Diabetes can be classified into the following general categories:
  1. Type 1 diabetes (due to β-cell destruction, usually leading to absolute insulin deficiency)
  2. Type 2 diabetes (due to a progressive loss of insulin secretion on the background of insulin resistance)
  3. Gestational diabetes mellitus (GDM) (diabetes diagnosed in the second or third trimester of pregnancy that is not clearly overt diabetes)
  4. Specific types of diabetes due to other causes, e.g., monogenic diabetes syndromes (such as neonatal diabetes and maturity-onset diabetes of the young [MODY]), diseases of the exocrine pancreas (such as cystic fibrosis), and drug- or chemical-induced diabetes (such as with glucocorticoid use, in the treatment of HIV/AIDS or after organ transplantation)
- Type 1 diabetes and type 2 diabetes are heterogeneous diseases in which clinical presentation and disease progression may vary considerably. Classification is important for determining therapy, but some individuals cannot be clearly classified as having type 1 or type 2 diabetes at the time of diagnosis.

- Criteria for screening for presence of diabetes:
  - By clinical symptoms:
    - obvious signs and symptoms of diabetes (polydipsia, polyuria, polyphagia, weight loss)
    - an incomplete clinical picture, such as glucosuria or equivocal elevation of random plasma glucose level or A1C
  - Other criteria:
    - age ≥45 years (typically for type 2 diabetes)
    - body mass index (BMI) ≥25 kg/m^2 or ≥23 kg/m^2 in Asian Americans and one or more additional risk factors for diabetes (typically for type 2 diabetes)
    - consider in children and adolescents who are overweight or obese and who have two or more additional risk factors for diabetes
    - relatives of patients with type 1 diabetes but only in the setting of a clinical trial (e.g., www.diabetestrialnet.org)
- Diagnosis of diabetes
  - typically when diabetes is fully evolved,
    - 8-h fasting plasma glucose levels are ≥126 mg/dL (>7.0 mmol/L),
    - 1 random plasma glucose level ≥200 mg/dL (>11.1 mmol/L) with symptoms,

- 2 or more random plasma glucose levels ≥200 mg/dL (>11.1 mmol/L),
- A1C is ≥6.5% (48 mmol/mol). (A1C elevation may not occur in the presence of certain hemoglobinopathies),
- 2-h plasma glucose ≥ 200 mg/dL (11.1mmol/L) during an OGTT (oral glucose tolerance test).
- any one of these criteria, shown twice, would be sufficient for diagnosis of diabetes
- the OGTT is rarely needed to diagnose type 1 diabetes
- delayed diagnosis is a serious, sometimes fatal, problem, especially among younger children
  - approximately 30% of children who present with newly diagnosed type 1 diabetes are ill with diabetic ketoacidosis; those <3 years of age are at highest risk, and may die from rapid metabolic decompensation and/or delayed diagnosis due to lack of suspicion of diabetes.
- type 1 diabetes generally presents with unequivocal hyperglycemia, although natural history studies, such as the Diabetes Prevention Trial of Type 1 (DPT-1) and the multinational TrialNet study, have shown that onset can be indolent and early diabetes can be relatively asymptomatic.
- Type 1 diabetes accounts for 5–10% of diabetes. Type 1 diabetes remains the most common form of diabetes in childhood, accounting for approximately three-quarters of new diagnoses of diabetes in patients ≤18 years of age in the U.S., despite the increasing rate of type 2 diabetes.

- The highest prevalence of type 1 diabetes is seen in non-Hispanic white youth, followed by African American, Hispanic, Asian-Pacific Islanders, and American Indian youth (2.55, 1.62, 1.29, 0.6, and 0.35 cases per 1,000 children 0–19 years old, respectively).
- The age of presentation of childhood onset type 1 diabetes has a bimodal distribution, with one peak at 4–6 years of age and a second in early puberty (10–14 years of age). Overall, about 45% of children present before 10 years of age. Incidence is similar in males and females. Type 1 diabetes has been increasing 3–4% per year in children and youth, and even more in young children under the age of 5 years.

CLINICAL PRESENTATION OF TYPE 1 DIABETES

- Fasting hyperglycemia occurs when β-cell mass is reduced by 80–90%. Typical symptoms of diabetes (i.e., polyuria, polydipsia) appear once hyperglycemia exceeds the renal threshold of ~180 mg/dL (~10.0 mmol/L) glucose.
- After diagnosis and correction of acute metabolic abnormalities, some individuals experience a "remission" or "honeymoon" phase, a temporary period when there is preservation of endogenous insulin secretion as determined by C-peptide levels, the need for exogenous insulin is diminished, glycemic control is improved, and glycemic variability is reduced. Multiple interventions have been studied to preserve β-cell function, but none has been shown to be effective in reversing the autoimmune destruction of β-cells.

PATHOGENESIS

- The primary defect in type 1 diabetes is inadequate insulin secretion by pancreatic β-cells.
- Genetic predisposition, which can be determined by the presence of certain genetic alleles (HLA-DR/DQ alleles can be either predisposing or protective), clearly plays a role in the development of type 1 diabetes. However, a host of environmental triggers, including infectious agents and food antigens, may be involved in initiating the autoimmune process, which is initially detected by the presence of autoantibodies to islet cell components (GAD, GAD65, or GADA; ICA512 or IA-2A, zinc transporter 8 or ZnT8A, and insulin autoantibodies or IAA). This is followed over months to years by the progressive loss of insulin secretion due to β-cell destruction, particularly in those with persistent, multiple autoantibodies.
- Within 5–10 years after clinical presentation, β-cell loss is significant, C-peptide secretion is low to undetectable, and circulating islet cell antibodies might not be detected. The diminution of antibodies may be attributable to loss of antigenic stimuli.

Diagnosis and Classification/Pathogenesis

Diabetes is a chronic disorder that is *1*) characterized by hyperglycemia; *2*) associated with major abnormalities in carbohydrate, fat, and protein metabolism; and *3*) accompanied by a propensity to develop relatively specific forms of renal, ocular, neurologic, and premature cardiovascular diseases. Diabetes encompasses a wide clinical spectrum, and the classification consists of four main categories including gestational diabetes mellitus (GDM) and specific types of diabetes due to other causes. However, the vast majority of cases of diabetes fall into two broad etiopathogenetic categories:

- type 1 diabetes, which is due to deficiency of insulin secretion from pancreatic β-cell destruction, and
- type 2 diabetes, which is due to a combination of resistance to insulin action and inadequate compensatory insulin secretion.

Diabetes may also occur because of conditions such as diseases of the exocrine pancreas (including cystic fibrosis), endocrinopathies (including Cushing's syndrome and acromegaly), resection, inflammation, or trauma of the pancreas, and use of certain drugs or chemicals (such as glucocorticoids after organ transplantation or drugs for HIV/AIDS). Less commonly, specific genetic defects (such as maturity-onset diabetes of the young [MODY]) and rare monogenic diabetes syndromes (such as neonatal diabetes) may be the etiology for diabetes.

Although type 1 diabetes accounts for ~5–10% of all diagnosed cases of diabetes, its immediate risks and stringent acute treatment requirements demand rapid recognition, early diagnosis, and effective management. This chapter explores characteristics that differentiate type 1 diabetes from other forms of diabetes, discusses criteria for correct diagnosis (Table 1.1), and illustrates various clinical presentations.

CRITERIA FOR DIAGNOSIS

The criteria for diagnosing diabetes include two or more of the following on different days: *1*) fasting (for at least 8 h) plasma glucose concentration ≥126 mg/dL (7.0 mmol/L), *2*) 2-h glucose after a 75-g oral glucose tolerance test (OGTT) ≥200 mg/dL, *3*) A1C ≥6.5%, or *4*) random plasma glucose level ≥200 mg/dL (11.1 mmol/L) in the presence of classic signs and/or symptoms of diabetes including polyuria, polydipsia, and unexplained weight loss, or hyperglycemic crisis. Unless

Table 1.1   Criteria for Diagnosis of Diabetes

Diagnosis of diabetes in nonpregnant patients should be restricted to those who have one of the following:

■ Symptoms of diabetes plus casual plasma glucose concentration greater than or equal to 200mg/dL (11.1 mmol/L). The classic symptoms of diabetes include polyuria, polydipsia, and unexplained weight loss. Casual refers to any time of day without regard to time since last meal.

or

■ Fasting plasma glucose greater than or equal to 126mg/dL (7.0 mmol/L). Fasting is defined as no caloric intake for at least 8 h.

or

■ 2-h plasma glucose greater than or equal to 200 mg/dL (11.1 mmol/L) during an oral glucose tolerance test (OGTT).* The test should be performed using a glucose load containing the equivalent of 75 g anhydrous glucose dissolved in water.

or

■ A1C greater than or equal to 6.5% in a laboratory using a method that is NGSP certified and standardized to the DCCT (Diabetes Control and Complications Trial) assay.

In the absence of unequivocal hyperglycemia with acute metabolic decompensation, these criteria should be confirmed by repeat testing on a different day.

*An OGTT is rarely needed to diagnose type 1 diabetes and is not recommended for routine clinical use.

there is a clear clinical diagnosis (meeting criterion number 4), a second test is required to confirm the diagnosis of diabetes.

The clinical signs and/or symptoms that accompany diabetes are due to persistent hyperglycemia and include polyuria, polydipsia, fatigue, polyphagia, weight loss, and blurred vision. If there is ketosis or ketoacidosis, then abdominal pain, vomiting, dehydration, and/or altered level of consciousness can occur. In the young child or infant, these signs or symptoms are frequently missed until the child presents as significantly ill due to ketoacidosis associated with dehydration, acidosis, and/or develops a severe candidal diaper rash.

An elevated glycated hemoglobin (A1C) confirms the presence of significant preexisting hyperglycemia (barring the presence of a hemoglobin variant). Prediabetes (previously known as impaired glucose tolerance or impaired fasting glucose), as distinguished from diabetes, refers to abnormal plasma glucose values that do not meet the established criteria to diagnose diabetes. Screening for prediabetes is generally reserved for those with risk factors for type 2 diabetes; however, prediabetes may be seen prior to the onset of type 1 diabetes due to autoimmune destruction of the β-cell mass. This has been observed in the context of research protocols in which high-risk relatives undergo screening and close follow-up (such as TrialNet; www.trialnet.org). As clinical type 1 diabetes is preceded by an asymptomatic phase that can be identified by serum islet autoantibodies, the possibility of broader screening of islet autoantibodies as biomarkers of impending type 1 diabetes has been proposed.

DISTINGUISHING TYPE 1 DIABETES FROM OTHER FORMS

Type 1 Diabetes

Type 1 diabetes can develop at any age. Although most cases are diagnosed before the patient is 20 years old, it also occurs in older individuals. Because patients with type 1 diabetes are insulinopenic, insulin therapy is essential to prevent rapid and severe dehydration, catabolism, ketoacidosis, and death (Table 1.2). Patients who are diagnosed with symptoms are usually lean and have experienced significant weight loss, polyuria, polydipsia, and fatigue before presentation. Some patients are diagnosed without any or with more subtle symptoms and they may be overweight, reflecting the secular trend of increasing obesity among adults and children. At presentation, there is often significant elevation of A1C levels, providing evidence of weeks, if not months, of hyperglycemia. In addition, 85–90% have circulating autoantibodies directed against one or more islet cell components (islet cell autoantibodies—typically multiple autoantibodies, autoantibodies to insulin [IAA], GAD [also called GAD65 or GADA], tyrosine phosphatases IA-2A [ICA512] and IA-2B, and zinc transporter 8 [ZnT8]). C-peptide levels, which typically fall to undetectable levels over time, may be in the low normal range at diagnosis. Profound insulinopenia occurs even though the pancreas from patients with long-standing type 1 diabetes shows that most retain some islet tissue, while others have a pattern of lobular destruction with destroyed and normal-appearing islets.

Distinguishing Characteristics

Type 1 diabetes and type 2 diabetes are heterogeneous diseases in which clinical presentation and disease progression may vary considerably. Classification is important for determining therapy, but some individuals cannot be clearly classified as having type 1 or type 2 diabetes at the time of diagnosis. The traditional paradigms of type 2 diabetes occurring only in adults and type 1 diabetes only in children are no longer accurate, as both diseases occur in both cohorts. Occasionally, patients with type 2 diabetes may present with diabetic ketoacidosis (DKA). Children with type 1 diabetes typically present with the hallmark symptoms of polyuria/polydipsia and approximately one-third with DKA. The onset of type 1 diabetes may be more variable in adults, and they may not present with the classic symptoms seen in children. Although difficulties in distinguishing diabetes type may occur in all age-groups at onset, the true diagnosis becomes more obvious over time.

Patients with secondary and other types of diabetes have certain associated conditions or syndromes (see Table 1.3).

Patients with gestational diabetes mellitus have onset or discovery of glucose intolerance during the second or third trimester of pregnancy, whereas women meeting the criteria for diagnosis of diabetes during the first trimester of pregnancy are classified as having preexisting diabetes (usually type 2).

Type 2 Diabetes

In contrast, patients with type 2 diabetes are less likely to develop ketoacidosis unless severely stressed physiologically, are generally but not always obese, may

Table 1.2 Distinguishing Characteristics of the Major Types of Diabetes

Diabetes can be classified into the following general categories:

1. Type 1 diabetes—due to β-cell destruction, usually leading to absolute insulin deficiency, autoimmune etiology
   —Idiopathic—no known etiologies. Permanent insulinopenia and are prone to ketoacidosis, but have no evidence of β-cell autoimmunity
   —Latent Autoimmune Diabetes in Adults (LADA)—gradual-onset antibody-positive diabetes in adults. Controversy exists as to whether LADA and adult-onset type 1 diabetes are the same clinical entity.

2. Type 2 diabetes—due to a progressive loss of insulin secretion on the background of insulin resistance

3. Gestational diabetes mellitus (GDM)—diabetes diagnosed in the second or third trimester of pregnancy that is not clearly overt diabetes

4. Specific types of diabetes due to other causes, e.g., monogenic diabetes syndromes (such as neonatal diabetes and maturity-onset diabetes of the young [MODY]), diseases of the exocrine pancreas (such as cystic fibrosis), and drug- or chemical-induced diabetes (such as with glucocorticoid use, in the treatment of HIV/AIDS or after organ transplantation)

be asymptomatic or only mildly symptomatic, and usually have a family history of diabetes. Once referred to as adult-onset diabetes, type 2 diabetes has emerged in youth as a consequence of the worldwide increase in childhood obesity. Type 2 diabetes generally presents after age 30, but an increasing number of obese adolescents and young adults have been developing type 2 diabetes, especially among African Americans, American Indians/Native Alaskans, Hispanics, and Asian/Pacific Islanders. Note that some of these patients present in ketoacidosis, or with hyperosmolar nonketotic coma, both of which can be fatal. The discrimination between type 2 and type 1 diabetes is becoming increasingly difficult in many cases, as patients with a type 2 phenotype may present in ketoacidosis but later become insulin-independent. Conversely, more type 1 patients are overweight or obese at the time of presentation.

Patients with type 2 diabetes are not absolutely dependent on exogenous insulin for survival, although insulin therapy is often used to lower blood glucose levels, since there appears to be progressive β-cell failure in type 2 diabetes as well (Table 1.2). The development of type 2 diabetes in youth has significant public health consequences. The TODAY (Treatment Options for Type 2 Diabetes in Adolescents and Youth) Study demonstrated that type 2 diabetes may have a much more aggressive course in youth, with early and rapid deterioration of β-cell function and faster progression to diabetes complications.

Not Quite Type 1 or Type 2 Diabetes

For some patients the diagnosis of type 1 versus type 2 diabetes is more challenging. The routinely available laboratory tests that help differentiate between the two types are serum C-peptide levels and measurements of autoantibodies to islet cell components; however, even these tests can be problematic. Although almost all patients with long-standing type 1 diabetes will have C-peptide values below the lower limit of normal for that assay method, with most being undetectable, at diagnosis, C-peptide may be in the normal range while there is still a viable β-cell mass. Approximately 15% of patients with clinical type 1 diabetes do not have autoantibodies at the time of diagnosis. Ten to fifteen percent of youth with clinical type 2 diabetes do have autoantibodies. There are numerous names being used for children who clinically appear to have type 2 diabetes but have autoantibodies, such as double diabetes, type 1.5 diabetes, or type 1 diabetes with insulin resistance (what we prefer). Although not routinely used in the clinical arena, markers of insulin resistance, such as adiponectin—which is elevated in type 1 and decreased in type 2—and lipoprotein concentrations, may help differentiate between diabetes types.

With absent availability of measurement of autoantibodies or C-peptide, if a patient is <20 years old, not obese, and has signs and symptoms of diabetes and an elevated fasting plasma glucose, the physician should assume type 1 diabetes and treat with insulin. The presence of moderate ketonuria with hyperglycemia in an otherwise unstressed individual strongly supports a diagnosis of type 1 diabetes, whereas absent or modest ketonuria is of no diagnostic value.

Clinicians should also be aware that in some cases, typically with adults, patients initially diagnosed with type 2 diabetes may subsequently be discovered to have antibody-positive, insulin-requiring diabetes (i.e., type 1 diabetes). In these individuals, autoantibodies to islet cell components may indicate the eventual need for insulin therapy. These patients are usually lean, and their insulin requirements increase as they develop manifestations of complete insulin deficiency. The condition has been referred to as Latent Autoimmune Diabetes in Adults (LADA) and studies suggest that genes associated with type 1 and type 2 diabetes coexist in these patients. It remains unclear whether LADA is *1*) a late manifestation of type 1 diabetes, *2*) an amalgamation of type 1 and type 2 diabetes, or *3*) a completely separate and distinct form of diabetes.

In contrast, occasionally some adolescents and young adults who initially present with typical signs and symptoms of type 1 diabetes, particularly ketosis, later require no or only intermittent insulin treatment. Commonly referred to as idiopathic type 1 diabetes or ketosis-prone diabetes mellitus, this occurs mainly in obese African Americans with a strong family history of diabetes, negative autoimmune markers, and lack of genetic association with human leukocyte antigen (HLA) markers. At presentation, they have markedly impaired insulin secretion, but intensified diabetes management results in significant improvement in β-cell function and eventual discontinuation of insulin therapy in many cases.

Table 1.3 illustrates specific conditions often associated with other forms of diabetes and glucose intolerance. Further studies are required to determine the pathophysiology of these conditions.

Genetic Defects Presenting with Childhood Onset

Several forms of diabetes are associated with monogenetic defects in β-cell function. These forms of diabetes are frequently characterized by onset of mild hyperglycemia at an early age, generally before the age of 25 years with no signs related to the autoimmune process or insulin resistance. They were formerly referred to as maturity-onset diabetes of the young (MODY), and are characterized by impaired insulin secretion with minimal or no defects in insulin action. However the term "MODY," which was introduced several decades ago, actually referred to a heterogeneous group of disorders that included monogenic diabetes, cases of what we now term type 2 diabetes occurring in childhood or adolescence, and rare forms of diabetes resulting from mitochondrial defects or mutations of the insulin receptor. MODY currently refers to monogenic diabetes, which is inherited in an autosomal-dominant pattern. MODY 3 (HNF1-alpha or HNF1A) is reported to be the most common form of monogenic diabetes, accounting for up to 5% of diabetes cases diagnosed prior to age 45 years. MODY patients are commonly misdiagnosed as having type 1 or type 2 diabetes.

Mutations in several genes involved in β-cell development or insulin secretion can cause MODY. MODY-causing genes are still being defined, and their

Table 1.3 Other Specific Types of Diabetes

Genetic Defects of β-Cell Function

Examples: Kir6.2 (KCNJ11), SUR1 (ABCC8) (permanent neonatal diabetes, PNDM); chromosome 12, HNF1A (hepatocytenuclear factor, MODY3); chromosome 7p, glucokinase (MODY2); chromosome 20q, HNF4A gene (MODY1); chromosome 13, in the insulin promoter factor-1 gene (IPF-1, MODY4); chromosome 17, HNF1B (MODY5); chromosome 2, *Neuro*D1 (MODY6)

Genetic Defects in Insulin Action

Examples: type A insulin resistance, leprechaunism, Rabson-Mendenhall syndrome, lipoatrophic diabetes

Diseases of the Exocrine Pancreas

Examples: pancreatitis, trauma or pancreatectomy, neoplasia, cystic fibrosis, hemochromatosis, fibrocalculous pancreatopathy

Endocrinopathies

Examples: acromegaly, Cushing's syndrome, glucagonoma, pheochromocytoma, hyperthyroidism, somatostatinoma, aldosteronoma

Drug- or Chemical-Induced Diabetes

Examples: Vacor, pentamidine, nicotinic acid, glucocorticoids, diazoxide, interferon-α tacrolimus, second-generation antipsychotics, certain protease inhibitors (PIs) and nucleoside reverse transcriptase inhibitors (NRTIs)

Infections

Examples: congenital rubella, cytomegalovirus, HIV

Uncommon Forms of Immune-Mediated Diabetes

Examples: "stiff man" syndrome, anti-insulin receptor antibodies

Genetic Syndromes Sometimes Associated with Diabetes

Examples: Down syndrome, Klinefelter syndrome, Turner syndrome, Wolfram syndrome, Friedreich's ataxia, Huntington's chorea, Laurence-Moon-Bardet-Biedl syndrome, myotonic dystrophy, porphyria, Prader-Willi syndrome

Table 1.4   MODY Subtypes: Gene Mutations, Pathophysiology, and Clinical Characteristics

MODY	Gene	Pathophysiology	Clinical Characteristics
1	HNF4A	Transcription factor; decreased insulin secretion	Rare (5%) neonatal hyperinsulinemia, low triglycerides, tendency for microvascular complications, sensitivity to sulfonylureas
2	GCK	Decreased glucose sensitivity due to phosphorylation defect; decreased glycogen storage	Common (30–50%); increased fasting glucose, increased likelihood of glucose <55 mg/dL on oral glucose tolerance test; mild diabetes that generally does not require anti-diabetes medication
3	HNF1A	Transcription factor; decreased insulin secretion, progressive β-cell damage	Common (30–50%), high penetrance; glycosuria, microvascular complications, sensitivity to sulfonylurea
4	PDX1/ IPF1	Impaired pancreas development; homozygotes experience pancreas agenesis	Rare (1%); mean age at diagnosis 35 years, requires oral anti-diabetes treatment (and insulin)
5	HNF1B	Transcription factor; decreased insulin secretion	Rare (5%); extra pancreatic signs (renal cysts or dysplasia, genital abnormalities in females, azoospermia in males) with diabetes; variable phenotype; requires insulin treatment
6	*NEUROD1*	Abnormal development of β-cell functions	Very rare (<1%); adult-onset diabetes
7	KLF11	Tumor-suppressor gene; decreased glucose sensitivity of β-cells	Very rare (< 1%); phenotype resembling type 2 diabetes
8	CEL	Decreased endocrine and exocrine pancreas functions (pathophysiology?)	Very rare (<1%); typically autosomal dominant diabetes
9	PAX4	Transcription factor affecting apoptosis and proliferation of β-cells	Very rare (<1%); possible ketoacidosis
10	INS	Heterozygous mutation of the insulin gene	Very rare (<1%); diabetes onset before 20 years of age; sulfonylurea or insulin treatment is generally required
11	BLK	Heterozygous mutation affecting insulin secretion	Very rare (<1%); increased penetrance with higher body mass indexes
12	ABCC8	ATP-sensitive potassium channels dysfunction	Very rare (<1%); clinical phenotype is similar to *HNF1A/4A-MODY*
13	KCNJ11	ATP-sensitive potassium channels dysfunction	Very rare (<1%); clinical phenotype is heterogenous

roles in the pathogenesis of diabetes are being investigated. Table 1.4 includes MODY subtypes with associated gene mutations, pathophysiology, and clinical characteristics.

Neonatal diabetes (NDM) is a rare, monogenic form of diabetes that occurs typically in the first 6 months of life. Incidence rates are 1 in 100,000–500,000 live births. Clinically, NDM subgroups include transient (TNDM) and permanent (PNDM). TNDM often develops within the first few weeks of life and remits by a few months of age; however, relapse occurs in 50% of cases, typically in adolescence or adulthood. Low birth weight and failure to thrive may be associated with NDM. PNDM most commonly results from mutations to one of the two subunits of the ATP-sensitive potassium channel of the β-cell: *1*) KCNJ11, which encodes Kir6.2 (inwardly rectifying potassium channel) or *2*) ABCC8, which encodes SUR1 (the type 1 subunit of the sulfonylurea receptor, a member to the ATP-binding cassette transporter family). SUR1 and ABCC8 defects can be treated with oral sulfonylureas, as can MODY 1, 3, and 4. Mutations involving other genes including INS (encoding the preproinsulin molecule) or GCK (encoding glucokinase) can also lead to PNDM.

Point mutations in mitochondrial DNA have been found to be associated with diabetes and deafness. In Wolfram Syndrome (referred to as DIDMOAD), diabetes and deafness are also associated with diabetes insipidus and optic atrophy. There are also unusual causes of diabetes that result from genetically determined abnormalities of insulin action. Leprechaunism and the Rabson-Mendenhall syndrome are two pediatric syndromes that have mutations in the insulin receptor gene with subsequent alterations in insulin receptor function and extreme insulin resistance. The former has characteristic facial features and is usually fatal in infancy, whereas the latter is associated with abnormalities of teeth and nails and pineal gland hyperplasia.

CONCLUSION

Patients with type 1 diabetes are dependent on insulin for as long as they live. Any lean individual <20 years of age with typical signs and symptoms of hyperglycemia accompanied by weight loss should be assumed to have type 1 diabetes. A high index of suspicion is needed to diagnose diabetes in very young children or elderly patients.

BIBLIOGRAPHY

American Diabetes Association. Standards of medical care in diabetes—2016. *Diabetes Care* 2016;39(Suppl. 1):S1–S112

Anik A, Çatlı G, Abacı A, Böber E. Maturity-onset diabetes of the young (MODY): an update. *J Pediatr Endocrinol Metab* 2015;28:251–263

Balasubramanyam A, Garza G, Rodriguez L, Hampe CS, Gaur L, Lernmark A, Maldonado MR. Accuracy and predictive value of classification schemes for ketosis-prone diabetes. *Diabetes Care* 2006;29:2575–2579

Bonifacio E. Predicting type 1 diabetes using biomarkers. *Diabetes Care* 2015;38:989–996

Chiang JL, Kirkman MS, Laffel LM, Peters AL, Type 1 Diabetes Sourcebook Authors. Type 1 diabetes through the life span: a position statement of the American Diabetes Association. *Diabetes Care.* 2014;37:2034–2054

DIAMOND Project Group: Incidence and trends of childhood type 1 diabetes worldwide 1990–1999. *Diabet Med* 2006;23:857–866

Expert Committee on the Diagnosis and Classification of Diabetes Mellitus. Report of the expert committee on the diagnosis and classification of diabetes mellitus. *Diabetes Care* 2003;26(Suppl. 1):S5–S20

Groop LC, Bottazzo GF, Doniach D. Islet cell antibodies identify latent type 1 diabetes in patients aged 35–75 years at diagnosis. *Diabetes* 1986;35:237–41

Lindstrom T, Frystykt J, Hedman CA, Flyvbjerg A, Arnqvist HJ. Elevated circulating adiponectin in type 1 diabetes is associated with long diabetes duration. *Clin Endocrinol* 2006;65:776–782

Michels AW, Eisenbarth GS. Immune intervention in type 1 diabetes. *Semin Immunol* 2011;23:214–219

The National Institute of Diabetes and Digestive and Kidney Diseases. Monogenic forms of diabetes: neonatal diabetes mellitus and MODY. Available from: www.diabetes.niddk.nih.gov/dm/pubs/mody

Naylor RN, Greeley SA, Bell GI, Philipson LH. Genetics and pathophysiology of neonatal diabetes mellitus. *J Diabetes Investig* 2011;2:158–169

Rewers A, Klingensmith G, Davis C, et al. Presence of diabetic ketoacidosis at diagnosis of diabetes mellitus in youth: the SEARCH for Diabetes in Youth Study. *Pediatrics* 2008;121:e1258–e1266

Rosenbloom AL, Silverstein JH, Amemiya S, Zeitler P, Klingensmith GJ. Type 2 diabetes in children and adolescents. *Pediatr Diabetes* 2009;10(Suppl. 12):17–32

SEARCH for Diabetes in Youth Study Group, Liese AD, D'Agostino RB Jr, Hamman RF, Kilgo PD, et al. The burden of diabetes mellitus among US youth: prevalence estimates from the SEARCH for Diabetes in Youth Study. *Pediatrics* 2006;118:1510–1518

Silverstein J, Klingensmith G, Copeland K, et al. Care of children and adolescents with type 1 diabetes: a statement of the American Diabetes Association. *Diabetes Care* 2005;28:186–212

Stenström G, Gottsäter A, Bakhtadze E, Berger B, Sundkvist G. Latent autoimmune diabetes in adults: definition, prevalence, β-cell function, and treatment. *Diabetes* 2005;54(Suppl. 2):S68–S72

Thomas CT, Philipson LH. Update on diabetes classification. *Med Clin North Am* 2015;99:1–16

TODAY Study Group. Lipid and inflammatory cardiovascular risk worsens over 3 years in youth with type 2 diabetes: the TODAY clinical trial. *Diabetes Care* 2013;36:1758–1764

TODAY Study Group. Rapid rise in hypertension and nephropathy in youth with type 2 diabetes: the TODAY clinical trial. *Diabetes Care* 2013;36:1735–1741

TODAY Study Group. Retinopathy in youth with type 2 diabetes participating in the TODAY clinical trial. *Diabetes Care* 2013;36:1772–1774

Vaziri-Sani F, Delli AJ, Elding-Larsson H, et al. A novel triple mix radiobinding assay for the three ZnT8 (ZnT8-RWQ) autoantibody variants in children with newly diagnosed diabetes. *J Immunol Methods* 2011;371:25–37

Wu J, Yang X, Chen B, Xu X. Pancreas β cell regeneration and type 1 diabetes (Review). *Exp Ther Med* 2015;9:653–657

CLINICAL PRESENTATION OF TYPE 1 DIABETES

The presentation of type 1 diabetes covers a broad range, from mild, nonspecific symptoms or no symptoms to coma. In children, establishing the correct diagnosis is often delayed because the presenting symptoms are ascribed to another process. For example, vomiting and lethargy may be felt to be due to gastroenteritis. Because adequate urine output continues as the result of osmotic diuresis, the child is often not considered to be dehydrated and in need of medical care. Polyuria may be incorrectly attributed to urinary tract infection or enuresis; anorexia rather than polyphagia may occur; and fatigue, irritability, weight loss, deterioration of school performance, and secondary enuresis are ascribed to emotional problems. In some cases, "failure to thrive" may be an overlooked indication of diabetes in a young child.

Approximately 75% of cases are diagnosed within 1 month of the onset of symptoms; ~30% of patients with previously undiagnosed type 1 diabetes present in diabetic ketoacidosis (DKA). Delayed diagnosis continues to be a serious and occasionally fatal problem, especially among poor and younger children. DKA rates approach 40% in children under 3 years of age and 60% in children under 2 years of age at diagnosis. The symptoms of polyuria are less obvious in young children and are frequently missed until metabolic decompensation has occurred. These very young children frequently present with severe dehydration, metabolic acidosis, and a clinical history that is inconsistent with the severity of their clinical appearance (e.g., absence of diarrhea or significant vomiting). Because of the delay in the diagnosis of the younger child, the frequency of coma as a presenting feature is considerably greater in children <2 years of age than in older children, adolescents, and adults. In young adults, the presentation is often less acute, although an absolute requirement for insulin becomes evident with time.

CLINICAL ONSET OF DIABETES SYMPTOMS AND METABOLIC DECOMPENSATION

When ongoing destruction has reduced β-cell mass by 80–90%, the individual's insulin secretory capacity becomes insufficient to normally regulate hepatic glucose production (Figure 1.1). Initially, only postprandial hyperglycemia occurs, reflecting a failure to adequately suppress hepatic glucose production during meal absorption together with some decrease in peripheral glucose utilization. As insulin secretion is further compromised, progressive fasting hyperglycemia occurs as a result of increased basal hepatic glucose production and decreased glucose uptake by peripheral tissue. Hyperglycemia per se may further compromise glucose utilization by reducing the number and/or activity of glucose transporters available on both insulin-dependent and non-insulin-dependent tissues, a phenomenon known as "glucose toxicity."

When the plasma glucose concentration exceeds the renal threshold of ~180 mg/dL (10.0 mmol/L), glucosuria results in an osmotic diuresis, generating the classic symptoms of polyuria and a compensatory polydipsia. If untreated, the symptoms usually progress as the hyperglycemia and glucosuria increase. With evolving insulin deficiency, weight loss occurs as body fat and protein stores are reduced because of increased rates of lipolysis and proteolysis, and calories are lost in the urine. With the superimposed metabolic abnormalities of diabetes itself or with a minor viral or bacterial infection, plasma concentrations of glucagon, growth hormone, epinephrine, and cortisol increase. These hormones antagonize insulin's effect, further promoting hepatic glucose production (by stimulating both glycogenolysis and gluconeogenesis), lipolysis, ketogenesis, and proteolysis. As long as fluid intake is sufficient to offset the fluid losses resulting from the combined diuresis of both glucosuria and ketonuria, some individuals can remain compensated for weeks, if not months. Should the individual be unable to consume adequate amounts of fluid as a result of nausea from the ketosis or because of a concurrent illness, rapid and severe losses of both intra- and extracellular fluid and electrolytes can ensue and, in the course of hours, lead to a clinical presentation of severe ketoacidosis.

REMISSION OR HONEYMOON PHASE

At initial presentation with symptomatic hyperglycemia and/or ketosis, circulating insulin concentrations are low, and there is no significant β-cell response to any of the usual insulin secretagogues. Initially, exogenous insulin requirements are relatively large, due not only to the reduced insulin secretion but also to insulin resistance and counterregulatory hormone elevation.

After the correction of dehydration, hyperglycemia, metabolic acidosis, and ketosis, endogenous insulin secretion improves from the residual, albeit small, β-cell population (Figure 1.1). During this time, exogenous insulin requirements may decrease dramatically. During the remission or 'honeymoon period,' which may last for up to 1 year or longer, good metabolic control may be easily achieved with intensive insulin therapy. The need for increasing exogenous insulin replacement is inevitable and should always be anticipated. Evidence from the Diabetes Control and Complications Trial (DCCT) follow-up cohort suggests that intensive insulin therapy from early diagnosis prolongs C-peptide secretion, a measure of endogenous insulin secretion, and thus creates less major hypoglycemia and fewer microvascular complications 10 years after diagnosis. As a result, intensive insulin therapy with strict attention to diet and self-monitoring of blood glucose should be initiated at diagnosis and maintained. Having diabetic ketoacidosis (DKA) at presentation of diabetes adversely affects the remission phase duration. In general, the honeymoon period for children is shorter than it is for adults, whose clinically significant endogenous insulin production is often lost over the course of several years.

PATHOGENESIS

Type 1 diabetes is the immune-mediated form of diabetes resulting from T cell–mediated destruction of β-cells within pancreatic islets. The immune-mediated destruction results in abnormal glucose homeostasis with decreased insulin secretion by pancreatic β-cells. This defect accounts for hyperglycemia, polyuria, polydipsia, weight loss, dehydration, electrolyte disturbance, and ketoacidosis observed in patients presenting for the first time with type 1 diabetes. The capacity of normal pancreatic β-cells to secrete insulin is far in excess of that normally needed to control carbohydrate, fat, and protein metabolism. As a result, clinical onset is preceded by an extensive asymptomatic period during which β-cells are inexorably destroyed. The evolving process of β-cell destruction reaches a point where insufficient insulin is secreted to maintain normal plasma glucose concentrations, which causes the broadly predictable abnormalities in carbohydrate, fat, and protein metabolism characterizing the uncontrolled diabetic condition.

The majority of the discussion in this section focuses on immune-mediated type 1 diabetes. However, some forms of type 1 diabetes have no evidence of autoimmunity or other known etiology and are labeled "idiopathic." Some of these patients have permanent insulin deficiency and are prone to ketoacidosis. Although only a minority of patients with type 1 diabetes fall into the idiopathic category, of those who do, most are of African, Asian, or Hispanic origin. Individuals with this form of diabetes often suffer from episodic ketoacidosis and exhibit varying degrees of insulin deficiency between episodes. This form of diabetes is strongly inherited, lacks immunological evidence for β-cell autoimmunity, and is not associated with human leukocyte antigen (HLA) genes, which confer significant risk for immune-mediated type 1 diabetes development. A requirement for insulin replacement therapy in affected patients may come and go.

PATHOPHYSIOLOGY OF THE CLINICAL ONSET OF TYPE 1 DIABETES

Insulin is the primary hormone that suppresses hepatic glucose production, lipolysis, and proteolysis. It increases the transport of glucose into adipocytes and myocytes and stimulates glycogen synthesis. In the presence of adequate plasma amino acids, insulin maintains or perhaps stimulates whole-body protein anabolism. As such, insulin is the primary hormone of anabolism of meal-derived nutrients (Table 1.5).

In the fasting state, the plasma concentration of glucose is maintained in a narrow range (80–95 mg/dL [4.4–5.3 mmol/L]) by precise regulation of hepatic glucose release and peripheral glucose utilization. Basal plasma insulin concentrations maintain hepatic glucose release at a rate of 1.9–2.1 mg/kg/min (10–12 µmol/L/kg/min). This is of critical importance to provide adequate glucose for the brain, which accounts for nearly 50% of total glucose utilization under these conditions. With prolonged fasting, the plasma insulin concentration decreases even further, permitting increased mobilization of free fatty acids (FFAs) from adipose tissue. The resulting increase in circulating FFA concentration and glucagon, accompanied by a hormonal milieu conducive to ketogenesis, drives hepatic ketogenesis, which results in ketosis. Increased availability of plasma FFAs, β-hydroxybutyrate, and acetoacetate provides alternative metabolic fuels to glucose and reduces the rates of glucose utilization by peripheral tissues and the brain.

After ingestion of a mixed meal (carbohydrates, protein, and fat), nearly 85% of ingested glucose enters the systemic circulation. The increasing arterial glucose concentration stimulates the secretion of insulin into the portal vein. About half of the secreted insulin is extracted by the liver, which signals the suppression of hepatic glucose release. The unextracted insulin enters the systemic circulation, where it stimulates glucose uptake, primarily by muscle and adipose tissue, and decreases lipolysis and proteolysis. This facilitates continuous entry of glucose into the systemic circulation by permitting a switch from endogenous glucose production to exogenous glucose. As dietary glucose entry decreases with the absorption of the meal-derived carbohydrate, plasma glucose decreases, as does the secretion and plasma concentration of insulin. When plasma glucose reaches or even falls slightly below basal concentrations, hepatic glucose production is again increased by both the decrease in plasma insulin and an increase in plasma glucagon concentration (Table 1.5).

Amylin, a glucoregulatory hormone, is produced in the pancreatic β-cell and co-secreted with insulin. Amylin regulates postprandial glucose concentrations by

Table 1.5   Physiological Effects of High- vs. Low-Insulin States

	High-Insulin (Fed) State	Low-Insulin (Fasted) State
Liver	Glucose uptake	Glucose production
	Glycogen synthesis	Glycogenolysis
	Lipogenesis	Absent lipogenesis
	Absent ketogenesis	Ketogenesis
	Absent gluconeogenesis	Gluconeogenesis
Muscle	Glucose uptake	Absent glucose uptake
	Glucose oxidation	Fatty acid, ketone oxidation
	Glycogen synthesis	Glycogenolysis
	Sustained protein synthesis	Proteolysis and amino acid release
Adipose tissue	Glucose uptake	Absent glucose uptake
	Lipid synthesis	Lipolysis and fatty acid release
	Triglyceride uptake	Absent triglyceride uptake

slowing gastric emptying, suppressing postprandial glucagon secretion, and reducing food intake. Amylin complements the effects of insulin, and both act together to regulate postprandial glucose concentrations. Type 1 diabetes is considered an amylin-deficient state.

PROGRESSION OF METABOLIC ABNORMALITIES DURING ONSET

The insulin secretory reserves of the normal pancreas are considerable. Therefore, individuals destined to develop type 1 diabetes go through a variable interval of months to years of autoimmune β-cell destruction before abnormalities in insulin secretion or glucose metabolism can be detected (Figure 1.1). During this time period, amylin secretion is also diminished and then lost.

The earliest detectable abnormality in insulin secretion is a progressive reduction of the immediate (first-phase) plasma insulin response during intravenous glucose tolerance testing. This impairment alone has little deleterious effect on overall glucose homeostasis: fasting plasma glucose concentrations remain normal, and the response to an oral glucose tolerance test (OGTT) is virtually unimpaired. At this stage of the disease, most affected individuals have circulating autoantibodies in their serum directed against their own insulin (IAA) and to other β-cell proteins (e.g., glutamic acid decarboxylase [GAD], islet tyrosine phosphatases [IA-2A], and zinc transporter 8 [ZnT8A]). These are markers of an ongoing autoimmune process, termed islet autoimmunity, which precede the development of clinical type 1 diabetes. There can be variability in the autoantibody pattern during the years prior to diagnosis; however, most individuals will develop multiple autoantibodies within a short time frame (months) and approximately 90% of all patients with type 1 diabetes have islet autoantibodies. Insulin autoantibodies, IAA, are more prevalent in young children, while adult-onset type 1 diabetes is typically characterized by GAD and IA-2A. The presence and then persistence of two or more autoantibodies is highly predictive for the development of type 1 diabetes (Figure 1.1). Given enough time, nearly 100% of children with two or more islet autoantibodies will develop clinical type 1 diabetes.

RISK OF DEVELOPING TYPE 1 DIABETES

Although type 1 diabetes is much less common in the general population than type 2 diabetes, type 1 diabetes is by no means rare among children and young adults. Three-quarters of all cases of type 1 diabetes are diagnosed in individuals less than 18 years old. Data derived from the SEARCH for Diabetes in Youth study in the U.S. showed that 0.78 per 1,000 children under the age of 10 years have diabetes. Type 1 accounts for more than 80% of these cases. In youths 10–19 years of age, 2.80 per 1,000 have diabetes, and of these cases 85.1% of white youths have type 1, with a lower percentage among other ethnic/racial groups—53.9% in Hispanic youth, 42.2% in non-Hispanic blacks, 30.3% in Asian/Pacific Islanders, and 13.8% in American Indian youth.

Type 1 diabetes has been increasing 3–4% per year in youths, and even more in young children under the age of 5 years. This makes diabetes one of the most

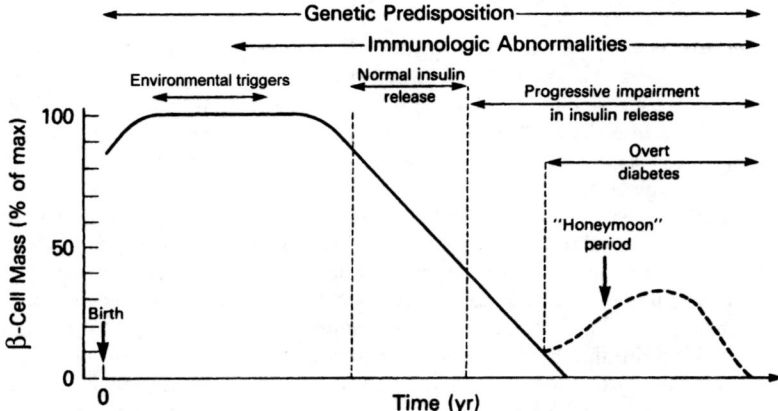

Figure 1.1 Proposed scheme of natural history of type 1 diabetes. Timing of trigger in relation to immunologic abnormalities is unknown. Note that overt diabetes is not apparent until insulin secretory reserves are <10–20% of normal.

common childhood diseases, with a much higher incidence rate than other chronic childhood diseases, such as cystic fibrosis, juvenile rheumatoid arthritis, nephrotic syndrome, muscular dystrophy, or leukemia.

The annual incidence of type 1 diabetes decreases after the age of 20 years. In those over 20 years old, incidence is similar in men and women, and it is lower in African Americans, Hispanics, Asian Americans, and American Indians than in whites, as is found in the younger age range.

Type 1 diabetes has strong HLA (human leukocyte antigen) associations. HLA genes contribute approximately half of the genetic risk for type 1 diabetes with the majority of the risk within the HLA-DQ-DR loci. As DQ and DR genes are located very close to one another on chromosome 6, there is linkage disequilibrium between the HLA-DQ and -DR genes. HLA-DR/DQ alleles can either be predisposing or protective, and the general population and family members can be assessed for risk by genetic evaluation. Most whites with type 1 diabetes carry HLA-DR3 or HLA-DR4 alleles, in blacks it is HLA-DR7, and in Japanese people it is HLA-DR9. The statistical risk of a family member developing type 1 diabetes is linked to the genetic similarities of the family members. For example, when one identical twin develops diabetes, the risk to the other twin may be as high as 65%. This is in contrast to a 0.4% risk in the general population, a 15% risk in HLA-identical siblings, and a 1% risk in HLA-nonidentical siblings. Without knowing HLA type, in general, the risk for type 1 diabetes in a first-degree family member is ~5%.

Relatives of patients with type 1 diabetes can have the opportunity to be tested for type 1 diabetes risk but only in the setting of a clinical research study (www.diabetestrialnet.org). There is evidence to suggest that early diagnosis may limit acute complications.

GENETICS AND IMMUNOLOGY OF TYPE 1 DIABETES

Type 1 diabetes is a genetically influenced and immunologically mediated disease with a prolonged asymptomatic phase (pre–type 1 diabetes), which eventually results in progressive β-cell destruction, insulin deficiency, and overt clinical symptoms. The identity of the initiating event(s) remains speculative. Viruses, food antigens, and intestinal microbes have been proposed as environmental triggers of β-cell autoimmunity.

The familial predisposition to type 1 diabetes has long been known. A specific mode of genetic transmission has not been established. Predisposition to type 1 diabetes is inherited as a heterogeneous polygenic trait with low penetrance and gender biases. There is a higher concordance rate for type 1 diabetes in monozygotic twins than in dizygotic twins. The initial estimate for monozygotic twins was 30–45%, but when examined longitudinally, the cumulative incidence of diabetes among monozygotic twins initially discordant for diabetes was 65% (95% confidence interval 39–91%). The empirical risk of type 1 diabetes is increased in first-degree relatives of probands with the disease (Table 1.6). There is an even greater risk for offspring of fathers with type 1 diabetes, especially those who were diagnosed at a young age.

Greater than 50% of the genetic predisposition to type 1 diabetes is conferred by genes on the short arm of chromosome 6, either within or in close proximity to the Class II HLA region of the major histocompatibility complex (MHC). At least 40 other loci have been suggested to be involved, with the largest contribution (about 10% of the genetic predisposition) being accounted for by the flanking region of the insulin gene on chromosome 11, INS-VNTR. Shorter forms of a variable number tandem repeated in the insulin promoter are associated with susceptibility, while longer forms are associated with protection. Other genes associated with T-cell activation and regulation have been identified: cytotoxic T lymphocyte antigen-4 (CTLA-4) and protein tyrosine phosphatase N22 (PTPN22) and multiple genes in the interleukin (IL-2) and IL-2 receptor (IL-2R) pathways. HLA, CTLA-4, and PTPN22 are associated with other autoimmune diseases.

The Class II MHC DR and DQ molecules are composed of alpha and beta chains, which present processed antigens to T cells. The HLA-DR beta chain along with DQ alpha and beta chains are polymorphic and commonly typed;

Table 1.6 Approximate Familial Risk of Type 1 Diabetes

Relationship to proband	Risk (%)
Sibling	10–15
Identical twin	65
Father	6
Mother	3
Offspring of father	12
Offspring of mother	1–4
General population	0.3–0.4

HLA-DR alpha chains are not polymorphic. The relationship between type 1 diabetes and specific MHC Class II region alleles is complex. There is a strong positive relationship with HLA-DR3/DQ2 and -DR4/DQ8 and a strong negative relationship with -DQ6 (DQB1*0602). DR and DQ alleles are in close linkage disequilibrium on chromosome 6. Indeed, more than 90% of Caucasians with type 1 diabetes have HLA-DR3/DQ2 and/or -DR4/DQ8, while 30% of children who develop type 1 are heterozygous for these haplotypes. Within families, the risk for diabetes is highest for those who have both DR3/DQ2 and DR4/DQ8 and who have inherited identical HLA haplotypes as their sibling with diabetes. There is an even stronger relationship of type 1 diabetes when DQ loci (DQα and DQβ) are considered together with DR loci, i.e., the predisposition to type 1 diabetes in Caucasians is associated with HLA-DR3, DQB1*0201, and with HLA-DR4, DQB1*0302, with the strongest association being the DQα-DQβ combination DQA1*0501-DQB1*0302. Other DQ alleles confer protection from type 1 diabetes, e.g., DQB1*0602 provides protection even in the presence of DQ susceptibility alleles. This suggests that protection is dominant over susceptibility. Because MHC class II genes regulate the immune response, the susceptibility and protective alleles could be involved differentially in antigen presentation of peptides that establish and maintain tolerance or influence the immune response.

Autoantibodies and Autoantigens

The identification of circulating autoantibodies to β-cell proteins in those who have developed diabetes and subsequently in nondiabetic first-degree relatives has made it possible to detect the preclinical disease. Numerous circulating autoantibodies have been identified, including cytoplasmic islet cell antibodies (ICAs) detected by immunofluorescence, insulin autoantibodies (IAAs), autoantibodies directed against the enzyme GAD (GAD65 or GADA), autoantibodies against islet tyrosine phosphatase (IA-2A [ICA512] and IA-2B), zinc transporter 8 A (ZnT8A) and several others. The four most frequently measured antibodies, referred to as biochemical islet autoantibodies, are IAA, GAD, IA-2A, and ZnT8. All four of these islet autoantibodies are now available as commercial assays. Most (>90%) newly diagnosed patients with type 1 diabetes have one or another of these circulating antibodies. The presence of two or more antibodies is highly predictive of increased risk of type 1 diabetes within 5 years.

These autoantibodies generally are not thought to mediate β-cell destruction by humoral mechanisms. Rather, it is likely that as β-cells are destroyed, multiple antigens are presented to CD4+T cells (helper T cells), which activate B-cells to form plasma cells and generate antibodies directed against these components. Thus, these autoantibodies are markers of immune activity or of β-cell damage and herald the disease process several years before overt clinical hyperglycemia. As β-cell function is lost and "total" diabetes evolves, ZnT8A, and IA-2A autoantibodies tend to decrease in titer and/or disappear, while GAD tends to persist the longest after diabetes diagnosis.

Association with Other Autoimmune Diseases

Depending on the gene type influencing type 1 diabetes, there can be increased shared risk for other autoimmune disorders, suggesting a common biological pathway. The range of additional autoimmune disorders varies from none to severe autoimmune polyglandular failure. In general, patients with type 1 diabetes are at increased risk for developing other autoimmune diseases, most commonly autoimmune thyroiditis and celiac disease. Other diseases that could potentially develop include Hashimoto's thyroiditis, Graves' disease, Addison's disease, vitiligo, autoimmune hepatitis, myasthenia gravis, and pernicious anemia. Adults who develop type 1 diabetes may develop autoimmune disorders, although the risk of coexisting autoimmunity is lower in adults than in youth with type 1 diabetes.

Autoimmune thyroid disease is the most common autoimmune disorder associated with diabetes, occurring in 17–30% of patients with type 1 diabetes. At the time of diagnosis, about 25% of children with type 1 diabetes have thyroid autoantibodies; their presence is predictive of thyroid dysfunction, most commonly hypothyroidism, although hyperthyroidism occurs in ~0.5% of cases. Thyroid function tests may be misleading (euthyroid sick syndrome) if performed at time of diagnosis owing to the effect of previous hyperglycemia, ketosis or ketoacidosis, weight loss, etc. Therefore, thyroid function tests should be performed soon after a period of metabolic stability and good glycemic control. Subclinical hypothyroidism may be associated with increased risk of symptomatic hypoglycemia and reduced linear growth rate. Hyperthyroidism alters glucose metabolism and usually causes deterioration of metabolic control. Celiac disease is an immune-mediated disorder that occurs with increased frequency in patients with type 1 diabetes (1.6–16.4% of individuals with type 1 diabetes compared with 0.3–1% in the general population). Fewer than 1% of children with type 1 diabetes have autoimmune adrenalitis screened with an anti-21-hydroxylase antibody. Type 1 diabetes can be seen with polyglandular autoimmune disease, especially type II, in which adrenal insufficiency, autoimmune thyroid disease, and gonadal insufficiency are the other major components.

Pregnancy-related management of women having Hashimoto's disease, prepregnancy planning, and postpartum testing for thyroid function, as well as screening of children in relation to thyroidal autoimmunity and celiac disease, are discussed at a later point in the book.

Cell-Mediated Immunologic Dysfunction

The existence of insulitis (lymphocytic infiltration of the pancreas by mononuclear cells) has been known for decades and was the earliest evidence for the autoimmune nature of type 1 diabetes. There is evidence of a role for both T- and B-cells in the pathophysiology of β-cell destruction in both human and animal models. However, type 1 diabetes in most spontaneous animal models of autoimmune diabetes is considered a T cell–mediated disorder because adoptive transfer occurs with T cells but not with autoantibodies. The underlying immunologic abnormalities in type 1 diabetes are an active area of research as are type 1 diabetes resistance mechanisms. To better understand the pathogenesis of human type 1 diabetes, the Network for Pancreatic Organ Donors (nPOD) has been formed to procure pancreata and lymph organs from at-risk and type 1 diabetes organ donors to study the etiopathogenesis of the disease within the target organs.

Environmental Triggers

The incomplete concordance rate of diabetes in identical twins suggests that environmental factors may be important in the pathogenesis of type 1 diabetes.

Viral infections, e.g., enteroviruses such as Coxsackie B4, rotavirus, and congenital rubella, have been inconsistently implicated as triggers for the immunologic process. The gut microflora may play a pathophysiological role through a variety of potential mechanisms including a chronic low-grade inflammation and altered intestinal barrier function. Exposure to substances toxic to the β-cells accounts for only a very small number of cases. Prolonged breast-feeding is reported to lower the incidence rates for type 1 diabetes. Substitution of highly hydrolyzed milk formula may reduce the risk for development of β-cell autoimmunity by reducing the adverse effect of early exposure to complex dietary proteins such as cow's milk. Little direct evidence exists to link any specific factor(s) to triggering autoimmune destruction of the β-cells in type 1 diabetes in humans. Currently, there is a large-scale prospective international study, The Environmental Determinants of Diabetes in the Young (TEDDY), ongoing with the goal of identifying environmental determinants of islet autoimmunity (development of islet autoantibodies) and eventually clinical type 1 diabetes.

Screening and Intervention Trials

Humoral autoantibodies allow for the identification of individuals who are at high risk for developing type 1 diabetes, and play a role in clinical research trials directed at the preservation of β-cell function. Screening of high-risk individuals (e.g., first-degree relatives of someone with type 1 diabetes) is done through research trials, most notably the National Institutes of Health (NIH)–sponsored Natural History Study conducted through Type 1 Diabetes TrialNet. Because type 1 diabetes is increasing in incidence and can be predicted with measurement of islet autoantibodies, and since ~85% of all patients diagnosed with type 1 diabetes do not have a family history, it is rational to consider general population screening for type 1 diabetes risk. At the current time, only screening of high-risk individuals (e.g., first-degree relatives of an individual with type 1 diabetes) is done through research trials. All subjects who screen positive for islet autoantibodies should be counseled about potential clinical intervention trials to delay the onset of diabetes and their risk of developing diabetes with follow-up offered.

Attempts to Preserve β-Cell Mass

A number of therapies have been tested to prevent the destruction of the β-cell mass, both prior to and after the diagnosis of type 1 diabetes. The trials are divided into primary, secondary, and tertiary prevention. Primary prevention clinical trials are in place targeting neonates at high genetic risk in an attempt to prevent islet autoimmunity (the development of islet autoantibodies). Interventions are, by necessity, benign as they target very young children who have no evidence of pathology. These interventions include randomization to cow's milk formula versus hydrolyzed casein formula, introduction of DHA (to deliver omega-3 fatty acids), and oral/intranasal insulin. To date, no intervention has delayed the development of islet autoimmunity or clinical type 1 diabetes.

Secondary prevention studies target those at high risk for developing clinical type 1 diabetes, i.e., those individuals with two or more islet autoantibodies. Two large, multicenter intervention trials involving either low-dose subcutaneous insulin therapy (Diabetes Prevention Trial-Type 1 [DPT-1]) or nicotinamide (ENDIT Trial) as immunoregulatory agents in the pre–type 1 diabetes state showed no benefit in delaying or preventing the onset of type 1 diabetes. A second arm of the DPT-1 using oral insulin in those deemed to be of moderate risk (25–50% risk) of developing diabetes showed that a subset of subjects with high-titer insulin autoantibodies had a several-year delay in progression to diabetes, and this is being evaluated now in the multinational Type 1 Diabetes TrialNet consortia that was developed after DPT-1.

Tertiary prevention trials occur in those individuals newly or recently diagnosed with type 1 diabetes. The outcome measure for these trials is the C-peptide area under the curve response to a standardized mixed-meal tolerance test (stimulus containing carbohydrate, protein, and fat). Early therapeutic attempts centered mainly on general immune suppression. Although effective in small pilot studies in prolonging the honeymoon period, none resulted in permanent remission.

TrialNet has completed multiple trials on a number of agents in new-onset type 1 diabetes, including rituximab (a B-cell depleting antibody) and abatacept (CTLA-4 Ig, which blocks T-cell costimulation), with both showing an attenuation in loss of C-peptide over the first year of the disease due to an initial response followed by a decline in C-peptide that mirrored the control group. Studies of anti-CD3 monoclonal antibodies (targeting the CD3 receptor on T cells) at onset of type 1 diabetes have found some preservation of C-peptide for at least 1 year, but failed to meet primary endpoints in large phase 3 trials. Combination therapy with mycophenolate mofetil (an inhibitor of purine synthesis) plus daclizumab (anti-CD25) was also evaluated and showed no benefit in preserving C-peptide. Antigen-specific therapy with GAD-alum was also evaluated in new-onset type 1 diabetes, again showing no preservation of endogenous insulin production. Additional interventions being evaluated include anti-thymocyte globulin plus G-CSF, heat shock protein DiaPep277, α-1 antitrypsin, imatinib, low dose IL-2, infusion of autologous regulatory T cells, and methyldopa. Methyldopa is an interesting therapy as it represents the first precision/personalized medicine approach to treating the underlying immunology in type 1 diabetes; methyldopa is being used to block HLA-DQ8 (present in ~60% of all type 1 diabetes patients) antigen presentation and subsequently $CD4^+T$-cell activation.

These intervention trials offer an opportunity to preserve a significant mass of β-cells and potentially prevent or delay overt diabetes and modify its course. Potential therapeutic modalities must be approached with caution and should be utilized only in conjunction with carefully defined scientific studies. Individuals at risk for diabetes because of family history and those newly diagnosed should be informed about available clinical trials designed to attempt to interdict the type 1 process.

CONCLUSION

Type 1 diabetes is an autoimmune, or alternatively idiopathic (autoimmune in the more common form of type 1 diabetes), disorder characterized by the progressive loss of β-cells in subjects at increased genetic risk. The resultant insulin deficiency is associated with intracellular abnormalities of metabolism in both liver and muscle tissue, leading to excessive hepatic glucose production, decreased muscle glucose uptake, frank glucose intolerance, and, if untreated, ketoacidosis. With irreversible insulin deficiency, patients are dependent on lifelong exogenous insulin treatment. Type 1 diabetes is increasing in incidence and is now predictable with the measurement of serum islet autoantibodies. There is a wealth of research into the pathogenesis and prevention of type 1 diabetes with the hope that the disease will one day be prevented and ultimately cured.

BIBLIOGRAPHY

Aly TA, Ide A, Jahromi MM, Barker JM, Fernando MS, Babu SR, Yu L, Miao D, Erlich HA, Fain PR, Barriga KJ, Norris JM, Rewers MJ, Eisenbarth GS. Extreme genetic risk for type 1A diabetes. *Proc Natl Acad Sci U S A* 2006;103:14074–14079

American Diabetes Association. (2) Classification and diagnosis of diabetes. *Diabetes Care* 2016;39(Suppl. 1):S13–S22

American Diabetes Association. Prevention of type 1 diabetes mellitus. *Diabetes Care* 2003;26(Suppl. 1):S140

Atkinson MA, Eisenbarth GS, Michels AW. Type 1 diabetes. *Lancet* 2014;383: 69–82

Bluestone JA, Herold K, Eisenbarth G. Genetics, pathogenesis and clinical interventions in type 1 diabetes. *Nature* 2010;464:1293–1300

Chase P, Gottlieb P, Eisenbarth GS. Chapter 12: Clinical Trials for the Prevention of Type 1 Diabetes (updated 6/2009). In *Type 1 Diabetes: Cellular, Molecular & Clinical Immunology*. Online Edition version 3.0. Eisenbarth GS, Ed. http://www.barbaradaviscenter.org. Accessed 30 September 2016

Dabelea D, Mayer-Davis EJ, Saydah S, Imperatore G, Linder B, Divers J, Bell R, Badaru A, Talton JW, Crume T, Liese AD, Merchant AT, Lawrence JM, Reynolds K, Dolan L, Liu LL, Hamman RF, SEARCH for Diabetes in Youth Study. Prevalence of type 1 and type 2 diabetes among children and adolescents from 2001 to 2009. *JAMA* 2014;311:1778–1786

Diabetes Prevention Trial - Type 1 Diabetes Study Group. Effects of insulin in relatives of patients with type 1 diabetes mellitus. *N Engl J Med* 2002;346:1685–1691

Eisenbarth GS. Chapter 11: Prediction of Type 1A Diabetes: TheNatural History of the Prediabetic Period (updated 9/2012). In *Type 1 Diabetes: Cellular, Molecular & Clinical Immunology*. Online Edition version 3.0. Eisenbarth GS, Ed. http://www.barbaradaviscenter.org. Accessed 30 September 2016

Eisenbarth GS. Type 1 diabetes: molecular, cellular and clinical immunology. *Adv Exp Med Biol* 2004;552:306–310

Fonseca VA, Kirkman MS, Darsow T, Ratner RE. The American Diabetes Association diabetes research perspective. *Diabetes Care* 2012;35:1380–1387

Genuth SM. Diabetic ketoacidosis and hyperglycemic hyperosmolar coma. *Curr Ther Endocrinol Metab* 1997;6:438–447

Hagopian WA, Lernmark A, Rewers MJ, Simell OG, She JX, Ziegler AG, Krischer JP, Akolkar B. TEDDY—The Environmental Determinants of Diabetes in the Young: an observational clinical trial. *Ann N Y Acad Sci* 2006;1079: 320-326

Haller MJ, Atkinson MA, Schatz DA. Efforts to prevent and halt autoimmune beta cell destruction *Endocrinol Metab Clin North Am* 2010;39:527–539

Handelsman Y, Bloomgarden ZT, Grunberger G, Umpierrez G, Zimmerman RS, Bailey TS, Blonde L, Bray GA, Cohen AJ, Dagogo-Jack S, Davidson JA, Einhorn D, Ganda OP, Garber AJ, Garvey WT, Henry RR, Hirsch IB, Horton ES, Hurley DL, Jellinger PS, Jovanovič L, Lebovitz HE, LeRoith D, Levy P, McGill JB, Mechanick JI, Mestman JH, Moghissi ES, Orzeck EA, Pessah-Pollack R, Rosenblit PD, Vinik AI, Wyne K, Zangeneh F. American Association of Clinical Endocrinologists and American College of Endocrinology—clinical practice guidelines for developing a diabetes mellitus comprehensive care plan—2015. *Endocr Pract* 2015;21(Suppl. 1):1–87

Harjutsalo V, Reunanen A, Tuomilehto J. Differential transmission of type 1 diabetes from diabetic fathers and mothers to their offspring. *Diabetes* 2006;55:1517–1524

Knip M, Virtanen SM, Seppä K, Ilonen J, Savilahti E, Vaarala O, Reunanen A, Teramo K, Hämäläinen AM, Paronen J, Dosch HM, Hakulinen T, Akerblom HK; Finnish TRIGR Study Group. Dietary intervention in infancy and later signs of beta-cell autoimmunity. *N Engl J Med* 2010;363:1900–1908

Lebovitz HE. Autoimmune polyglandular syndromes: interplay between the immune and the endocrine systems leading to a diverse set of clinical diseases and new insights into immune regulation. *Diabetes Technol Ther* 2013;15 (Suppl. 2):S2-21–S2-28.

Michels AW, Eisenbarth GS. Immune intervention in type 1 diabetes. *Semin Immunol* 2011;23:214–219

Patterson CC, Dahlquist GG, Gyürüs E, Green A, Soltész G; EURODIAB Study Group. Incidence trends for childhood type 1 diabetes in Europe during 1989-2003 and predicted new cases 2005-20: a multicentre prospective registration study. *Lancet* 2009;373:2027–2033

Pugliese A, Yang M, Kusmarteva I, Heiple T, Vendrame F, Wasserfall C, Rowe P, Moraski JM, Ball S, Jebson L, Schatz DA, Gianani R, Burke GW, Nierras C, Staeva T, Kaddis JS, Campbell-Thompson M, Atkinson MA. The Juvenile Diabetes Research Foundation Network for Pancreatic Organ Donors with Diabetes (nPOD) Program: goals, operational model and emerging findings. *Pediatr Diabetes* 2014;15:1–9

Redondo MJ, Jeffrey J, Fain PR, Eisenbarth GS, Orban T. Concordance for islet autoimmunity among monozygotic twins. *N Engl J Med* 2008;359:2849–2850

Redondo MJ, Yu L, Hawa M, Mackenzie T, Pyke DA, Eisenbarth GS, Leslie RDG. Heterogeneity of type I diabetes: analysis of monozygotic twins in Great Britain and the United States. *Diabetologia* 2001;44:354-362 [Erratum, *Diabetologia* 2001;44:927]

Rewers M, Norris J, Kretowski A. Chapter 9: Epidemiology of Type 1 Diabetes (updated 11/2010). In *Type 1 Diabetes: Cellular, Molecular & Clinical Immunology*. Online Edition version 3.0. Eisenbarth GS, Ed. http://www.barbaradaviscenter.org. Accessed 30 September 2016

Skyler JS. Prevention and reversal of type 1 diabetes—past challenges and future opportunities. *Diabetes Care* 2015;38:997–1007

Smyth DJ, Plagnol V, Walker NM, Cooper JD, Downes K, Yang JH, Howson JM, Stevens H, McManus R, Wijmenga C, Heap GA, Dubois PC, Clayton DG, Hunt KA, van Heel DA, Todd JA. Shared and distinct genetic variants in type 1 diabetes and celiac disease. *N Engl J Med* 2008;359:2767–2777

Sosenko JM1, Skyler JS, Palmer JP, Krischer JP, Cuthbertson D, Yu L, Schatz DA, Orban T, Eisenbarth G; Diabetes Prevention Trial–Type 1 and Type 1 Diabetes TrialNet Study Groups. A longitudinal study of GAD65 and ICA512 autoantibodies during the progression to type 1 diabetes in Diabetes Prevention Trial–Type 1 (DPT-1) participants. *Diabetes Care* 2011;34:2435–2437

Steck AK, Pugliese P, Eisenbarth GS. Chapter 7: Type 1 Diabetes Mellitus of Man: Genetic Susceptibility and Resistance (updated 10/2012). In *Type 1 Diabetes: Cellular, Molecular & Clinical Immunology*. Online Edition version 3.0. Eisenbarth GS, Ed. http://www.barbaradaviscenter.org. Accessed 30 September 2016

TEDDY Study Group. The Environmental Determinants of Diabetes in the Young (TEDDY) study: study design. *Pediatr Diabetes* 2007;8:286–298

Writing Team for the Diabetes Control and Complications Trial/Epidemiology of Diabetes Interventions and Complications Research Group. Effect of intensive therapy on the microvascular complications of type 1 diabetes mellitus. *JAMA* 2002;287:2563–2569

Wu J, Yang X, Chen B, Xu X. Pancreas β cell regeneration and type 1 diabetes (Review). *Exp Ther Med* 2015;9:653–657

Ziegler AG, Rewers M, Simell O, Simell T, Lempainen J, Steck A, Winkler C, Ilonen J, Veijola R, Knip M, Bonifacio E, Eisenbarth GS. Seroconversion to multiple islet autoantibodies and risk of progression to diabetes in children. *JAMA* 2013;309:2473–2479

Diabetes Standards and Education

Highlights
Diabetes Standards and Education

PHILOSOPHY AND GOALS

- The main factors that influence the treatment regimen a patient will adopt and the likelihood of achieving treatment goals are:
  - patient centeredness and patient engagement
  - the diabetes management team's ability to tailor education, support, and treatment to the patient/family
  - diabetes team/patient/family alignment of goals and ability to work collaboratively to implement and sustain self-management skills and behaviors
- The goals of treatment are to:
  - promote and maintain day-to-day clinical and psychological well-being
  - avoid severe hypoglycemia, symptomatic hyperglycemia, and ketoacidosis
  - avoid long-term microcirculatory and macrovascular complications and comorbid conditions
  - promote normal growth and development in children
  - develop plan for continuing care
    - Foster patient empowerment and the successful facilitation of the behavior change necessary to achieve the best possible glycemic control and prevent, delay, or arrest long-term diabetes complications while minimizing

hypoglycemia and excess weight gain or disordered eating.
  - The physician and patient must set treatment goals together with the diabetes management team and family. Glycemic goals should be set as close to optimal as possible given the patient's abilities and presence of risk factors and comorbidities.
- Initial and long-term clinical goals are presented in Clinical Goals. They focus on:
  - metabolic stabilization
  - restoration and maintenance of desirable body weight
  - elimination of hyperglycemic symptoms and minimization of severe hypoglycemia

PATIENT SELF-MANAGEMENT EDUCATION AND SUPPORT

- The goal of diabetes self-management education and support is to provide patients with the knowledge, skills, and motivation to incorporate diabetes self-management into their daily lives and to engage in active collaboration with their health-care team. The process includes:
  - teaching of information needed for diabetes self-management

- training in skills needed for treatment procedures
- guidance and empowerment of the patient, incorporating his or her experiences and preferences in devising strategies for behavior change to fit the diabetes treatment regimen into the individual's lifestyle in order to optimize his/her quality of life

■ Diabetes self-management education and support is a planned process that includes:
- assessment to identify the patient's individual education needs
- setting a diabetes self-management goal or goals
- effective implementation of education
- evaluation of learning
- reassessment(s) for new needs over time and across the life span
  - To be effective, diabetes self-management education and support must be individualized, provided in the context of a team approach to diabetes care, and continued across the life span of the individual with diabetes. When indicated, family members and caregivers should be included. Patients hospitalized with newly diagnosed or uncontrolled diabetes should receive education in the inpatient setting as part of a comprehensive diabetes care plan.

■ Newly diagnosed patients with type 1 diabetes need to learn the basic skills that will enable them to implement their treatment regimen at home. Initial education should focus on teaching survival skills, with more in-depth information and additional topics added after the patient has had time to adjust to diabetes self-care. Written patient guidelines for detecting and treating hypoglycemia and for managing mild illnesses reinforce self-management skills that are not routinely needed and should be part of survival skills education.

■ Patient education is essential for the management of type 1 diabetes. Therefore, physicians who treat type 1 diabetes patients need to provide diabetes self-management training opportunities for their patients. Physicians can incorporate diabetes patient education into their clinical practice by:
- including diabetes educators as an integral part of the diabetes team in the office and/or by developing a team relationship with diabetes educators working in the community
- referring patients to diabetes education programs recognized by the American Diabetes Association or American Association of Diabetes Educators (AADE) as meeting the National Standards for Diabetes Self-Management Education and Support
- becoming knowledgeable about other diabetes education resources online (i.e., technology-assisted tools including Internet-based social networks, distance learning, DVD-based content, and mobile applications) and in their communities

Diabetes Standards and Education

Type 1 diabetes is a chronic disease in which the goal of treatment has been well defined—to achieve the best glycemic control possible with the least associated risk of hypoglycemia. The diabetes management team must work with the patient to determine which treatment strategies will best achieve the desired outcomes. The diabetes management team comprises a consortium that includes (but is not limited to) the endocrinologist (or other health-care provider with expertise in type 1 diabetes management), nurse, dietitian, social worker, mental health professional, pharmacist, parent/peer advisors and mentors, and other health-care specialists. The diabetes management team interfaces with the primary care provider, who helps coordinate care and establishes the patient's medical home. Three factors that strongly influence treatment are:

- the diabetes management team's ability to assess the optimal, individualized regimen for patient/family
- the patient/family's self-care attitudes and abilities
- the diabetes team–patient/family alignment of goals and ability to work collaboratively

The primary goals of treatment are *1*) to promote and maintain day-to-day clinical and psychological well-being; *2*) to avoid severe hypoglycemia, symptomatic hyperglycemia, and ketoacidosis; *3*) to avoid long-term microcirculatory and macrovascular complications; and *4*) to promote normal growth and development in children. The secondary goal of treatment is patient empowerment and the successful facilitation of the necessary behavior change to achieve the best possible glycemic control to prevent, delay, or arrest long-term diabetes complications while minimizing hypoglycemia and excess weight gain or disordered eating. The primary goals are clearly achievable at variable degrees of cost, inconvenience, and risk; the secondary goal, although more difficult, should be attainable by most patients.

GLYCEMIC CONTROL AND COMPLICATIONS: A SUMMARY OF EVIDENCE

Evidence relating hyperglycemia and/or other metabolic consequences of insulin deficiency to the development of vascular complications comes from animal studies, from older epidemiologic studies of European and North American patients with type 1 diabetes, and from more recent controlled clinical trials from Scandinavia and North America.

Animal Studies

Strong experimental support for an association between metabolic abnormalities and vascular complications is found in animal studies. Animals that are rendered insulin deficient and hyperglycemic develop pathologic changes resembling early human retinopathy, kidney disease, and neuropathy. These changes can be prevented or ameliorated and, in some instances, reversed by early intensive insulin treatment, by curing diabetes via pancreas or islet transplantation, or by transplanting the affected organ into a nondiabetic animal.

Other Causes of Diabetes

Microvascular disease also develops in some patients with diabetes resulting from removal or destruction of the islets caused by pancreatectomy, chronic pancreatitis, or toxicity (e.g., from the rodenticide Vacor). These observations further support the theory that loss of insulin secretion or some consequent metabolic derangement is responsible for microvascular abnormalities in patients with immune-mediated type 1 diabetes. Genetic predisposition may influence the development of microvascular, neuropathic, and other complications; however, hyperglycemia is a prerequisite to development of these complications.

Kidney Transplantation Observations

Normal kidneys transplanted into recipients with type 1 diabetes begin to show pathologic changes resembling diabetic kidney disease after several years. Normal kidneys transplanted into patients with successful whole-pancreas transplantation have less glomerulopathy than kidneys transplanted into patients treated with conventional therapy. These observations point to a causative role for the diabetic metabolic milieu.

DYSGLYCEMIA AND COMPLICATIONS FROM POPULATION-BASED DATA

In data from 1,066 individuals aged >40 years from the 2005–2006 National Health and Nutrition Examination Survey, the relationship between fasting plasma glucose (FPG), A1C, and retinopathy has shown that retinal lesions do not develop before measures of glycemia become elevated. These data on a specific and early clinical complication of diabetes point to the causative role of even minimal hyperglycemia. Several epidemiologic studies in patients with type 1 diabetes suggest that the higher the glucose level, the greater the incidence of microvascular disease.

Prospective Clinical Trials

The Diabetes Control and Complications Trial (DCCT) examined whether intensive treatment with the goal of maintaining glucose concentrations close to the normal range could decrease the frequency and severity of diabetes complications. Investigators studied 1,441 patients with type 1 diabetes—726 with no retinopathy and 715 with mild retinopathy at baseline. Patients were randomly assigned to intensive therapy administered with insulin pumps or multiple injections of insulin guided by blood glucose monitoring, or to conventional therapy with one or two insulin injections per day. The mean A1C in the conventional group was 9.1% while the mean A1C achieved in the intensive therapy group was 7.4%. The patients were followed a mean of 6.5 years. Results showed that in the primary intervention cohort, intensive therapy reduced the mean risk of developing retinopathy by 76%. In the secondary intervention group, intensive therapy slowed the progression of retinopathy by 54% and reduced the development of proliferative retinopathy by 47%. In both groups combined, intensive therapy reduced the occurrence of albumin levels >40 mg/24 h by 39% and albumin levels >300 mg/24 h by 54%. Clinical neuropathy was reduced by 60%. However, the reductions in microvascular complications were achieved at the expense of a threefold increase in severe hypoglycemia. Comparable results were seen in the Stockholm Diabetes Intervention Study after 5 and 8 years.

After completion of the DCCT, most of the participants were enrolled in a long-term observational study entitled the Epidemiology of Diabetes Interventions and Complications (EDIC) study. The difference in the median A1C values between the conventional therapy and intensive therapy groups narrowed during follow-up (at 4 years, the median was 8.2% and 7.9%, respectively). Despite this small difference in glycemic control between the two groups, the marked reduction in the risk of progressive retinopathy and kidney disease that resulted from intensive therapy persisted in the EDIC study at 4 years of follow-up. Furthermore, subsequent publications from the EDIC follow-up study showed a significant difference in the progression of the carotid intima-media thickness (a measure of atherosclerosis) between groups at 6 years of follow-up. After an average of 17 years of follow-up from the DCCT through EDIC, the number of cardiovascular disease (CVD) events in the conventional group was more than double that of intensive-therapy subjects. Intensive therapy reduced the risk of any CVD event by 42% and the risk of nonfatal myocardial infarction (MI), stroke, or death by 57%. Finally, over a median follow-up of 23 years and after adjustment for baseline factors in the DCCT, intensive therapy was associated with a reduction in the risk of any diabetes-related ocular surgery by 48% (95% confidence interval [CI], 29 to 63; P<0.001) and a reduction in the risk of all such ocular procedures by 37% (95% CI, 12 to 55; P=0.01). The beneficial effects of intensive therapy were fully attenuated after adjustment for mean glycated hemoglobin levels over the entire follow-up period.

An analysis of longitudinal data from DCCT/EDIC and from the observational study of type 1 patients from Allegheny County, Pennsylvania (Pittsburgh Epidemiology of Diabetes Complications Experience [EDC]), conducted from 1983–2005, reveals the effect of glycemic control on the rate of diabetes complications 30 years after diagnosis. In the DCCT conventional treatment group, the cumulative incidence of proliferative retinopathy, kidney disease, and cardiovascular disease was 50%, 25%, and 14%, respectively, while in the EDC cohort, the cumulative incidence was 47%, 17%, and 14%, respectively. The cumulative incidence of these microvascular complications was substantially lower in the DCCT intensive therapy group: 21%, 9%, and 9%, respectively. Furthermore, fewer than 1% of individuals became blind, required kidney replacement therapy, or had a diabetes-related amputation during this time.

These follow-up findings strongly support the implementation of intensive therapy and lowering of A1C as early as is safely possible, and the maintenance of such therapy for as long as possible, with the expectation that a prolonged period of near-normal blood glucose levels will result in a lasting reduction in the risk of both microvascular and macrovascular complications in patients with type 1 diabetes.

GOALS OF TREATMENT

The physician and patient, with the diabetes management team and family, must set treatment goals together. Although this concept seems obvious, overlooking this step often leads to failure of the treatment plan. The physician, convinced of the importance of stringent glycemic control in every case, will be frustrated by a patient who does not understand the need for, or is unable to accept the goal or methods used to achieve, glycemic control. Conversely, the patient who wants blood glucose levels to be normal all the time and is truly willing to work for it will be frustrated by a physician who lacks the time, facilities, or training to help achieve this goal or who is unable to guide the patient to achieve this goal safely.

An aligned diabetes management team–patient treatment goal and plan requires open communication and appropriate patient education. At the tightest end of the treatment spectrum, the patient must have a sophisticated and practical understanding of physiology, pharmacology, and technology when striving to maintain normal glucose levels when, for example, exercising strenuously. At the looser end, knowledge may be more rudimentary, but patients must at least know that to avoid diabetic ketoacidosis (DKA), they may have to take extra insulin on sick days when appetite is poor, though common sense seems to dictate the reverse. Treatment must always be individualized. Success in achieving small incremental steps is more likely to lead to a greater improvement over the long term.

The physician and other team members should avoid seeming autocratic, moralistic, or judgmental. They should work with the patient to try to understand why goals are not met and empathize with the challenges faced by the patient in paying daily attention to the never-ending demands of diabetes self-care combined with other aspects of the patient's life. It is paramount to work with the patient to identify obstacles to the treatment plan so the patient can actively participate in addressing them. It is important to encourage the best incremental steps that are achievable without demanding the impossible, unsafe, or impractical.

The process of setting individual patient glycemic targets should take into account the results of prospective randomized clinical trials, most notably the DCCT. This trial conclusively demonstrated that, in patients with type 1 diabetes, the risk of development or progression of retinopathy, kidney disease, and neuropathy is reduced 50–75% by intensive treatment regimens when compared with conventional treatment regimens. These benefits were observed with an A1C of 7.2% in intensively treated groups of patients compared with an average A1C of 9.0% in conventionally treated groups of patients. The reduction in risk of these complications correlated continuously with the reduction in A1C produced by intensive treatment. This relationship implies that complete normalization of glycemic levels may prevent complications. The nondiabetic reference range for A1C in the DCCT was 4.0–6.0%.

Glycemic targets for nonpregnant adults are listed in Table 2.1, for children in Table 2.2, and for women who are pregnant in Table 2.3.

As the DCCT only included pediatric patients aged ≥13 years (195 adolescents aged 13–17 years at entry), treatment guidelines for pediatric patients have been based nearly exclusively on professional, expert advice. The ADA's blood glucose and A1C goals traditionally have been developmentally or age based in the pediatric population and rooted in earlier thought that severe, recurrent hypoglycemia was associated with neurocognitive dysfunction. More recent and

Table 2.1 Summary of Glycemic Recommendations for Nonpregnant Adults with Diabetes

A1C	<7.0% (53 mmol/mol)*
Preprandial capillary plasma glucose	80–130 mg/dL* (4.4–7.2 mmol/L)
Peak postprandial capillary plasma glucose†	<180 mg/dL* (10.0 mmol/L)

*More or less stringent glycemic goals may be appropriate for individual patients. Goals should be individualized based on duration of diabetes, age/life expectancy, comorbid conditions, known CVD or advanced microvascular complications, hypoglycemia unawareness, and individual patient considerations.

†Postprandial glucose may be targeted if A1C goals are not met despite reaching preprandial glucose goals. Postprandial glucose measurements should be made 1–2 h after the beginning of the meal, generally peak levels in patients with diabetes.

Table 2.2 Blood Glucose and A1C Goals for Type 1 Diabetes across All Pediatric Age-Groups

Blood glucose goal range			
Before meals	Bedtime/overnight	A1C	Rationale
90–130 mg/dL	90–150 mg/dL	<7.5%	A lower goal (<7.0% [53 mmol/mol]) is reasonable if it can be achieved without excessive hypoglycemia
(5.0–7.2 mmol/L)	(5.0–8.3 mmol/L)	(58 mmol/mol)	

Key concepts in setting glycemic goals:

- Goals should be *individualized*, and lower goals may be reasonable based on a benefit–risk assessment.

- Blood glucose goals should be modified in children with frequent hypoglycemia or hypoglycemia unawareness.

- Postprandial blood glucose values should be measured when there is a discrepancy between preprandial blood glucose values and A1C levels and to assess preprandial insulin doses in those on basal–bolus regimens.

Source (Tables 2.1 and 2.2): American Diabetes Association. Standards of medical care in diabetes—2016. *Diabetes Care* 2016;39(Suppl. 1):S43, S87.

Table 2.3 Optimal Target Blood Glucose Levels in Pregnancy

Time of Measurement	Blood Glucose (mg/dL [mmol/L])
Fasting	<90–95 (5.0–5.3)
1-h postprandial	<130–140 (7.2–7.8)
2-h postprandial	≤120 (6.7)
A1C*	<6.0–6.5%

* <6% may be optimal if this can be achieved without significant hypoglycemia, but target may be relaxed to <7% if necessary to prevent hypoglycemia.

If pregnant women cannot achieve the glycemic targets listed above without significant hypoglycemia, the American Diabetes Association suggests consideration of slightly higher targets: fasting <105 mg/dL, 1-h postprandial <155 mg/dL, and 2-h postprandial <130 mg/dL. The American College of Obstetricians and Gynecologists (ACOG) recommends the following targets for pregnant women with diabetes: fasting <90 mg/dL, preprandial <105 mg/dL, 1-h postprandial <130–140 mg/dL, and 2-h postprandial <120 mg/dL. Until harmonization of these guidelines is achieved, the ADA recommends setting targets based on clinical experience while individualizing care as needed.

Source: Adapted from American Diabetes Association. Standards of medical care in diabetes—2016. *Diabetes Care* 2016;39(Suppl. 1):S96.

ongoing research (such as DirecNet), has dispelled concerns regarding hypoglycemia and neurocognitive dysfunction. Also, there is some evidence that elevated blood glucose levels and glycemic variability in young children may produce adverse outcomes, at least in the short term, on neurocognitive function and the central nervous system. Therefore, an A1C goal of <7.5% is recommended across all pediatric age-groups, keeping in mind that glycemic variability plays a role. The individualization of goals while minimizing the risk of severe hypoglycemia and hyperglycemia and maintaining normal growth and development is paramount (see Table 2.2).

Self-monitoring of blood glucose (SMBG) targets in the DCCT were 70–120 mg/dL (3.9–6.7 mmol/L) before meals and at bedtime and <180 mg/dL (<10.0 mmol/L) when measured 1.5–2.0 h postprandially. Intensive insulin therapy (at that time, a combination of human regular and human intermediate-acting insulins, or pump therapy with human regular) was associated with a threefold increased risk of severe hypoglycemia.

Since the DCCT, the introduction of insulin analogs, enhanced provider experience, the widespread use of multiple daily injections and insulin pumps giving smaller more frequent doses of insulin, and the use of continuous glucose monitoring (CGM) appears to have decreased the severe hypoglycemia rates found in the DCCT while also decreasing A1C values.

Individual treatment goals should take into account the patient's capacity to understand and carry out the treatment regimen, the patient's risk for severe hypoglycemia, and other patient factors that may increase risk or decrease benefit, e.g., very young or old age, end-stage renal disease, advanced cardiovascular or cerebrovascular disease, or other coexisting diseases that will materially affect quality of life or shorten life expectancy. The benefits of interventions such as stringent glycemic control may not apply to those with advanced complications of diabetes or to those with a life expectancy of less than the anticipated time frame of benefit. Conversely, the risks of interventions such as tight glycemic control (hypoglycemia, treatment burden) may be greater in older patients. Although individualization is critical, in general, older patients with a long life expectancy and little comorbidity should have treatment targets similar to those of middle-aged or younger adults. In more frail patients, treatment targets might reasonably be relaxed, while symptomatic hyperglycemia or the risk of DKA should still be avoided. A framework for considering treatment goals for glycemia, blood pressure, and dyslipidemia in older adults with diabetes is outlined in Table 2.4.

The desired outcome of glycemic control in type 1 diabetes is to lower glycated hemoglobin (A1C or an equivalent measure of chronic glycemia) so as to achieve maximum prevention of complications with regard for patient safety.

CLINICAL GOALS

Initial Goals
- Assessment of disease, psychosocial status, and overall health
- Correct hyperglycemia, ketosis, DKA
  - replenish fluid losses slowly
  - insulin management
  - electrolyte replacement
  - avoid cerebral edema
  - treat any other underlying/precipitating issues (coexistent autoimmunity, vaginitis or balanitis, recurrent infections, etc.)
- Confirm diagnosis
- Team-based approach
  - educate (initially survival skills)
  - aligned goals
  - support

Additional Goals
- Age-appropriate and special situation medical, psychosocial, and education care
- Glycemic control
  - optimize and individualize glucose and A1C targets to achieve best possible control on an assessment of potential risks and benefits (Tables 2.1 and 2.2)
  - day-to-day fluctuations in blood glucose level are unavoidable, and both patients and providers should focus on patterns to improve glycemic variability as safe as possible
  - minimize short- and long-term complications
    —minimize severe hypoglycemia
    —minimize severe hyperglycemia

Table 2.4   Framework for Considering Treatment Goals for Glycemia, Blood Pressure, and Dyslipidemia in Older Adults with Diabetes

Patient characteristics/ health status	Rationale	Reasonable A1C goal‡	Fasting or preprandial glucose	Bedtime glucose	Blood pressure	Lipids
Healthy (few coexisting chronic illnesses, intact cognitive and functional status)	Longer remaining life expectancy	<7.5% (58 mmol/ mol)	90–130 mg/dL (5.0–7.2 mmol/L)	90–150 mg/dL (5.0–8.3 mmol/L)	<140/90 mmHg	Statin unless contraindicated or not tolerated
Complex/intermediate (multiple coexisting chronic illnesses* or 2+ instrumental ADL impairments or mild-to-moderate cognitive impairment)	Intermediate remaining life expectancy, high treatment burden, hypoglycemia vulnerability, fall risk	<8.0% (64 mmol/ mol)	90–150 mg/dL (5.0–8.3 mmol/L)	100–180 mg/dL (5.6–10.0 mmol/L)	<140/90 mmHg	Statin unless contraindicated or not tolerated
Very complex/ poor health (LTC or end-stage chronic illnesses** or moderate-to-severe cognitive impairment or 2+ ADL dependencies)	Limited remaining life expectancy makes benefit uncertain	<8.5%† (69 mmol/ mol)	100–180 mg/dL (5.6–10.0 mmol/L)	110–200 mg/dL (6.1–11.1 mmol/L)	<150/90 mmHg	Consider likelihood of benefit with statin (secondary prevention more so than primary)

This represents a consensus framework for considering treatment goals for glycemia, blood pressure, and dyslipidemia in older adults with diabetes. The patient characteristic categories are general concepts. Not every patient will clearly fall into a particular category. Consideration of patient and caregiver preferences is an important aspect of treatment individualization. Additionally, a patient's health status and preferences may change over time. ADL, activities of daily living; LTC, long-term care.

‡ A lower A1C goal may be set for an individual if achievable without recurrent or severe hypoglycemia or undue treatment burden.

* Coexisting chronic illnesses are conditions serious enough to require medications or lifestyle management and may include arthritis, cancer, congestive heart failure, depression, emphysema, falls, hypertension, incontinence, stage 3 or worse chronic kidney disease, myocardial infarction, and stroke. By "multiple," we mean at least three, but many patients may have five or more.

** The presence of a single end-stage chronic illness, such as stage 3–4 congestive heart failure or oxygen-dependent lung disease, chronic kidney disease requiring dialysis, or uncontrolled metastatic cancer, may cause significant symptoms or impairment of functional status and significantly reduce life expectancy.

† A1C of 8.5% (69 mmol/mol) equates to an estimated average glucose of ~200 mg/dL (11.1 mmol/L). Looser A1C targets above 8.5% (69 mmol/mol) are not recommended as they may expose patients to more frequent higher glucose values and the acute risks from glycosuria, dehydration, hyperglycemic hyperosmolar syndrome, and poor wound healing.

Source: American Diabetes Association. Standards of medical care in diabetes—2016. *Diabetes Care* 2016;39(Suppl. 1):S83.

- General health
  - maintain normal growth and development
  - maintain weight within a desirable range
  - maintain maximum exercise tolerance and stamina
  - screen and treat any coexisting autoimmune conditions
  - screen and treat for complications
- Psychosocial
  - maintain a sense of psychosocial well-being and normal initiative in self-care
  - sustain normal family and marital relationships and sex life
  - prevent a diabetes-dictated or diabetes-oriented lifestyle (i.e., diabetes controlling the patient rather than vice versa)
- Educate and Support
  - self-management skills
  - different management approaches (pens, pumps, CGM, etc.)
  - Special situations (sick day, exercise, driving, transitioning, pregnancy, etc.)

Assessment of A1C

During diabetes visits, glycemic control is assessed by results of glycohemoglobin tests. Many different types of glycohemoglobin assay methods were available in the past, differing considerably with respect to the glycated components measured, interferences, and nondiabetic range. Glycated hemoglobin A_{1c} (A1C) has become the preferred standard for assessing glycemic control, and in 1996, the National Glycohemoglobin Standardization Program (NGSP) was formed to standardize the A1C test to DCCT values. Since then, A1C measurements in North America have been almost universally standardized to the DCCT assay range.

The International Federation of Clinical Chemistry (IFCC) developed a standard for A1C that results in a measurement of concentration (mmol A1C/mol HbA) rather than percent and a reference range that is different than the DCCT standard. A consensus between the IFCC and world diabetes organizations, including the American Diabetes Association, suggests that in medical journals and in the clinical arena, A1C results will be reported in both ways: the IFCC concentration and the DCCT-standardized A1C (as percent). Mmol/mol is the Système International (SI) unit. In the U.S., most lab reports do not use SI units, so it is unclear whether clinically these units will become more common. Although small studies had suggested this to be the case for type 1 populations, a multicenter study in subjects with type 1, type 2, and no diabetes; of multiple ethnic groups; and on multiple types of diabetes therapies confirmed that there is a close association of A1C with the mean blood glucose over the prior 2–3 months across the entire study population. This has led some laboratories in the U.S. to report, on request, both A1C as a percentage and estimated average glucose (eAG).

In the past, when data compiled from diabetes specialty clinics in North America and Europe were analyzed, patients with type 1 diabetes have shown median A1C values (DCCT standard) of 8.0–9.0%. These correspond to mean blood glucose levels of ~200 mg/dL (~11.1 mmol/L). Adolescents with type 1 diabetes generally average 0.5–1.0% higher values and a blood glucose that is 20–40 mg/dL (1.1–2.2 mmol/L) higher than adults. Hemoglobin variants have the potential to cause falsely low or high A1C readings, especially with older assays. A list of assays and whether or not they are accurate in patients with hemoglobin variants can be found on the NGSP website (www.ngsp.org/interf.asp).

Assessment and Goals of Glycemic Control

In addition to A1C, during diabetes visits, individual glucose values from SMBG and CGM can be obtained from logbooks, uploading glucose meters and CGM devices, or glancing through the stored data on the meter and CGM screens. Diabetes control is assessed by the patient at home via SMBG, CGM, and urine or blood ketones. As the ability to have more daily blood glucose information has increased, teaching patients to interpret estimated A1C by average blood glucose can really help connect patients and providers around diabetes control.(See Table 2.5 below for corresponding A1C/eAG values).

Results of Optimal Control

At an optimal level of control, patients are entirely asymptomatic and may perceive a very good or excellent sense of well-being, energy, and exercise capacity and less disease-related anxiety compared with maintenance at poor control. They may also express a greater sense of control over the management of the disease if they use a flexible, individualized management program. However, they may experience increased mild self-treated and also severe hypoglycemic episodes. Some patients may feel excessively burdened by the required frequent monitoring, insulin administration methods, and constant dietary adherence. Negotiation (and renegotiation) of mutually acceptable goals will reduce the chances that patients will abandon reasonable self-care. In fact, treatment of type 1 diabetes always involves a negotiated therapeutic alliance between patient (and family) and the diabetes management team.

Table 2.5 Corresponding A1C and eAG Values

A1C (%)	eAG (mg/dL)	eAG (mmol/L)
5	97	5.4
6	126	7.0
7	154	8.6
8	183	10.2
9	212	11.8
10	240	13.4
11	269	14.9
12	298	16.5

Source: American Diabetes Association, eAG/A1C Conversion Calculator [webpage]. Available from http://professional.diabetes.org/diapro/glucose_calc. Accessed 6 September 2016.

CONCLUSION

For patients with type 1 diabetes, the long-term benefits of optimal diabetes management appear extremely promising. A flexible, individualized diabetes management program that utilizes the principles of intensive insulin therapy should be encouraged in almost all type 1 diabetes patients from onset. The benefits of optimal management must be balanced in each patient against actual risks and costs. The diabetes management team together with the patient should set treatment goals on the basis of their own best judgment regarding individual patient capabilities and understanding.

BIBLIOGRAPHY

American Diabetes Association. Standards of medical care in diabetes—2016. *Diabetes Care* 2016;39(Suppl. 1):S23–S35

Chiang JL, Kirkman MS, Laffel LM, Peters AL; Type 1 Diabetes Sourcebook Authors. Type 1 diabetes through the life span: a position statement of the American Diabetes Association. *Diabetes Care* 2014;37:2034–2054

DCCT Research Group. The effect of intensive treatment of diabetes on the development and progression of long-term complications in insulin-dependent diabetes mellitus. *N Engl J Med* 1993;329:977–986

DCCT Research Group. The relationship of glycemic exposure (HbA$_{1c}$) to the risk of development and progression of retinopathy in the Diabetes Control and Complications Trial. *Diabetes* 1995;44:968–983

DCCT/EDIC Research Group. Retinopathy and nephropathy in patients with type 1 diabetes four years after a trial of intensive therapy. *N Engl J Med* 2000;342:381–389

DCCT/EDIC Research Group, Nathan DM, Zinman B, Cleary PA, Backlund JY, Genuth S, Miller R, Orchard TJ. Modern-day clinical course of type 1 diabetes mellitus after 30 years' duration: the Diabetes Control and Complications Trial/Epidemiology of Diabetes Interventions and Complications and Pittsburgh Epidemiology of Diabetes Complications Experience (1983–2005). *Arch Intern Med* 2009;169:1307–1316

DCCT/EDIC Research Group, Aiello LP, Sun W, Das A, Gangaputra S, Kiss S, Klein R, Cleary PA, Lachin JM, Nathan DM. Intensive diabetes therapy and ocular surgery in type 1 diabetes. *N Engl J Med* 2015;372:1722–1733

Goldstein DE, Little RR, Lorenz RA, Malone JI, Nathan DM, Peterson CM; American Diabetes Association. Tests of glycemia in diabetes. *Diabetes Care* 2003;26(Suppl. 1):S106–S108

Kitzmiller JL, Block JM, Brown FM, et al. Managing preexisting diabetes for pregnancy: summary of evidence and consensus recommendations for care. *Diabetes Care* 2008;31:1060–1079

Klein R. Hyperglycemia and microvascular and macrovascular disease in diabetes. *Diabetes Care* 1995;18:258–268

Nathan DM, Lachin J, Cleary P, Orchard T, Brillon DJ, Backlund JY, O'Leary DH, Genuth S; Diabetes Control and Complications Trial/Epidemiology of Diabetes Interventions and Complications Research Group. Intensive diabetes therapy and carotid intima-media thickness in type 1 diabetes. *N Engl J Med* 2003;348:2294–2303

Nathan DM, Cleary PA, Backlund JY, Genuth SM, Lachin JM, Orchard TJ, Raskin P, Zinman B; DCCT/EDIC Study Research Group. Intensive diabetes treatment and cardiovascular disease in patients with type 1 diabetes. *N Engl J Med* 2005;353:2643–2653

National Cholesterol Education Program (NCEP) Expert Panel on Detection, Evaluation, and Treatment of High Blood Cholesterol in Adults. Executive summary of the Third Report of the National Cholesterol Education Program (NCEP) Expert Panel on Detection, Evaluation, and Treatment of High Blood Cholesterol in Adults (Adult Treatment Panel III). *JAMA* 2001;285:2486–2497

Pirart J. Diabetes mellitus and its degenerative complications: a prospective study of 4,400 patients observed between 1947 and 1973. *Diabetes Care* 1978;1:252–263

Reichard P, Nilsson BY, Rosenqvist U. The effect of long-term intensified insulin treatment on the development of microvascular complications of diabetes mellitus. *N Engl J Med* 1993;329:304–309

Rohlfing CL, Wiedmeyer HM, Little RR, England JD, Tennill A, Goldstein DE. Defining the relationship between plasma glucose and HbA(1c): analysis of glucose profiles and HbA(1c) in the Diabetes Control and Complications Trial. *Diabetes Care* 2002;25:275–278

Santiago JV. Lessons from the Diabetes Control and Complications Trial. *Diabetes* 1993;42:1549–1554

Silverstein J, Klingensmith G, Copeland K, Plotnick L, Kaufman FR, Laffel L, Deeb L, Grey M, Anderson B, Holzmeister LA, Clark N; American Diabetes Association. Care of children and adolescents with type 1 diabetes: a statement of the American Diabetes Association. *Diabetes Care* 2005;28:186–212

Skyler JS. Tactics for type 1 diabetes. *Endocrinol Metab Clin North Am* 1997;26:647–657

PATIENT SELF-MANAGEMENT EDUCATION AND SUPPORT

Diabetes management is a team effort. Physicians, nurses, dietitians, pharmacists, and other health-care professionals contribute their expertise to the design of therapeutic regimens that will enable patients to achieve the best possible metabolic control. The patient is at the center of the team and, supported by his or her family, is responsible for the day-to-day implementation of the treatment plan. In the case of children, the caregivers take on this responsibility. Therapy will be most effective if the patient understands the regimen, is not ambivalent about the value, and has mastered the skills to do required tasks correctly. Therefore, the clinical management of diabetes relies heavily on patient self-management.

The importance of patient education and support is underscored by the DCCT, which demonstrated that intensive treatment of diabetes, with great demands in patient self-management, can prevent or delay the long-term complications of diabetes. Because intensive therapy brings an increased risk of hypoglycemia, patient education and support are critical to providing safety. In addition, diabetes self-management training has been shown to improve A1C with as much as a 0.76% reduction immediately after education is delivered. The effect of diabetes education and support on A1C is directly correlated to the amount of contact time spent between the educator and the patient; 23.6 h of educator contact has been shown to decrease A1C by 1%, an amount known to be associated with a dramatic reduction in microvascular disease.

This section provides an overview of diabetes patient education and support, including information on the principles, process, content, and guidelines for incorporating education and support into clinical practice. Several terms, including "diabetes self-management education and support" and "diabetes self-management training," are used to describe patient education and support in diabetes. They will be used interchangeably in this manual. However, for reimbursement purposes, "diabetes self-management training" is the preferred terminology.

GENERAL PRINCIPLES

The goal of diabetes self-management education and support is to provide patients with the knowledge, skills, motivation, and support to incorporate ongoing diabetes self-care into their daily lives and to actively collaborate with their diabetes health-care team in managing the disease. To meet this goal, diabetes education and support must include teaching patients the new information they need to know about the diabetes disease process, training them in the various skills they need for their prescribed treatment plan and procedures, assisting them in developing strategies to fit the regimen into their lifestyle, and helping them reconcile diabetes care with their quality of life so they are motivated to manage their disease. To accomplish this, diabetes self-management education and support should be responsive to the unique and individual needs of the patient and equally accessible to all patients regardless of economic, social, and environmental circumstances.

Ideally, a diabetes management team should be involved in patient education and support. In the Diabetes Attitudes, Wishes and Needs (DAWN) study, a survey conducted among patients, nurses, and physicians, it was found that nurses provide better education and support, spend more time with patients, are better listeners, and get to know patients better than physicians. In addition, patients had better outcomes when they had access to a nurse, but less than 50% of patients surveyed said they had such access. Many physicians do not have a diabetes education and support team available in their practice setting. They need to refer patients, if possible, to a diabetes education and support program or to diabetes educators. Physicians can develop a team approach by collaborating with diabetes educators working in diabetes education and support programs. The American Diabetes Association's Education Recognition Program and the American Association of Diabetes Educators identify diabetes education and support programs that meet the National Standards for Diabetes Self-Management Education and Support through a Medicare-approved accreditation process. A list of active American Diabetes Association–recognized programs is available on the Association's website and can be accessed at www.diabetes.org/findaprogram.

Diabetes self-management education and support is a planned process that requires resources, including time, materials, space, and professional expertise (Table 2.6). The knowledge and skills patients need to implement their treatment regimen and sustain a lifetime of living with diabetes cannot be acquired during a quick interaction on the day of diagnosis or in a single instructional session in a physician's office or any other setting. Moreover, patient education and support is an ongoing component of diabetes care, not a one-time encounter. Despite this emphasis on diabetes education and support, a number of studies have found that self-management programs are underutilized, with relatively fewer patients having ongoing contact with educators.

For the newly diagnosed patient, a staged approach to education and support should be used, with the initial teaching focused on the critical information or

Table 2.6 Process of Diabetes Self-Management Education and Support

Assessment	Gathering information, both subjective and objective, to identify a patient's individual education and support needs
Planning	Designing education and support for the patient based on the assessment, including topics, goals for education and support, and selection of teaching/learning strategies
Implementation	Providing the planned education and support in an environment that supports learning
Documentation	Documenting the educational activities to inform other members of the diabetes management team and to record the care provided
Evaluation	Measuring the impact of education and support by testing knowledge and skills and by evaluating behavioral and metabolic outcomes
Reassessment	Periodically reviewing clinical and nonclinical information about the patient to identify new needs and re-educate as needed

"survival skills" that will enable the individual, or caregiver, to implement the regimen at home (Table 2.7). Once the patient is comfortable with the fundamental components of the regimen, teaching can be expanded to provide more in-depth information and to introduce additional topics. Continuing education and support across the life span provides opportunities for learning new management techniques; for making adjustments in the regimen to accommodate lifestyle changes, growth, and aging; to consider adding new therapies or technologies; and to sustain the positive clinical and quality-of-life outcomes achieved.

To be effective, diabetes self-management education and support must be individualized. Teaching methods, however, need not be limited to individual instruction. Group classes and self-study methods can supplement individual instruction and offer advantages in meeting different learning styles and in efficient use of teaching time. Information from all sources must be consistent, whether provided by different health professionals or from diverse instructional materials. Therefore, all members of the diabetes management team need to be aware of the content of the education and support program.

SELF-MANAGEMENT EDUCATION AND SUPPORT PROCESS

Diabetes self-management education and support is a systematic process that starts with an assessment of individual educational needs to guide the planning of teaching/learning strategies, followed by implementation of the plan and documentation of the process, and concluding with evaluation of learning as evidenced by behavior change and health outcomes. Although terms may be different, the process mimics the traditional steps clinicians use to diagnose and treat patients.

Table 2.7 Basic Education and Support at Diagnosis: Survival Skills

Topics and the critical knowledge and skills patients need to manage their diabetes at home include:

General facts	Explain the need for daily insulin injections and that treatment of diabetes involves insulin, diet, exercise, and SMBG
Medications	Measure insulin dosage accurately, inject correctly, and understand timing of injections and how to handle insulin and supplies
Nutrition	Explain the relationship of food to insulin and blood glucose and the amount of food, type of food, and times to eat to maximize blood glucose control
Exercise	Explain the relationship of exercise, food, and insulin and how to prevent hypoglycemia from exercise
Monitoring	Perform accurate SMBG and urine or blood ketone test
Hyperglycemia and hypoglycemia	Differentiate between the signs and symptoms of high and low blood glucose levels and know what actions to take for each situation; know when to seek immediate medical assistance for intercurrent illness, hyperglycemia, or ketonuria
Use of the health-care system	Identify how to obtain insulin supplies, whom to call for professional advice, and how to get help in an emergency

Understanding the commonalities of patient education and support and medical care facilitates integration of education and support into the clinical management of diabetes.

There are guiding principles for diabetes education and support. These principles are supported by numerous studies and include:

1. Diabetes education and support is effective in improving clinical outcomes and quality of life,
2. Diabetes self-management education and support has evolved from didactic presentations to theoretically based empowerment models,
3. There is no one best methodology, and effective programs have incorporated behavioral and psychosocial strategies, culture- and age-specific programming, and individual and group sessions,
4. Ongoing support is important for sustained benefit, and
5. Behavioral goal-setting is an effective strategy to support self-management behaviors

Assessment

The first step in the education and support process is an assessment, which obtains clinical, psychosocial, and educability data to determine an individual education and support plan. Information obtained in this assessment can guide both treatment and education and support decisions. For example, if assessment shows that the individual has limited learning skills, treatment with a simple insulin regimen versus a complex algorithm of dose adjustments would be appropriate, with educational strategies including selection of pictorial instructional materials, return demonstration, and a plan for evaluating accurate performance at home.

The education and support assessment also focuses on the three key areas of the learning process: cognitive/knowledge, psychomotor/skills, and affective/attitude. To develop effective teaching strategies, the educator needs to evaluate each patient to determine specific knowledge that needs to be acquired; skills that need to be mastered; personal attitudes toward diabetes, health care, and life skills, and experiences that will predict behavior change potential since most aspects of diabetes self-care and management require behavior changes.

As a general framework, the educational assessment should include:

- demographic information: age, gender, level of education, occupation, and family status; and for children, this information must be obtained about parents or caregivers as well
- medical history: height; weight; BMI; blood pressure; blood glucose values (A1C, fasting, plasma glucose, and self-monitoring results); blood lipid values; medications (prescribed and over-the-counter); allergies; other medical problems; general health status, including smoking, alcohol consumption, sexual activity, and use of social drugs; health service or resource utilization; and for children, developmental capabilities, prior growth records, and pubertal stage
- diabetes history: type of diabetes; duration of diabetes; current treatment plan, including medication, diet, exercise, monitoring, and problems with

adherence; acute and chronic complications; family history; previous diabetes education; and for children, diabetes management plan at school or child care
- dietary habits: meal times and locations, snacking patterns, food preferences, resources for food preparation, patterns suggestive of disordered eating, food allergies/intolerances, and previous diet instructions (note that medical nutrition therapy includes a more detailed history; see Nutrition, page 125)
- physical activity: work/school activity, recreational activity, time of day of activity, duration and intensity
- social history: information on household, extended family, social network, cultural factors, religious practices, health beliefs, beliefs about insulin, and current health practices
- economic profile: income, health insurance, transportation resources, and neighborhood environment
- lifestyle: activities of daily living, including work, school, and leisure time; for children, information on after-school, weekend, and summer activities
- psychosocial status: feelings about diabetes; personal relationships (with spouse, partner, parents, family, peers); developmental stages in life-cycle; history of sleep or eating disorders, stress, anxiety, or depression; health goals
- education factors: functional health literacy, computational skills, readiness to learn, preferred learning methods, visual acuity, hearing loss, dexterity, life experiences, and for children, developmental stage
- knowledge and skill level in each of the nine content areas of the National Standards for Diabetes Self-Management Education and Support

Additional information will be required to develop educational plans to meet the idiosyncratic needs of individual patients. However, the extent and completeness of the assessment will be determined by the patient as he or she presents for education and support. For example, a newly diagnosed patient overwhelmed by the diagnosis may not be ready to digest the need for acquiring all these data before a session. The ultimate goal is to completely assess the patient over time. Parts of the complete assessment can be deferred until the patient is fully able to participate and provide the most beneficial information for education and support planning. Assessment should therefore be dynamic, ongoing, and dictated by patient readiness, in order to obtain the most beneficial information to guide education and support. Also, as is the case with medical nutrition therapy, each member of the diabetes management team will use a more extensive assessment specific to their area of expertise.

Patient autonomy should be supported by understanding the patients' diabetes-related priorities and needs, acknowledging patients' feelings and experiences, facilitating meaningful self-management choices, offering relevant information, and avoiding controlling patients' behavior.

Planning Educational Strategies

The assessment identifies the topics that need to be included in the education and support plan and the teaching methods that would be most effective. From this analysis, educational goals are developed for each patient. The educational goals must correspond with the therapeutic goals established by the diabetes management team and the diabetes management goals set by the patient. If the diabetes management team is focused on normalization of blood glucose and the patient is focused on making a minimum number of lifestyle changes, teaching will not be effective until there is agreement. Once goals are established, measurable behavioral objectives are developed with the patient to clearly identify steps that will be used to achieve these goals.

The education and support plan delineates what is to be taught when, how, where, and by whom. There are numerous teaching strategies that can be used with a patient (Table 2.8). For a newly diagnosed patient, the plan would specify topics that need to be covered immediately to provide the patient with the "survival skills" necessary to manage his or her diabetes at home (Table 2.7). Teaching methods could include:

- one-on-one sessions with the dietitian to develop a meal plan
- one-on-one sessions with the diabetes educator to learn insulin injection and monitoring techniques

Table 2.8   Teaching Strategies

Methods

- Individual instruction: education and support can be tailored to individual learning needs and focused on specific details of a patient's self-management plan; can also accommodate patient-specific learning barriers like vision problems or cognitive challenges
- Group classes: efficient use of educator time, patients benefit from social support and peer learning
- Self-study: flexible, allows patient to pace learning, educator should monitor and evaluate progress
- Can be mastery-based

Techniques

- Short lecture: effective for presenting new information
- Discussion: allows patients to personalize information, ask questions, disclose feelings, and share experiences
- Skills training: provides "hands on" learning; educator demonstrates, patient practices then performs a return demonstration and receives feedback from educator
- Problem-solving: allows patients to integrate information on several topics, such as diet, insulin, and exercise, and to test their knowledge in hypothetical situations
- Role-playing: can be used to reinforce learning (patient plays educator role), to practice social skills (explaining diabetes to friends), and to explore personal problems (family stress)
- Case studies: provide an objective approach to learning that can be used for planning, for problem-solving, and to help patients identify errors they are making in their diabetes self-management

- observation of patient injection and monitoring skills by staff nurses
- a videotape describing pathophysiology
- Internet education modules

The plan would include methods for evaluating learning accomplished in the initial phase, steps to reinforce what has been taught, and resources for obtaining in-depth education and support within a reasonable time frame.

Implementation

Teaching can take place in a classroom, at bedside, in an office, in the home, in the cafeteria, in a community facility, or in a number of other settings, as well as remotely via online coaching and webinars. Whatever space is used, it is critical that the environment support learning and reinforce the importance of the educational process as part of diabetes care. There should be adequate lighting and furnishings and minimal distractions. Education and support sessions should be scheduled at specific times. Scheduling will help ensure that teaching and learning take place and help establish the concept that education and support is a specific part of diabetes care. The same measures used to reinforce routine clini-

- Self-assessment: blood glucose records, food diaries, and exercise logs can be used to help patients recognize problems in their diabetes self-management and often to identify solutions
- Contracting/goal-setting: used to get patient buy-in on the specifics of changing behavior. Patient-driven, plan for reevaluating contracts or goals to assess degree of achievement, acknowledge successes, and reinforce needed information. AADE-7 is a framework for contracting/goal-setting
- Demonstrate projects: dining out, cooking classes, supermarket trips offer practical ways to apply complex information

Materials
- Printed materials: can be used to reinforce teaching, for self-study, and as an information resource for future needs (e.g., sick-day guidelines)
- Audio and visual aids: slides, films, overheads, audiotapes and videotapes, food models and labels, sample diabetes products, and dolls and puppets are effective in enhancing learning
- Interactive learning programs: available in printed, audio, visual, and computer formats; allow individuals to learn at their own pace, with frequent evaluation to provide feedback on learning
- Games: crossword puzzles, board games, and group games introduce fun into the educational process while enhancing participant learning
- Mobile applications, electronic games, and other technologies
- A case study with questions to evaluate learning and problem-solving skills
- Conversation maps: very effective in stimulating "conversation" and directing teaching to patient-expressed needs

cal appointments should be used for education and support sessions, including written information giving the appointment time, location (with directions if needed), and the name(s), telephone number(s), or Internet addresses of the educator(s). Text messaging can be used to send reminders and to encourage/motivate patients.

Documentation

Documentation of education and support is as important as documentation of treatment procedures. It provides a means of communication among the diabetes management team as well as a means of substantiating the provision of educational care. Documentation can also provide a reference for reinforcing educational and behavioral objectives necessary to accomplish treatment goals by other members of the diabetes team.

Documentation can be included in progress notes in the patient's medical chart or electronic medical record, maintained in education and support charts or an electronic database, or written in correspondence and reports. Whatever method of documentation is used, a permanent record of a patient's educational experience must be maintained.

Evaluation

The effectiveness of the educational plan is evaluated in several ways. First, assessment of learning will provide measures of knowledge gained, skills acquired, and changes in attitudes. This type of evaluation often is included in the implementation process to allow for reinforcement in areas where the patient exhibits weaknesses. It is typically done in the short run, in the immediate post-education and support phase. Periodic reassessments will provide measures of lapses in knowledge, skills, or attitudes that can be remedied with a refresher course. Another evaluation procedure measures changes in behavior. This evaluation takes place some time after education and support (1–3 months) to measure whether the short-term attitude changes and behavior modifications are maintained and have resulted in sustained behavior change. The behavioral objectives developed during the planning phase may be used, or a different set of objectives can be set at the completion of education and support as an outgrowth of the learning process. A third approach evaluates the effectiveness of education and support by examining treatment goals, such as lower A1C, improvement in quality of life evidenced by minimal hypoglycemia, or absence of ketoacidosis. All forms of evaluation yield an assessment of additional educational needs of the patient.

CONTENT OF DIABETES SELF-MANAGEMENT EDUCATION AND SUPPORT

Topics to be included in diabetes patient education and support are numerous and vary according to type of diabetes, patient age, and other individual characteristics. The National Standards for Diabetes Self-Management Education and Support specify that programs should be equipped to provide information in nine core content areas. The suggested topics are listed below with basic teaching points for type 1 diabetes:

- **Describing the diabetes disease process and treatments:** Type 1 diabetes is a chronic metabolic disorder in which the body no longer produces insulin required to use food for energy. The loss of insulin production is due to an autoimmune process that results from an interaction of genes and environmental triggers. Lack of insulin can be life threatening. Daily insulin administration is essential and needs to be balanced with meals and physical activity to manage diabetes. Understanding the interactions among the three (food, insulin, and physical activity) and their impact on blood glucose levels is important to making self-management decisions. Self-monitoring values provide information that can be used to make adjustments in one or more of the three therapeutic agents.
- **Incorporating nutritional management into lifestyle:** Food is an important part of diabetes treatment and health. The amount, type, and timing of meals and snacks must be balanced with insulin and exercise to maintain good blood glucose control. Meal planning should be individualized to reflect food preferences and daily schedules, provide optimum nutrition, maintain a healthy weight, and make diabetes self-care as effective as possible.
- **Incorporating physical activity into lifestyle:** Physical activity is recommended for health and diabetes management. Physical activity can affect blood glucose levels and other health parameters like blood pressure, weight, and stress, usually by lowering them. For the purposes of diabetes education and support, exercise can be characterized as any tolerable increase in baseline activity. Planning for exercise can prevent hypoglycemia that may occur during or after exercise.
- **Using medication(s) safely and for maximum therapeutic effectiveness:** Insulin must be taken daily as prescribed. It is important to know the type and amount of insulin to be taken and the times to administer insulin and to understand the action and duration of the prescribed insulin. Correct techniques for drawing up and injecting insulin with a syringe or pen device, or use of an insulin inhalation device are critical to ensure that the dose is accurate. There are different types of insulin regimens, from fixed 2–3 injections, to basal bolus therapy with multiple daily injections or insulin pump therapy. Family members, close friends, coaches, teachers, co-workers, and others who closely interact with the diabetes patient on insulin need to know how to administer glucagon in the event of severe hypoglycemia.
- **Monitoring blood glucose and other parameters and interpreting and using the results for self-management decision-making:** Blood glucose monitoring results can be used to assess the effectiveness of the treatment regimen, identify low blood glucose levels requiring treatment to prevent hypoglycemia, indicate high blood glucose levels possibly associated with illness, show the effect of different meals and activities on blood glucose, and guide decisions on when to contact health-care providers. Proper technique, including ensuring that hands are clean and dry before using the blood glucose meter, is crucial to achieving reliable results. The downloading of meter data can help with data management. CGM has an additional role in showing trends and patterns and alerting at set or predictive thresh-

olds. Urine or blood testing for ketones is required during times of sickness or unexplained hyperglycemia and may be necessary during pregnancy.

- **Preventing, detecting, and treating acute complications (hypoglycemia, hyperglycemia, and illness):** Hypoglycemia comes on quickly. Therefore, it is important to recognize the signs and symptoms of hypoglycemia and to know how to prevent and treat it (Table 2.9). Use of glucagon in appropriate situations needs to be reinforced. Hyperglycemia that cannot be explained by diet or another aspect of the regimen (e.g., decrease in exercise or inadequate insulin delivery or amount) may indicate illness. Patients with type 1 diabetes can develop diabetic ketoacidosis when ill. Therefore, guidelines for sick days need to be followed carefully (Table 2.10). Family members, friends, coworkers, and teachers need to know how to respond in case of emergencies.

- **Preventing, detecting, treating, and rehabilitation of chronic complications:** Chronic complications are a serious concern in diabetes. Steps that can reduce the risk of complications include: maintaining blood glucose levels as near to normal as feasible, not smoking, having annual eye exams, controlling blood pressure and blood lipid levels, assessing urine microalbumin excretion, and taking preventive care of feet.

- **Developing personal strategies to address psychosocial issues:** Fear, anger, and denial are common responses to the diagnosis of diabetes and other stages of the disease process. The day-by-day demands of diabetes management can be frustrating. Stress may cause problems with blood glucose control. Coping skills, stress reduction techniques, and professional counseling can help the patient handle the psychosocial impact of diabetes. Type 1 diabetes affects the whole family. Family members, friends, coworkers, and teachers need to know about diabetes and how to support the treatment regimen. Adolescents must not be left to manage diabetes without some degree of parental supervision, even when they have the skills to manage diabetes on their own. Camps, awareness walks, bike rides, and support groups, including online diabetes networks, can help with denial and isolation.

- **Developing personal strategies to promote health and behavior change:** Most aspects of diabetes management require changes in behavior. Behavior change is not simply willpower. Strategies such as goal setting, contracting, and developing problem-solving techniques based on patient experience are helpful in changing habits to reduce health risks and improve diabetes control. Risk factors for diabetic complications, including cardiovascular disease, should be addressed. Achieving optimal glucose control may deter the complications of diabetes, including those occurring during pregnancy. Women with type 1 diabetes need to achieve excellent blood glucose control before becoming pregnant (optimally for 3 months before conception) and maintain tight glucose control throughout pregnancy; however, tight control brings an increased risk of hypoglycemia. Individuals with diabetes need to be responsible for their diabetes management, which includes working with their diabetes management team to select the treatment plan that meets their personal goals for health. Because changing behavior underlies most aspects of diabetes self-management, presenting the content areas in action-oriented, behavioral terms will help to underscore the importance of active patient participation in diabetes care and management.

ADDITIONAL TOPICS OF IMPORTANCE FOR TYPE 1 DIABETES

■ Using the health-care system and community resources: People with diabetes need to be good consumers of the health-care system and of community resources. Ongoing versus episodic care is important. Contact information—including phone numbers and Internet addresses of diabetes management team members and emergency services—should be readily available for use by family and friends as well as the individual with diabetes. Identifying accessible resources in the community, through mobile

---

Table 2.9 Sample Patient Guidelines for Treating Mild* Hypoglycemia: 15/15 Rule

If blood glucose falls below 70 mg/dL:

■ Eat 15 g carbohydrate, preferably in the form of glucose products

■ Wait 15 min—retest, and if blood glucose remains <70 mg/dL, treat with another 15 g carbohydrate

■ Repeat testing and treating until blood glucose returns to normal range

■ If >1 h to next meal, add additional 15 g carbohydrate to maintain blood glucose in normal range

Sources of carbohydrate	
Glucose products (preferred):	
Glucose tablets	4–5 g/tablet
Glucose gel	15 g/dose
Insta-glucose gel	24 g tube/one-dose tube
Food/beverages (use if above products are not available), 15-g carbohydrate portions:	
Graham crackers	3
Saltine crackers	6
Raisins	2 Tbsp
Syrup or honey	1 Tbsp
Juice (apple/orange)	1/2 cup
Ginger ale	3/4 cup
Soft drink (regular)	1/2 cup
Skim milk	1 cup

* Severe hypoglycemia needs to be treated by someone knowledgeable about diabetes. Guidelines should be available in schools and at work sites. If the patient cannot swallow well, glucagon must be used instead of oral treatment.

Table 2.10 Sample Patient Guidelines for Sick-Day Management

Illness can make diabetes more difficult to manage. Even when you do not feel well, you must take your insulin, test blood glucose and urine or blood ketones, drink fluids, and eat if you can. Eating food is less important. You will need ketone strips and fluids that can be a source of glucose and electrolytes. Therefore, planning ahead for sick days is important. The following guidelines will help you during mild illnesses.

Monitoring
Blood glucose and urine (or blood) ketones need to be tested frequently during illness, often every 24 h. Test for ketones if you have unexplainable high blood glucose values >250 mg/dL or if you feel ill, even if blood glucose values are normal. Write down the values and call a member of your diabetes management team when premeal blood glucose values stay >250 mg/dL and/or when you measure moderate or large ketones.

Insulin
Never stop taking long-acting insulin even if vomiting and unable to eat. Your body often needs more insulin during illness. Therefore, your health-care professional may ask you to take additional insulin (a correction bolus) according to results of blood glucose monitoring.

Food and fluid intake
Eat small meals and eat more frequently when you are ill. Soft foods or liquids are often tolerated best. Eating about 10–15 g carbohydrate every 1–2 h is usually sufficient. Foods and beverages containing about 15 g carbohydrate include:

1/2 cup regular gelatin	3/4 cup regular ginger ale
1/2 cup vanilla ice cream	1/2 cup regular soft drink
1/2 cup custard	1/2 cup orange or apple juice
1 regular double Popsicle	1 cup Gatorade
1/2 cup applesauce	1 cup clear soup
1/2 small banana	1/3 cup rice
1 slice toast	

Fluid intake is essential during illness. If vomiting, diarrhea, or fever is present, take small quantities of liquids every 15–30 min. Clear broth, tea, and other fluids can supplement liquids containing carbohydrate.

Seek medical attention when you have:
- Fever >100°F
- Persistent diarrhea
- Vomiting and are unable to take fluids for >4 h
- Blood glucose levels that are difficult to control, with or without ketones (see information above on monitoring)
- Severe abdominal pain
- Other unexplained symptoms
- Vomiting that persists over 24 h

Physician's #_____   Pharmacy #_____

apps, and on the Internet for supplies, services, information, and support groups makes day-to-day diabetes management easier and helps the patient to maintain positive outcomes over time.
- Wearing an identification bracelet or necklace: This is strongly encouraged and recommended at all times so that having diabetes can be quickly ascer-

tained in the event of acute crises such as unconsciousness or a motor vehicle accident.

■ Driving a motor vehicle: Special care should be taken to prevent hypoglycemia while driving a car, truck, motorboat, or any other powered vehicle. Blood glucose levels should be checked before driving, especially if the last meal was more than 3 h earlier or if the trip will be long, and low blood glucose values should be treated appropriately (Table 2.9). People with diabetes should not start to drive until blood glucose is >100 mg/dL. Supplies for SMBG and treating hypoglycemia should be carried in the vehicle at all times. If symptoms of hypoglycemia occur, driving should stop immediately and not be resumed until blood glucose levels are in the normal range for at least 10 min.

■ Traveling: Insulin and diabetes supplies 1.5 times a patient's projected needs should be sufficient for the entire trip to accommodate delays and other potential travel mishaps. Supplies should be carried with the traveler and not put into checked baggage. Food to treat hypoglycemia and for any meal that may be delayed by late arrival should also be carried with the patient. Additional prescriptions should be carried as well, in case the need to purchase supplies does occur.

■ Working: Some jobs have erratic schedules, shift work, long periods between meals, lack the flexibility to stop work and test blood glucose levels, or have other conditions that make diabetes management more challenging. The Americans with Disabilities Act (ADA) requires employers to make reasonable accommodations for employees with disabilities, including diabetes. The person with diabetes along with his or her supervisor and diabetes management team can identify ways to modify a job to accommodate the demands of work and diabetes management.

■ Orientation and continuing education and support for school personnel: Children with diabetes in school are protected by Section 504 of the Rehabilitation Act of 1973, the Americans with Disabilities Act, and the Individuals with Disabilities Education Act (IDEA) so that there is a medically safe environment and equal access to educational opportunities and school-related activities. The Diabetes Medical Management Plan, devised by the health-care team and the student/parents, outlines what must be done in school with regard to administration of medication, monitoring, nutrition, activity, and diabetes-related emergencies. Parents, students, school personnel, and the diabetes management team work together to create a safe and supportive environment for school-age children.

INCORPORATING PATIENT EDUCATION AND SUPPORT IN CLINICAL PRACTICE

Patient education and support is essential for management of type 1 diabetes. However, not all medical practice settings are equipped to provide diabetes self-management training. Moreover, the complexity of type 1 diabetes, particularly when treated with intensive therapy, requires health-care providers to have special expertise in diabetes. Physicians who specialize in the treatment of diabetes and who see many patients with type 1 diabetes can develop a team relationship with diabetes educators in the community, if hiring educators on a full- or part-time basis is not feasible. Systems such as health maintenance organizations, preferred provider organizations, telemedicine, and affiliations with hospitals offer potential resources for certified diabetes educators who can work with a number of physicians to maximize the economy of this specialized type of care. Physicians practicing in an area where there are education and support programs that have achieved American Diabetes Association Recognition or are accredited by the American Association of Diabetes Educators may refer patients to programs that meet the National Standards for Diabetes Self-Management Education and Support. The local American Diabetes Association office maintains a list of recognized programs in their area, and this list is also available on the Association's website (visit www.diabetes.org/findaprogram).

To establish a team approach to diabetes self-management education and support, health-care professionals should 1) share a common philosophy toward diabetes management and 2) develop efficient methods for communicating about patient care and education and support to ensure that a consistent message is given to the patient. Forms, handwritten or electronic, can be helpful in documenting the educational process in a concise format that allows team members to keep abreast of each others' activities and to reinforce all areas of education and support. Communication by fax, computers (i.e., via HIPAA-compliant e-mail or electronic medical record messages), and HIPAA-compliant text messaging offers the opportunity for expedient transfer of information among health professionals not working in the same location. Forms, if placed in the front of a chart or a similar place routinely used in providing patient care, or in the electronic medical record, can serve as a prompt to educate while providing routine medical care.

Diabetes education and support materials can be obtained from the American Diabetes Association, from companies manufacturing pharmaceuticals or diabetes equipment and supplies, and through a number of additional resources available through the National Diabetes Information Clearinghouse website at www.diabetes.niddk.nih.gov.

CONCLUSION

Patients with type 1 diabetes need self-management education and support to be able to implement their treatment regimen. Education and support should be individualized to reflect the diabetes treatment regimen and learning characteristics of each patient. Self-management training is a systematic patient care process that requires educators with expertise in diabetes and resources of time and materials. Physicians should use a team approach to manage individuals with type 1 diabetes with self-management education and support integrated into the clinical care of the patient.

BIBLIOGRAPHY

American Association of Diabetes Educators. Diabetes Education Curriculum: A Guide to Successful Self-Management, 2nd ed. Chicago, American Association of Diabetes Educators, 2016

American Diabetes Association. Standards of medical care in diabetes—2016. *Diabetes Care* 2016;39(Suppl. 1):S39-47, S83–S89

American Diabetes Association, Lorber D, Anderson J, Arent S, Cox DJ, Frier BM, Greene MA, Griffin J Jr, Gross G, Hathaway K, Hirsch I, Kohrman DB, Marrero DG, Songer TJ, Yatvin AL. Diabetes and driving. *Diabetes Care* 2014;37(Suppl. 1):S97–S103

Anderson BJ, Rubin RR (Eds.). *Practical Psychology for Diabetes Clinicians*. 2nd ed. Alexandria, VA, American Diabetes Association, 2003

Anderson RM. Taking diabetes self-management education to the next level. *Diabetes Spectrum* 2007;20:202–203

Anderson RM, Funnell MM, Burkhart N, Gillard ML, Nwankwo R. *101 Tips for Behavior Change in Diabetes Education*. Alexandria, VA, American Diabetes Association, 2002

Cheng YJ, Gregg EW, Geiss LS, Imperatore G, Williams DE, Zhang X, Albright AL, Cowie CC, Klein R, Saaddine JB. Association of A1C and fasting plasma glucose levels with diabetic retinopathy prevalence in the U.S. population: implications for diabetes diagnostic thresholds. *Diabetes Care* 2009;32:2027–2032

Chiang JL, Kirkman MS, Laffel LM, Peters AL; Type 1 Diabetes Sourcebook Authors. Type 1 diabetes through the life span: a position statement of the American Diabetes Association. *Diabetes Care* 2014;37:2034–2054

Funnell MM, Brown TL, Childs BP, Haas LB, Hosey GM, Jensen B, Maryniuk M, Peyrot M, Piette JD, Reader D, Siminerio LM, Weinger K, Weiss MA. National standards for diabetes self-management education. *Diabetes Care* 2012;35(Suppl. 1):S101–S108

Funnell MM, Brown TL, Childs BP, Haas LB, Hosey GM, Jensen B, Maryniuk M, Peyrot M, Piette JD, Reader D, Siminerio LM, Weinger K, Weiss MA. National standards for diabetes self-management education. *Diabetes Care* 2011;34(Suppl. 1):S89–S96

Funnell M, Peyrot M, Rubin RR, Siminerio L. Steering toward a new DAWN in diabetes management. *Diabetes Educ* 2005;31(Suppl.):1–18

Funnell MM (Ed.). *Life with Diabetes: A Series of Teaching Outlines by the Michigan Diabetes Research and Training Center*. 3rd ed. Alexandria, VA, American Diabetes Association, 2004

Kanzer-Lewis G. *Patient Education: You Can Do It! A Practical Guide to Teaching and Motivating Patients*. Alexandria, VA, American Diabetes Association, 2003

Kaufman F, Silverstein J, Kadohiro J, Arent S, Spiegel G, Marschilok C, Bobo N, Gallivan J, Linder B, Hoogstraten A, Greenberg R; National Diabetes Education Program. *Helping the Student with Diabetes Succeed: A Guide for School Personnel.* Available from https://www.niddk.nih.gov/health-information/ health-communication-programs/ndep/health-care-professionals/school-guide/Pages/publicationdetail.aspx. Accessed 2012

Michigan Diabetes Research and Training Center. *Teenagers with Type 1 Diabetes: A Curriculum for Adolescents and Families.* Alexandria, VA, American Diabetes Association, 2003

Seaquist ER, Anderson J, Childs B, Cryer P, Dagogo-Jack S, Fish L, Heller SR, Rodriguez H, Rosenzweig J, Vigersky R. Hypoglycemia and diabetes: a report of a workgroup of the American Diabetes Association and the Endocrine Society. *Diabetes Care* 2013;36:1384–1395

Siminerio L, McLaughlin S, Polonsky W. *Diabetes Education Goals.* 3rd ed. Alexandria, VA, American Diabetes Association, 2003

GENERAL ROUTINE CARE

As part of the comprehensive medical care of persons with type 1 diabetes, several non–glucose-specific aspects of health maintenance need to be addressed, including immunizations, counseling about tobacco use, periodontal care, and screening for hearing loss. These will be discussed briefly in this section.

Routine vaccinations are recommended for all children and adults with diabetes according to age-related guidelines. The most up-to-date recommendations can be found on the Centers for Disease Control and Prevention (CDC) website, which contains age-specific vaccine schedules (visit www.cdc.gov/vaccines/schedules/index.html). There are immunization schedules for individuals aged birth through 18 years that summarize recommendations for routine vaccines. The CDC website also contains other resources for health-care professionals such as versions of the schedules to give parents, including a version in Spanish. Recommendations are also available for adults over 18 years of age.

Influenza and pneumococcal pneumonia are common, preventable diseases, and influenza is associated with high mortality and morbidity in the young, the elderly, and individuals with chronic diseases. The CDC recommends influenza vaccines (starting at 6 months of age) and pneumococcal vaccines for all individuals with diabetes. For individuals age 2 years and older, the pneumococcal polysaccharide vaccine 23 (PPSV23) is advised, while the pneumococcal conjugate vaccine 13 (PCV13) and PPSV23 should be administered in series to all adults age 65 years and older. Hepatitis B vaccinations should be administered to all adults with diabetes; people with type 1 or type 2 diabetes have a higher rate of hepatitis B.

Evidence for the link between cigarette smoking and detrimental health effects—including increased risk of cardiovascular disease, premature mortality, and microvascular complications—makes the routine assessment of tobacco use an essential part of diabetes care, either for prevention or to encourage cessation. Brief counseling is efficacious and cost-effective. Pharmacologic therapy may be an option for motivated individuals. Available research regarding electronic cigarettes (e-cigarettes) is not strong and do not support this as a healthy alternative to smoking or an effective strategy for smoking cessation. Patients should be advised against the use of any tobacco products including cigarettes and e-cigarettes.

Periodontal disease is more severe in individuals with diabetes and adversely affects diabetes outcomes. However, evidence regarding the effects of treatment of periodontal disease on diabetes-related outcomes is mixed. Nonetheless, patients should be advised to undergo regular dental cleanings and examinations, with the awareness that periodontal disease and infections can worsen glucose control and may increase the risk for other diabetes complications.

Impaired hearing is approximately two-fold more prevalent in people with diabetes as compared with individuals without diabetes even after adjustment for age and other risk factors for hearing loss. Diabetes may confer a higher risk for hearing loss because of neuropathy and/or vascular disease. However, evidence for increased risk has not been able to distinguish differences (if any) between the relative incidence in type 1 diabetes versus type 2 diabetes. Awareness of the higher prevalence of this potentially hidden comorbidity is a key to detection, and clinicians caring for individuals with diabetes should have a lower threshold for recommending screening for hearing loss when suggested by the history and/or exam.

BIBLIOGRAPHY

American Diabetes Association: Standards of medical care in diabetes—2016. *Diabetes Care* 2016;39(Suppl. 1):S23–S35

Bainbridge KE, Hoffman HJ, Cowie CC. Diabetes and hearing impairment in the United States: audiometric evidence from the National Health and Nutrition Examination Survey, 1999 to 2004. *Ann Intern Med* 2008;149:1–10

Bhatnagar A, Whitsel LP, Ribisl KM, Bullen C, Chaloupka F, Piano MR, Robertson RM, McAuley T, Goff D, Benowitz N; American Heart Association Advocacy Coordinating Committee, Council on Cardiovascular and Stroke Nursing, Council on Clinical Cardiology, and Council on Quality of Care and Outcomes Research. Electronic cigarettes: a policy statement from the American Heart Association. *Circulation* 2014;130:1418–1436

Borgnakke WS, Ylöstalo PV, Taylor GW, Genco RJ. Effect of periodontal disease on diabetes: systematic review of epidemiologic observational evidence. *J Periodontol* 2013;84(Suppl.):S135–S152

Chiang JL, Kirkman MS, Laffel LM, Peters AL; Type 1 Diabetes Sourcebook Authors. Type 1 diabetes through the life span: a position statement of the American Diabetes Association. *Diabetes Care* 2014;37:2034–2054

Colquhoun AJ, Nicholson KG, Botha JL, Raymond NT. Effectiveness of influenza vaccine in reducing hospital admissions in people with diabetes. *Epidemiol Infect* 1997;119:335–341

Khader YS, Dauod AS, El-Qaderi SS, Alkafajei A, Batayha WQ. Periodontal status of diabetics compared with nondiabetics: a meta-analysis. *J Diabetes Complications* 2006;20:59–68

Kim DK, Bridges CB, Harriman KH; Centers for Disease Control and Prevention (CDC); Advisory Committee on Immunization Practices (ACIP); ACIP Adult Immunization Work Group. Advisory Committee on Immunization Practices recommended immunization schedule for adults aged 19 years or older—United States, 2015. *MMWR Morb Mortal Wkly Rep* 2015;64:91–92

Ranney L, Melvin C, Lux L, McClain E, Lohr KN. Systematic review: smoking cessation intervention strategies for adults and adults in special populations. *Ann Intern Med* 2006;145:845–856

Smith SA, Poland GA. Use of influenza and pneumococcal vaccines in people with diabetes. *Diabetes Care* 2000;23:95–108

Strikas RA; Centers for Disease Control and Prevention (CDC); Advisory Committee on Immunization Practices (ACIP); ACIP Child/Adolescent Immunization Work Group. Advisory Committee on Immunization Practices recommended immunization schedules for persons aged 0 through 18 years— United States, 2015. *MMWR Morb Mortal Wkly Rep* 2015;64:93–94

Suarez L, Barrett-Connor E. Interaction between cigarette smoking and diabetes mellitus in the prediction of death attributed to cardiovascular disease. *Am J Epidemiol* 1984;120:670–675

Valdez R, Narayan KM, Geiss LS, Engelgau MM. Impact of diabetes mellitus on mortality associated with pneumonia and influenza among non-Hispanic black and white US adults. *Am J Public Health* 1999;89:1715–1721

Voulgari C, Katsilambros N, Tentolouris N. Smoking cessation predicts amelioration of microalbuminuria in newly diagnosed type 2 diabetes mellitus: a 1-year prospective study. *Metabolism* 2011;60:1456–1464

Tools of Therapy

Highlights
Tools of Therapy

INSULIN TREATMENT

- Patients with type 1 diabetes are dependent on insulin to survive.
- The insulins primarily in use today are: recombinant human insulin, with the same amino acid sequence as native human insulin (with or without protamine to delay its absorption, onset, and duration of action) and recombinant human insulin analogs, in which the amino acid sequence of human insulin is altered to affect its absorption, onset, and duration of action.
- Insulin preparations are classified by duration of action (rapid, short, intermediate, and basal).
- The insulin regimen should be tailored to the needs of the individual patient. Adjustments in the insulin regimen or specific insulin doses should be based on actual glycemic values obtained from patient self-monitoring of blood glucose (SMBG) or continuous glucose monitoring (CGM) rather than on "textbook" predictions of insulin action.
- More physiological multiple-component "flexible" regimens emphasize the difference between basal and prandial (bolus) insulin. These insulin regimens consist of
  - three or more daily injections (prandial/bolus and basal insulins)
  - insulin pump therapy

- Insulin needs may fluctuate during the first weeks or months of treatment. If a honeymoon or remission phase occurs, the insulin dose must be appropriately reduced, occasionally to as little as 0.1–0.3 units/kg/day, but insulin should not be discontinued or replaced with an oral hypoglycemic agent.
- Continuous subcutaneous insulin infusion is an alternative that offers advantages in lifestyle flexibility and glycemic variability.
- Regimens using insulin algorithms place more demands on both patient and physician than does a fixed course of treatment, but they provide greater flexibility in lifestyle and improved control. All forms of intensive therapy require high degrees of long-term commitment and flexibility on the part of the patient, the family, and the diabetes management team.
- Common problems associated with insulin therapy are detailed in Common Problems in Long-Term Therapy (page 95).

ADJUNCTIVE THERAPY IN TYPE 1 DIABETES

- Non-insulin adjunctive therapy, many commonly used in type 2 diabetes, complements intensive insulin therapy by addressing a variety of physiologic disturbances in type 1 diabetes, offering potential for helping patients reach their glycemic targets and preventing diabetes-related complications. In order for these therapies to be considered for routine clinical practice, well-designed, randomized, placebo-controlled trials are needed to clearly demonstrate safety and efficacy. Aside from pramlintide, the non-insulin adjunctive therapies listed below do not have a U.S. Food and Drug Administration (FDA) indication for use in individuals with type 1 diabetes.

- Pramlintide is a soluble nonaggregating amylin analog that is an adjunct to patients receiving prandial insulin therapy. The clinical benefits of pramlintide are achieved by replacing the action of amylin, a naturally occurring β-cell hormone that is deficient in type 1 diabetes. Results from clinical studies showed that when pramlintide was added to insulin regimens, patients with type 1 diabetes had improved glycemic control with no increased body weight or severe hypoglycemia. Despite its approval by the FDA for use as an adjunctive therapy in type 1 diabetes, its availability, and its alternative mechanism of action and efficacy, in reality the utilization of pramlintide is currently extremely low.
- Glucagon-like peptide (GLP)-1 is an incretin that is normally secreted in response to nutrient ingestion to enhance insulin secretion, delay gastric emptying, suppress glucagon, and induce satiety. Although there are few studies of GLP-1 agonists as adjunctive therapy in type 1 diabetes, there is clearly potential for therapeutic benefit including improved glycemic control, lower insulin doses, and weight loss. Longer-duration clinical trials are currently underway to assess the potential benefit of GLP-1 agonists in inhibiting β-cell apoptosis and promoting β-cell regeneration.
- Sodium-glucose cotransporter-2 (SGLT2) inhibitors are highly selective, orally active agents that reduce renal glucose absorption in the proximal renal tubules. Off-label use of SGLT2 inhibitors as adjunct therapy in type 1 diabetes is increasing. Recently, the concern that SGLT2 inhibitors may predispose to ketoacidosis has been raised, and in May 2015 the FDA issued a warning to that end. Further study on the safety and efficacy of SGLT2 inhibitors is clearly needed.
- Metformin is an inexpensive and well-established oral glucose-lowering agent commonly used as first-line therapy for type 2 diabetes. A principal mode of metformin action is activation of the energy-regulating enzyme AMP-activated protein kinase principally in muscles and liver, with associated decreased hepatic glucose production. Evidence on the effects of metformin in type 1 diabetes is limited. Results vary surrounding its effect on glycemic control and whether there are benefits for cardiovascular outcomes. Metformin is generally well tolerated, although an increase in gastrointestinal side effects is possible.
- Sitagliptin, a dipeptidyl peptidase IV (DPP-4) inhibitor, increases endogenous GLP-1 levels by inhibiting its rapid metabolism through the DPP-4 enzyme. Further investigation with larger cohorts to assess the clinical efficacy of DPP-4 inhibitor use as adjunctive therapy in type 1 diabetes is needed.

- Miglitol is an alpha-glucosidase inhibitor that targets postprandial hyperglycemia via inhibition of digestion of carbohydrates (such as disaccharides, oligosaccharides, and polysaccharides) into monosaccharides, particularly in the upper small intestine. There are limited data of its use as adjunctive therapy in type 1 diabetes.
- Pioglitazone is a thiazolidinedione that works by increasing insulin sensitivity by activating peroxisome proliferator-activated receptors. There are limited data of their use as adjunctive therapy in type 1 diabetes.

MONITORING

- Patients can only manage type 1 diabetes effectively and safely if they self-monitor. This includes self-monitoring of blood glucose (SMBG) from the finger or an alternate site, alone or with the additional use of a continuous subcutaneous glucose sensor (CGM), as well as urine or blood ketone monitoring as needed and careful record keeping.
- Monitoring allows objective goals for therapy and is a means to measure the efficacy of changes in therapy.
- SMBG is the established monitoring method that allows:
  - detection and prevention of hypoglycemia and hyperglycemia
  - adjustment of insulin, diet, and physical activity to achieve target blood glucose levels
  - analysis of data (from both SMBG and CGM) to look at patterns and trends, daily means (and standard deviations), means (and standard deviations) by time of day, and percentages of values in the hypoglycemic and hyperglycemic ranges. This

can be done by keeping a logbook, or with programs that analyze and display the information.
- Minimum of four to six SMBG measurements every day—before breakfast, lunch, afternoon, exercise, supper, and bedtime—usually provide the necessary information sufficient to adjust insulin, activity, and diet. Tests are done before meals and at bedtime at a minimum. Additional testing may be warranted after meals (2 h after the start of the meal); in the middle of the night; before, during, and after exercising; on sick days; after an intervention to correct a high or low glucose value; or when a schedule change has occurred.
- Continuous or intermittent glucose monitoring of interstitial fluid is available to provide additional information to adjust insulin, activity, and diet to optimize glycemic control and prevent hypoglycemia.
- The concept of a closed-loop, automated insulin delivery system, with continuous glucose sensing and insulin delivery informed by a control algorithm without patient intervention, offers the potential to decrease the burden of daily diabetes management and to modify the significant glycemic excursions associated with conventional therapy. Closed-loop technology represents a change in the treatment paradigm for diabetes as the transition is made from primarily self-management behaviors to automated insulin therapy, potentially relieving the burden and guilt of suboptimal glucose control.
- A properly performed A1C provides the best available index of chronic glucose levels and is highly reliable.

NUTRITION

- The overall goal of medical nutrition therapy (MNT) for type 1 diabetes is to enable patients to attain blood glucose levels as near normal as possible by integrating exogenous insulin into their usual eating and activity patterns. The MNT prescription should be individualized based on nutrition assessment and treatment goals. In general, recommendations follow nutrition guidelines for the general population:
  - calorie levels should be prescribed to achieve and maintain healthy body weight
  - protein intake of 10–20% of calories is adequate to support health, and the evidence is inconclusive regarding consumption of a specific amount to optimize glucose control or reduce cardiovascular risk in individuals without renal disease. However, a protein intake of 0.8 g/kg/day is recommended for individuals with diabetic kidney disease as manifest by albuminuria and/or a reduced glomerular filtration rate.
  - fat consumption should be moderate (the former Institute of Medicine—now the Health and Medicine Division of the National Academies of Sciences, Engineering, and Medicine—defines an acceptable range of 20–35% of total calories from fat for adults, with no defined level of upper intake), and should emphasize elements of a Mediterranean-style diet rich in monounsaturated fatty acids such as those found in plant-based foods. Trans fat intake should be avoided altogether.
  - carbohydrate foods, such as grains, dried beans, legumes, vegetables, fruits, and nonfat dairy products are rich sources of vitamins, minerals, and/or dietary fiber and are preferred choices for carbohydrate-containing foods. For type 1 diabetes, the total amount of carbohydrate in a meal, rather than the source (sugar or starch), should guide the estimation of insulin dosage. The glycemic effect of foods may provide an additional benefit to using total carbohydrate.
  - vitamin and mineral requirements for individuals with diabetes are the same as for the general population. Supplementation is advised if conditions create a deficiency.
- Insulin therapy regimens using multiple daily doses of insulin allow greater flexibility in eating patterns than do conventional regimens. Blood glucose levels obtained by self-monitoring can be used to make adjustments in diet, activity, and insulin regimen to maximize blood glucose control.
- The complexity of integrating nutrition and insulin therapies and the importance of diabetes self-management education and support require a coordinated team approach to care for individuals with type 1 diabetes.
- MNT for diabetes is based on an assessment of the individual's metabolic and lifestyle parameters, implemented through a nutrition self-management plan, and evaluated through nutrition-related outcomes such as blood glucose and lipid levels and achievement of a healthy weight and normal growth in children. Patients and their families should be actively involved in setting nutrition goals, developing the self-management plan, and evaluating treatment effectiveness through SMBG levels.

- Registered dietitians have the expertise to design the nutrition intervention and to counsel patients on nutrition self-management. Nutritional counseling for newly diagnosed patients with type 1 diabetes should be provided in stages to allow the patient time to adjust to the treatment regimen. Nutritional care cannot be limited to diagnosis but must continue throughout the patient's life span. Follow-up may be appropriate every 3–6 months for children and every 6–12 months for adults.

EXERCISE

- Exercise should be an integral part of the treatment plan for patients with type 1 diabetes.
- Physiological responses to exercise in people without diabetes and in patients with type 1 diabetes are described in this section.
- Potential benefits of exercise are explained on page 152. Some people do not consider what they do to be exercise, but may be physically active because they use stairs, walk their dog, or do house cleaning or gardening. In this manner, physical activity, like regular exercise, can improve cardiovascular risk factors and may:
  - aid in achieving and maintaining a healthy weight
  - heighten sense of well-being
  - improve glucose control

- Potential risks of exercise include destabilization of metabolic control, e.g., hypoglycemia during or after exercise (most likely with sporadic or inconsistent exercise) or hyperglycemia and ketosis (if diabetes is uncontrolled or ketones are present before beginning activity).
- A pre-exercise medical evaluation should be performed regardless of the patient's age.
- Exercise should be prescribed with caution in patients with:
  - unstable blood glucose values
  - cardiovascular disease, neuropathy that results in loss of sensation, or proliferative retinopathy
  - hypoglycemia unawareness
- Guidelines for safe exercise are addressed in Table 3.17. They include:
  - monitoring blood glucose and taking appropriate action (when necessary)
  - altering food or insulin if needed
  - carrying short-acting carbohydrate and identification
  - monitoring intensity of exercise
  - avoiding trauma to joints, muscles, or ligaments as well as to the skin of the feet

Tools of Therapy

Type 1 diabetes is characterized by a near-absolute deficiency in endogenous insulin secretion within days or months after initial diagnosis. Affected patients are dependent on exogenous insulin to survive for the duration of their lives, and the insulin regimen must be individualized for each patient.

INSULIN PREPARATIONS

For the most part, insulin is no longer obtained from animal pancreas but rather it is made chemically identical to human insulin by recombinant DNA technology, then either provided in solution (human regular insulin) or complexed with protamine to delay its absorption and duration (human NPH insulin). In addition, there are a number of human insulin analogs, in which the amino acid sequence of the human insulin molecule has been modified to change its pharmacokinetics. Insulin preparations are generally classified by duration of action (rapid-, short-, intermediate-, and long-acting). Three rapid-onset, short-duration analogs (insulin lispro, insulin aspart, and insulin glulisine) are available. Human regular insulin and human NPH insulin are characterized as short- and intermediate-acting, respectively, and two long-acting or basal analogs (insulin glargine and insulin detemir) are available. A rapid-acting human insulin inhalation powder was approved for use in the U.S. in 2014. U-500 insulin is a five-fold more concentrated formulation of regular insulin, and has a peak that is similar to regular insulin but with a duration of action more similar to NPH insulin. U-300 is a three-fold more concentrated form of insulin glargine. Ultra-long-acting insulins are currently in development. Insulin degludec is an FDA-approved ultra-long-acting insulin, and has a flat, stable profile at steady state, with a duration of action greater than 40 h. In the BEGIN Basal-Bolus Type 1, phase 3 study, insulin degludec was noninferior to insulin glargine in glycemic control (A1C) with similar rates of hypoglycemia overall, and 25% reduction in nocturnal hypoglycemia. Insulin degludec is also available in a U-200 formulation which is two-fold more concentrated. LY2605541, a PEGylated insulin lispro, is another ultra-long-acting basal insulin in development, with estimated duration of action >36 h. Lente (intermediate-acting) and ultralente (long-acting) insulin are no longer available. More insulins of varied onset and duration are currently in development. Clinicians should familiarize themselves with several preparations and learn to use them rationally (see Tables 3.1 and 3.2).

Table 3.1   Insulins Available in the United States

Product	Manufacturer
Rapid acting	
Humalog (insulin lispro)*	Lilly
NovoLog (insulin aspart)*	Novo Nordisk
Apidra (insulin glulisine)†	sanofi-aventis
Afrezza (Technosphere insulin, inhaled)	MannKind
Short acting	
Humulin R (regular)	Lilly
Novolin R (regular)	Novo Nordisk
Intermediate acting	
Humulin N (NPH)†	Lilly
Novolin N (NPH)	Novo Nordisk
Humulin R U-500*	Lilly
Long acting	
Lantus (insulin glargine)*	sanofi-aventis
Levemir (insulin detemir)†	Novo Nordisk
Tresiba U-100 (insulin degludec)	Novo Nordisk
Tresiba U-200 (insulin degludec)	Novo Nordisk
Toujeo (insulin glargine U-300)	sanofi-aventis
Combinations	
Humulin 70/30 (70% NPH, 30% regular)†	Lilly
Humalog 75/25 (75% insulin lispro protamine suspension [NPL], 25% insulin lispro)†	Lilly
Humalog 50/50 (50% NPL, 50% lispro)†	Lilly
Novolin 70/30 (70% NPH, 30% regular)	Novo Nordisk
NovoLog 70/30 (70% insulin aspart protamine [NPA], 30% insulin aspart)	Novo Nordisk

*Available in prefilled disposable pen injectors and cartridges for pen injectors in addition to vials.
†Available in cartridges for pen injectors in addition to vials.

Species and Purity

In the U.S. today, insulin is prepared by recombinant DNA technology and no longer derived from animal sources. All insulin preparations sold in the U.S. are of the highest purity and contain less than one part per million of impurities. Such purification is associated with a reduced incidence of insulin antibodies, less insulin allergy, and less lipoatrophy at the injection site than previous less purified or more immunogenic animal preparations.

Duration of Action

Although insulins are classified into rapid-, short-, intermediate-, and long-acting preparations, actual insulin effects do not always coincide with such simple descriptions. For example, local subcutaneous tissue conditions not clearly understood may cause rates of absorption to vary by 20–40% from day to day in any

Table 3.2 Insulins by Comparative Action

	Onset (h)	Peak (h)	Effective duration (h)
Rapid acting			
Insulin lispro (analog)	<0.25–0.5	0.5–2.5	3–6.5
Insulin aspart (analog)	<0.25	0.5–1	3–5
Insulin glulisine (analog)	<0.25	1–1.5	3–5
Technosphere insulin	<0.25	0.25	3
Short acting			
Regular (soluble)	0.5–1	2–3	3–6
Intermediate acting			
NPH (isophane)	2–4	4–10	10–16
U-500	0.5–1	2–3	10–16
Long acting			
Insulin glargine (analog)	2–4	Relatively flat	20–24
Insulin detemir (analog)	0.8–2 (dose dependent)	Relatively flat	Dose dependent 12 h for 0.2 units/kg; 20 h for 0.4 units/kg; up to 24 h binds to albumin
Insulin glargine U-300 (analog)	1–2	12–16	32–36
Ultra-long acting			
Insulin degludec (analog)	1–2	7–9	36–42
Combinations			
70% NPH, 30% regular	0.5–1	Dual	10–16
75% NPL, 25% lispro	<0.25	Dual	10–16
50% NPL, 50% lispro	<0.25	Dual	10–16
70% aspart protamine, 30% aspart	<0.25	Dual	15–18

one patient. Furthermore, higher doses of administered insulin and higher insulin concentrations may result in longer duration of action. In light of the many other variables influencing insulin pharmacokinetics, the clinician is cautioned against relying too heavily on textbook descriptions of insulin action. Health professionals should base therapy adjustments on actual glycemic values obtained from the patient's self-monitoring of blood glucose (SMBG) or continuous glucose monitor (CGM).

Rapid- and short-acting insulins are relatively predictable on a day-to-day basis in onset and duration of action. Therefore, in the absence of hypoglycemia that is attributable to dose, they can be adjusted after a 2- to 3-day observation period to attempt to normalize postprandial glucose values. This adjustment can be made by changing a fixed dose or the insulin-to-carbohydrate ratio, the timing of insulin in relation to the meal, or the amount of insulin used to correct a glucose value above the target range (correction factor). In the case of hypoglycemia that has been attributed to dose of insulin, a single hypoglycemic event if otherwise unexplained is sufficient basis for an immediate downward dose adjustment the next time the specific component of therapy is due to be given. Any change in the dose of intermediate-acting (NPH) or long-acting (glargine or detemir) insulin requires a 2- to 5-day observation period before further dose adjustment because of the relatively slow absorption and long duration of action of these insulins and because of day-to-day variability in food, activity, and stress.

The use of SMBG to map out a profile of blood glucose values is invaluable in assisting the physician, patient, and diabetes management team with therapy. Blood glucose levels should be measured before and after meals and during the night, particularly when initiating or intensifying insulin therapy or when seeking the cause of hypoglycemia or hyperglycemia. CGM is an emerging technology that provides a continuous measure of interstitial glucose levels, providing real-time readings every 5 min. In addition to providing a more complete look at glucose patterns, CGMs provide glucose trends, alarms for hypoglycemia and hyperglycemia, and rate-of-change alarms for rapid glycemic excursions. Routine frequency of monitoring or use of CGM should be based on mutually defined goals, as described in Philosophy and Goals, beginning on page 33.

Insulin Pens and Apps

Most of the current human insulins and insulin analogs are available in insulin cartridges and/or disposable pens (see Table 3.1). Such devices aid the patient in insulin measurement and simplify insulin administration with minimal added cost to therapy. Several manufacturers of insulin pens and pen needles exist; pens are either durable or disposable, and some devices deliver insulin by half units or have a memory device that records the prior doses. Use of pen devices will not only facilitate the adaptation to basal-bolus therapy and enhance the compliance to intensive insulin therapy, but will also improve outcomes when using flexible regimens. Some versions of insulin pens record the most recent dose and time for extra reassurance. Applications on glucose meters and phones or computers can be used to record insulin doses as well.

Mixing Insulins

Mixing insulin is declining in the U.S. because fixed regimens are being replaced by flexible basal-bolus regimens and pen usage is increasing. Insulin glargine and insulin detemir should not be mixed with other insulins. Mixing short- or rapid-acting insulin with NPH in the same syringe is an accepted and convenient way to produce differently timed pharmacologic actions with a single injection. Stable premixtures of intermediate-acting and short- or rapid-acting insulins in fixed proportion (e.g., 70% NPH/30% regular, 75% insulin lispro protamine [NPL]/25% insulin lispro, 50% NPL/50% insulin lispro, and 70% insulin aspart protamine [NPA]/30% insulin aspart) are also available commercially. Premixed insulins are not suitable when daily variation in the dose of short-acting insulin is required, which is the case for most patients with type 1 diabetes.

TREATING NEWLY DIAGNOSED PATIENTS

Diagnosis and Stabilization

At diagnosis, initial objectives of therapy are dependent on the degree of illness (e.g., resolving DKA if it exists, eliminating symptomatic hyperglycemia, or initiating insulin therapy in the asymptomatic patient). The goal is to resolve hyperglycemia, fluid deficit, and electrolyte disturbance while avoiding hypoglycemia and cerebral edema (in children). Therefore, glycemic targets should be approached gradually. Depending on issues such as degree of acidosis and β-cell function, treatment typically begins with ~0.5–1 unit of insulin per kg of body weight per day. However, during the first week of therapy, this amount can be expected to increase to an average of 1.0–1.5 units/kg/day, because most patients are relatively insulin resistant at this time. Insulin recommendations for when a patient is in DKA are addressed in the Special Situations chapter.

Immediately after diagnosis or after ketoacidosis has been resolved, therapy should begin with the insulin program that is negotiated and agreed upon between the patient/family and health-care team, e.g., two or three daily insulin injections or a "flexible" intensive insulin program consisting of preprandial or bolus insulin at each meal and basal insulin once~ or twice per day. It is preferable to start with the flexible basal-bolus insulin program at the outset instead of learning twice-daily insulin injections. Although twice- or once-daily insulin may suffice for a short time in patients who retain some of their β-cell function, psychological acceptance of flexible intensive injection programs is easier for both patient and family if introduced as soon as possible after diagnosis, even if glycemic control could be adequate on a different program with fewer injections. Moreover, there is evidence from the Diabetes Control and Complications Trial (DCCT) and the Epidemiology of Diabetes Interventions and Complications study (EDIC) that intensive exogenous insulin helps preserve β-cell function and should be given in adequate doses so that the patient does not need to utilize endogenous insulin for routine glycemic control.

Although not recommended, some clinicians start with two or three insulin injections per day, to acquaint the patient with basic diabetes management principles, before initiating a flexible intensive program. With the two-dose regimen, about two-thirds of the insulin dose is given in the morning before breakfast, and one-third is given before dinner (supper). The two doses may consist of premixed insulins (sometimes the case for infants and very young children) or two doses of rapid- or short-acting and intermediate- or long-acting insulins. The pre-breakfast dose consists of about two-thirds NPH and one-third regular or insulin aspart, lispro, or glulisine. The pre-dinner dose is usually divided into equal amounts of NPH or insulin glargine or detemir, and regular insulin or insulin aspart, lispro, or glulisine. When giving glargine or detemir it will require two separate injections. For the three-dose regimen, the same routine is followed, however, the evening doses are split with the regular insulin or rapid-acting insulin before dinner and the NPH or insulin glargine or detemir before bed.

Patients and families should be taught the technique of blood glucose monitoring at diagnosis. They should determine blood glucose levels repeatedly under professional supervision to ensure the reliability of the readings. If premixed formulations (e.g., 70% NPH/30% regular; 75% NPL/25% insulin lispro) are used initially, patients should also have supplies of short- or rapid-acting insulins for use when needed, such as supplementation for sick days.

Remission or Honeymoon Phase

Within weeks after diagnosis, with resolution of ketosis and hyperglycemia, there may be some recovery of β-cell function, and consequently, exogenous insulin requirements often decrease for weeks to months. This honeymoon phase of type 1 diabetes may be marked by the appearance of recurrent hypoglycemia. A honeymoon phase occurs less frequently in younger children, and is more common in the late teenage years and in adults. During this period, insulin dosage must be appropriately reduced, occasionally to as little as 0.1–0.3 units/kg/day. Not all patients exhibit a profound honeymoon phase, but some period of stability in blood glucose levels is common, with low insulin requirements at 0.2–0.5 units/kg/day. Evidence suggests that the honeymoon phase could be prolonged if blood glucose levels are kept in the near-normal range with basal-bolus therapy. Any attempt to reduce or discontinue monitoring or insulin should be carefully weighed against the apparent benefits of even modest preservation of β-cell function and, most importantly, risk of DKA if the honeymoon phase is waning.

Type 1 Diabetes TrialNet is an international network of researchers in the U.S., Canada, Australia, and Europe, exploring methods to prevent, delay, and reverse the progression of type 1 diabetes. One goal of TrialNet is to preserve β-cell mass, as assessed by C-peptide secretion. TrialNet is actively investigating the use of immunosuppressive and immunomodulating agents, as well as intensive metabolic control in preventing, delaying, or reversing type 1 diabetes. Patients should be informed of this study at the time of diagnosis. Patients and families can be referred to the TrialNet website (www.diabetestrialnet.org), to determine whether or not they are interested and eligible for clinical studies.

Chronic Phase: Developing a Long-Term Treatment Plan

As the honeymoon period comes to an end with the progressive decrease of β-cell function, insulin requirements increase gradually over several months. Prepubertal children and adults usually require between 0.5 and 1.0 units/kg/day, and pubertal children may require up to 1.5 units/kg/day because of relative insulin resistance, increased caloric intake during rapid growth spurts, and changes in hormone secretory patterns. After puberty, insulin doses should decrease to <1.0 units/kg/day to prevent excessive weight gain. Dose requirements for pregnant patients vary with gestational duration and are discussed in the Pregnancy section (page 196) of Special Situations.

Careful balance of caloric and carbohydrate intake, activity, and insulin dosing is required for an insulin regimen to be successful. It is most desirable to vary insulin doses to match variations of food intake, activity, and prevailing blood glucose. On the other hand, if insulin dose is kept constant from day to day, food intake and activity should also be kept constant. The choice of insulin regimen should be based on the individual's characteristics, preferences, and habits, including age, stage of development, meal plans, and potential adherence to diabetes treatment. The diabetes management team should develop an acceptable and realistic treatment plan together with the patient/family. For example, an adolescent patient who is experiencing difficulties in following the treatment plan with frequent episodes of hyper-glycemia or ketoacidosis may have to be treated with two injections per day administered by a family member or visiting nurse until his or her problems are resolved. School can be used to administer one of the injections. On the other hand, the choice of insulin regimen should not be dictated by forces outside of the patient/family and health-care team. For school-age children, the school must accommodate the delivery of a lunchtime injection of insulin if the child/family and health-care team decide to use an intensive insulin regimen. Employed adults should similarly have flexibility for testing and injecting in the workplace.

After the initial dose adjustments, ongoing long-term and short-term adjust-ments are made on the basis of daily repeated blood glucose measurements and/ or the use of CGM. At a minimum, glucose levels should be assessed before meals, after meals, and at bedtime (HS) every day. At least once per week overnight basal insulin and blood glucose patterns should be reviewed and adjusted accordingly to ensure blood glucose levels stay in an individualized range. One method for overnight blood glucose checks would be to acquire three triplets of BG read-ings—at bedtime, midsleep, and upon arising—with the last food intake and insu-lin bolus being 3–4 h prior to the bedtime check. During times of more variability in insulin sensitivity and/or BG levels, overnight blood glucose should also be checked, such as in instances when there are changes in basal insulin, an increase in physical activity, recurrent daytime hypoglycemia, an assessment of dawn phe-nomenon, post alcohol consumption, or during illness. With time, education, and practice, patients and families are able to make adjustments with relative ease and become progressively independent of the diabetes management team; this includes determining how to adjust basal insulin, the carbohydrate-to-insulin ratio, and the insulin sensitivity factor (used to calculate the amount of insulin needed to correct a glucose level above the target range). In addition to long-term adjustments, insulin doses and waiting times between injections and food intake could be adjusted in response to high or low blood glucose levels, changes in food intake, activity level, or intercurrent illness. All of these adjustments can be made by patients who have been thoroughly trained and who can measure their blood glucose levels (or use CGM) and calculate dose changes precisely.

Patient education is time-consuming but essential and should be conducted by a skilled diabetes management team working together with the patient and his or her family. Many newly diagnosed patients will require an initial period of instruction of up to 10–12 h, with periodic review and follow-up sessions every few months until both patient and family feel comfortable with their knowledge and skills. Insulin regimens and blood glucose targets also should vary depending on the individual patient and should take into consideration the frequency and adherence to SMBG or CGM, the patient's ability to recognize and respond to hypoglycemic episodes, and the limitations imposed by what the patient and/or family are willing or ready to do. However, individualization should not prevent continued efforts toward the goal of achieving near-euglycemia while avoiding severe hypoglycemia.

A frequent problem in the management of diabetes is the disappointment that sets in at the end of the honeymoon period when patients or parents of children with type 1 diabetes realize that the efforts invested in the treatment are not rewarded by the achievement of euglycemia. Often, minor deviations from treatment or even no deviations at all result in unexplained fluctuations of glucose levels. Because these fluctuations are part of the nature of type 1 diabetes, even under the strictest and most flexible treatment conditions, such as with the use of multiple injections and insulin pumps, it is helpful at diagnosis to warn patients and families that the treatment of diabetes is imperfect and that glucose fluctuations are to be expected. Adequate explanations about the unpredictability of blood glucose levels and their relationship to daily variations of insulin absorption, food composition and absorption, and changes in the level of physical activity often help to prevent the development of feelings of guilt and incompetence that can plague patients and families. A useful attitude on the part of the diabetes management team is to stress the importance of overall blood glucose control, such as assessing the mean glucose from meter or CGM readings, rather than individual values. However, if individual values are used, relatively wide fluctuations (70–160 mg/dL [3.9–8.9 mmol/L] preprandial, up to 180–200 mg/dL [11.1 mmol/L] postprandial, and 90–180 mg/dL at bedtime and overnight [5.0–10.0 mmol/L]) can be accepted, even when narrower glycemic targets might be preferred.

A1C does not provide a measure of glycemic variability or hypoglycemia. In addition to genetic and environmental risks, high glycemic variability is thought to be a risk factor for vascular complications and should be a primary treatment target. For more information about glycemic variability, see Glycemic Variability under Patient-Performed Monitoring (page 114).

INSULIN REGIMENS

General Principles

Physiologic insulin secretion is characterized by continuous basal release, with superimposed bursts of additional insulin integrated precisely to the rise in glucose with food intake. Additionally, insulin is secreted into the portal vein and approximately half is cleared by the liver before entering the general circulation. Ideally, exogenous insulin treatment regimens should mimic all aspects of this pattern. Unfortunately, with the available means of treatment, this is not entirely possible. Therefore, insulin treatment regimens represent varying degrees of compromise to achieve near-normalization of blood glucose levels, one of the most important goals of diabetes management. Ideally, insulin regimens should have both basal and bolus components to mimic normal insulin secretion.

The normal prandial burst of insulin is best mimicked by administering rapid-acting insulin (lispro, aspart, or glulisine) before meals at the appropriate time, depending on the blood glucose level. Prandial insulin typically comprises ~50–60% of the total daily dose. Advantages of rapid-acting insulin analogs over human regular insulin are convenience, better postprandial control, and reduced risk of postprandial hypoglycemia occurring 3–6 h postinjection. Disadvantages of rapid-acting analogs are cost and inability to cover snacks without another bolus dose of insulin.

Basal insulin secretion comprises ~40% of the total daily insulin secretion. It can be mimicked best by giving long-acting insulin glargine or detemir once or twice a day, insulin degludec once a day (although this has not been FDA approved for use in children under the age of 18 years), or by delivering short- or rapid-acting insulin continuously by an insulin pump (continuous subcutaneous insulin infusion [CSII]). The basal insulin in CSII has the advantage of being variable and adjustable to cover the early morning rise in glucose levels (the dawn phenomenon) as well as periods of increased insulin sensitivity such as nighttime or during or after exercise. Compared to NPH, insulin glargine, detemir, and degludec have the advantage of being relatively peakless. Insulin glargine has an onset of action of ~1.5 h postinjection and mean duration of action of ~23.5 h after several days of injections. As a result, clinical studies in type 1 diabetes have shown better fasting blood glucose with less nocturnal hypoglycemia with glargine than NPH once, twice, or four times daily. In ~20% of individuals, glargine lasts <20 h and may have to be given twice daily, usually in a 50:50 format. Insulin detemir achieves its longer duration by binding insulin with albumin and is injected once or twice daily. It has an onset of action between 0.8–2 h and a duration that is dose dependent lasting ~12 h at 0.2 units/kg and ~20–24 h at 0.4 units/kg. Insulin degludec forms multi-hexamers upon injection into subcutaneous fat, with formation of a depot of insulin. The long duration of action is mainly due to delayed absorption into the systemic circulation and secondarily due to binding of insulin degludec to albumin. The onset of action is approximately 1–2 h and the duration of action ranges from approximately 36–42 h. Disadvantages of glargine and detemir over NPH are that they are only basal insulins and do not cover snacks without a bolus injection, they cannot be mixed with other insulins in the same syringe, and they are more costly. Long-acting insulin can be given once daily before breakfast, dinner, or bedtime or twice daily at breakfast and bedtime or at breakfast and dinner. With once-daily long-acting insulin given at breakfast, there is concern for rising glucose in the early morning (dawn phenomenon) for those individuals where the long-acting insulin lasts <20 h. The long-acting kinetics of insulin glargine require precipitation in the subcutaneous tissue; therefore, young and lean individuals should be carefully advised on injection technique, and short needles <8mm should be used to avoid intramuscular injections, which lead to unexpected rapid insulin action.

Though not recommended in this day and age, NPH can be used as a basal insulin and should be given twice daily at breakfast and bedtime. NPH has an onset of action ~2 h after the injection and produces peak levels ~6–10 h after injection. Morning NPH provides hyperinsulinemia, especially in mid- or late afternoon, when snacks may be needed to prevent hypoglycemia. Bedtime NPH provides progressive overnight basal hyperinsulinemia with peak serum insulin around breakfast time; giving the injection at bedtime rather than predinner reduces the risk of nocturnal hypoglycemia and may provide coverage for the dawn phenomenon. Of note, there is more thought that the dawn phenomenon is not consistent; therefore, continuous insulin therapy with CGM is ideal.

Starting Insulin Requirement

The starting insulin dose is usually based on body weight. On average, a patient will eventually require anywhere between 0.4–1.0 units/kg/day with higher amounts during puberty (generally 1.0–1.5 units/kg/day). It is best to start conservatively at 0.5 units/kg/day (or 1.0 units/kg/day during puberty) and increase insulin doses according to SMBG readings.

Two or Three Injections Daily

The twice-daily "split-mixed" insulin regimen (Figure 3.1) was the most commonly used treatment regimen before results of the DCCT. Morning short- or rapid-acting insulin (regular or insulin aspart/lispro/glulisine) has major action between breakfast and lunch, and its effect is reflected in the prelunch blood glucose levels. Morning intermediate-acting (NPH) insulin has major action between breakfast and dinner, and its effect is reflected in the predinner blood glucose levels. Evening short-acting insulin has major action between dinner and bedtime, and its effect is reflected in the bedtime tests. The evening intermediate-acting insulin has its major action overnight, and its effect is reflected in the blood glucose level on arising the next morning. The evening intermediate-acting insulin can be replaced with long-acting insulin. The initial dose can be divided (based on % of total daily insulin) into a morning injection containing ~40% NPH and ~15% insulin aspart/lispro/glulisine or regular at breakfast, plus an evening injection containing ~30% NPH (or long-acting insulin) and ~15% insulin aspart/lispro/glulisine or regular at dinner. In younger children, the proportions are closer to 80%/20% for both components.

The only advantages to this regimen are simplicity and a limited number of injections. The most frequent and serious disadvantage of this regimen is that, in many patients, attempts to achieve fasting normoglycemia result in nocturnal hypoglycemia (from midnight to 4:00 A.M.) and early-morning hyperglycemia (from 4:00 to 8:00 A.M., due to the dawn phenomenon). In these cases, it is better to move the intermediate-acting insulin to bedtime and thus reduce the peak effect of insulin from 2:00 to 4:00 A.M. and increase it at dawn (Figure 3.1B). In addition, postlunch hyperglycemia is often not controlled without the risk of daytime hypoglycemia from ratcheting up the morning NPH dose, and thus, an insulin injection at lunch or with an afternoon snack is often needed. Generally, it is challenging to achieve near-normal glycemic levels with two or three injections per day.

Multiple-Component Flexible Regimens

Basal insulin requirements typically account for ~35–45% of the patient's total daily dose. Basal insulin may be provided as glargine, detemir, degludec, or NPH insulin or as a rapid-acting insulin with multiple-dose insulin programs or as a basal infusion of insulin analog with CSII (regular insulin is infrequently used in insulin pump therapy) (Figure 3.2). The remaining ~55–65% of insulin is given as prandial insulin, using a rapid-acting insulin analog delivered before meals and/or snacks either by syringe, pen, or an insulin pump bolus. Short-acting regular insulin is less frequently used in multiple-component flexible regimens. The amount of prandial insulin can be determined by calculating the insulin-to-carbohydrate ratio (discussed below) or by using a typical starting distribution of ~25% of the total daily dose as a rapid-acting insulin bolus before breakfast, ~10% before lunch, and ~20% before dinner. These prandial boluses are varied based on the carbohydrate content of the meal as well as the blood glucose determined by SMBG at that time.

Glargine and detemir cannot be mixed in the same syringe with other insulin preparations. Another alternative is the combination of premeal injections (regu-

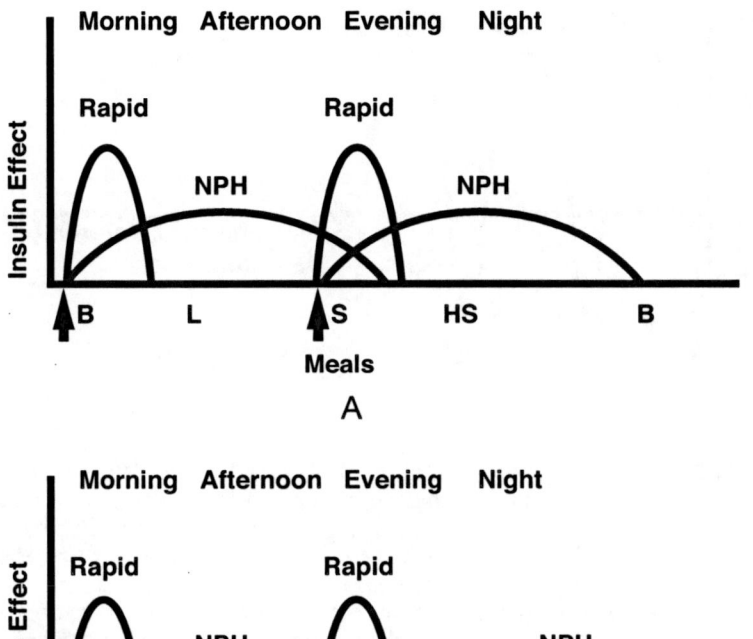

Figure 3.1 Schematic representation of idealized insulin effect provided by (A) "split-mixed" insulin regimen consisting of two daily injections of rapid- and intermediate-acting insulin given before breakfast and supper and (B) three daily injections with rapid- and intermediate-acting insulin before breakfast, rapid-acting insulin at supper, and intermediate-acting insulin at bedtime. B, breakfast; L, lunch; S, supper; HS, bedtime; *Arrow*, time of insulin injection, before meals. In this schematic representation, optimal relative dose sizes are not necessarily represented by the areas under the curves.

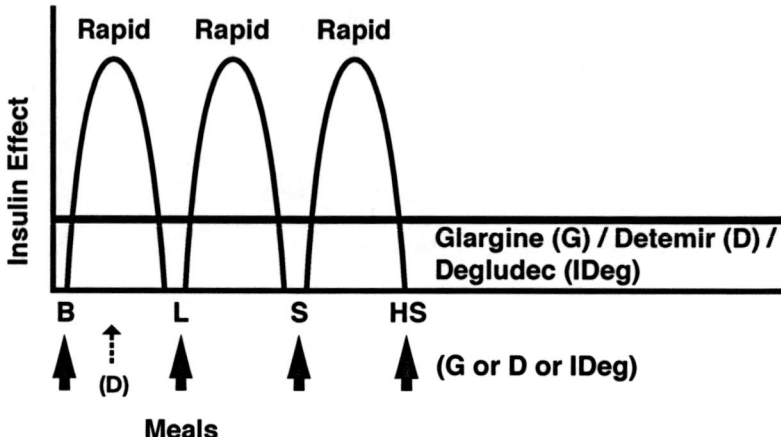

Figure 3.2 Schematic representation of idealized insulin effect provided by three daily injections with rapid-acting insulin at meals and once-daily insulin glargine, detemir, or degludec at bedtime. Detemir sometimes is given twice daily (dashed arrow). B, breakfast; L, lunch; S, supper; HS, bedtime; *Arrow,* time of insulin injection. Insulins glargine, detemir, and degludec may be administered in the morning or at other times, once daily, and insulins glargine and detemir may be administered twice daily as a split dose.

lar insulin or rapid-acting insulin analogs at breakfast, lunch, and dinner) with NPH at bedtime, or with a small amount of NPH before breakfast (Figure 3.3) or at every meal.

The combination of premeal rapid-acting insulin analogs with long-acting basal insulin (glargine or detemir) every 12 or 24 h is quite popular because, *1*) it offers flexibility in meal size and timing, *2*) it is very easily understood by most patients because each period of the day has a well-defined insulin component, *3*) the pharmacokinetics of analogs more closely mimics normal basal and prandial insulin secretion, and *4*) the introduction of insulin pens has made it very convenient. Dinner or bedtime administration of glargine, detemir, or degludec allows the easy titration of the fasting glucose to normal with minimal risk of nocturnal hypoglycemia. If predinner or bedtime glucose levels are high with normal post-lunch values and no afternoon snack, as well as after consideration of the insulin-to-carbohydrate ratio (hereafter referred to as the carb ratio) at supper, and the activity level and possible snacking after supper, then consider the use of glargine twice a day. Another basal option is basal insulin only in the morning with titration to obtain the fasting morning glucose levels in the normal range. If this is not successful due either to daytime hypoglycemia or fasting hyperglycemia, then basal insulin should be moved to the evening or given twice a day.

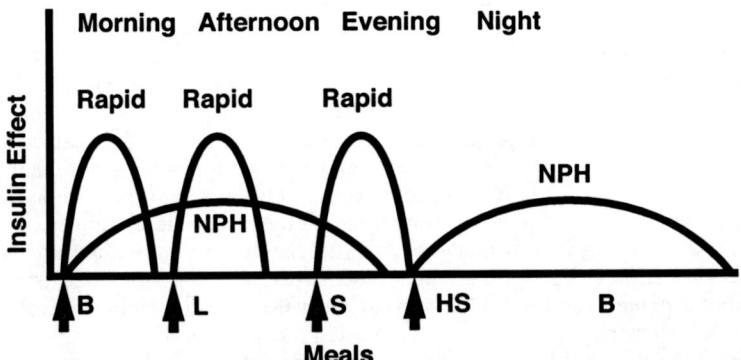

Figure 3.3 Schematic representation of idealized insulin effect provided by three daily injections with rapid-acting insulin at meals and two daily injections of intermediate-acting insulin at breakfast and at bedtime. B, breakfast; L, lunch; S, supper; HS, bedtime; *Arrow,* time of insulin injection. The areas under the curve are not necessarily quantitatively representative of the relative doses.

Continuous Subcutaneous Insulin Infusion

The most precise way to mimic normal insulin secretion clinically is to use an insulin pump in a program of continuous subcutaneous insulin infusion (CSII). Pump devices provide continuous insulin administration to control blood glucose levels throughout the 24-h period. Because insulin delivery is continuous, it can more or less mimic normal insulin secretion. The pump delivers microliter amounts (as low as 0.025 units depending on the manufacturer) of rapid-acting insulin on a continual basis, thus replicating basal insulin secretion. (Regular insulin is rarely used in CSII.) The basal rate may be programmed to vary at times of diurnal variation in insulin sensitivity. For example, the basal infusion rate may be programmed to decrease at night to avert nocturnal hypoglycemia and/or to increase in the early morning to counteract the dawn phenomenon or to accommodate the lifestyle of shift workers. More than one basal pattern can be set if there are marked variations in insulin needs on different days (such as differences in activity levels between the weekdays and weekends, or for women who experience a change in insulin requirements at different times in their menstrual cycle). Unique patterns of basal infusions may be needed by some patients, but most patients' circadian insulin requirements are met with two to four basal rates per day.

The pump is activated before meals to provide increments of rapid-acting insulin as meal "boluses" whenever a meal or snack is consumed. This allows flexibility in meal timing. Meal boluses with rapid-acting insulin analogs are generally given 10–30 min before eating a meal. It may be recommended to give the pre-meal bolus 30 min prior for glucose (mg/dL) in the 300s, 20 min prior for glucose in the 200s, 10 min prior for glucose in the 100s, and right at mealtime for glucose <100. For small children with erratic eating patterns, the meal bolus may be delivered immediately after the meal when the amount of food consumed is known. Alternatively, the dose may be split so that part of the dose is given prior to the meal and the remainder is given as a second bolus immediately after the meal. A similar strategy can be used for the patient who is anorexic or nauseated (e.g., in early pregnancy or during illness). If a meal is skipped, an insulin bolus may be given for correction of hyperglycemia as needed, but no carbohydrate coverage is necessary. If a meal is larger or smaller than usual, a larger or smaller insulin bolus is selected based on the carbohydrate content of the meal. Some pumps also offer variable bolus options including immediate delivery, extended delivery over a set amount of time (~2–5 h), or dual-wave delivery with both immediate and extended delivery together in a programmable percentage (e.g., 60% immediate and 40% of total bolus given over 4 h). Dual-wave delivery is useful for high-fat meals such as pizza and Mexican food, as well as for patients suspected of having gastroparesis. Recognizing patterns from frequent SMBG or continuous glucose monitor readings will help to determine the proper setting of the immediate and extended bolus. Thus, CSII patients have the potential of easily varying meal size, content, and timing, as well as the option of omitting meals if necessary.

The ability to program insulin pumps also allows a temporary reduction or suspension of basal insulin delivery with increased physical activity, which serves to reduce the risk of exercise-related hypoglycemia. Caution should be taken regarding the duration of suspension of the basal insulin delivery because hyperglycemia and ketosis may rapidly supervene if insulin delivery is interrupted for >2 h. Switching to a reduced temporary basal rate for a set amount of time may be preferable. The temporary basal rate reduction should ideally be initiated ~60 min prior to physical activity to mitigate risks of exercise-related hypoglycemia. Pump-activated threshold suspend will be discussed in a later section.

Insulin pumps are relatively small, lightweight, portable, battery-driven devices; they are either attached directly to the body (tubeless/patch pump) or worn on clothing or in a pouch (traditional pump). The patch pump is placed on the skin with adhesive and the small needle catheter is automatically inserted under the skin; after insertion they cannot be removed temporarily. The patch pump is controlled by a handheld personal digital assistant (PDA). The traditional pump is attached via plastic tubing to a small subcutaneous cannula that is taped to the skin. Most of these catheters offer a quick-release device to remove the pump for such activities as swimming, contact sports, showering, sexual activity, or dressing. The devices on the market have features such as alarms for low battery, blocked delivery, and low/empty reservoir. Other options found in pumps include calculating meal or correction boluses based on insulin-to-carbohydrate ratio and insulin sensitivity factors, setting glucose targets, correcting bolus delivery for low glucose, accounting for the duration of active insulin so as to avert hypoglycemia when giving multiple correction doses, alerting to recommend SMBG tests and changing the infusion sets at specified times, and wireless connections to blood glucose meters. Some insulin pumps can be integrated with continuous glucose monitors. The information from the pump or PDA memory can be electronically extracted for review of total daily insulin doses, number and timing of insulin boluses, carbohydrate input used in bolus calculations, pump settings, and glucose levels from SMBG or CGM by the patient, family, and the health-care team.

Treatment with insulin pumps is extremely effective in improving glucose control in patients with type 1 diabetes. As long- and rapid-acting insulin analogs have been developed, however, multiple-dose insulin regimens have become increasingly comparable to pump therapy in terms of the ability to mimic normal physiology. However, the results of a meta-analysis of 12 randomized controlled trials comparing pumps to optimized multiple daily injections (MDI) showed less insulin is used and glycemic control is better during pump therapy. Although the difference in glycemic control is small, it should be sufficient to reduce risk of microvascular disease. Disadvantages of pump therapy include cost and the need to overcome the psychological aversion some patients have to "always being hooked to something." In addition, due to the short duration of rapid-acting analogs and the lack of a subcutaneous depot of basal insulin, patients on pump therapy can develop severe hyperglycemia or ketosis rapidly with interruption of insulin delivery (such as kinking or disconnection of the subcutaneous cannula, empty insulin reservoir, or pump malfunction). Such episodes can be prevented or averted quickly with proper attention and education.

On initiating CSII therapy, the patient must receive additional detailed instruction from the diabetes management team on aspects of therapy including (though not limited to):

- accurate monitoring of capillary blood glucose at least before each meal, after each meal, at bedtime, and at mid-sleep
- knowing safe blood glucose targets during the day and night and the duration of active insulin to avoid hypoglycemia, the most frequent complication of intensive therapy
- learning strategies to reduce the risk of nocturnal hypoglycemia, if it occurs, including increasing the target fasting blood glucose to 100–140 mg/dL (5.6–7.8 mmol/L), decreasing the basal rate if 3:00 A.M. blood glucose levels are <80 mg/dL (<4.4 mmol/L), and daily measurements of blood glucose levels at bedtime followed by ingestion of carbohydrate (or carbohydrate in combination with protein and/or fat) or use of temporary basal rates if the values are ≤100 mg/dL (≤5.5 mmol/L)
- understanding how to avoid hypoglycemia during and after exercise by suspending or decreasing basal insulin infusion, decreasing bolus insulin, and/or ingesting additional carbohydrates
- caring for the infusion site with changes of the catheter every 2–3 days to avoid infection, inflammation, and loss of glycemic control
- understanding the urgency of preventing or reversing hyperglycemic crises from insulin underdelivery by taking the following steps with detection of moderate unexplained hyperglycemia: monitoring urine or blood ketones, changing the infusion set and taking an insulin injection immediately, contacting the medical team for persistent problems, and troubleshooting the reasons for insulin underdelivery (kinked cannula, leaking, obstruction, pump malfunction) after correcting the hyperglycemia
- knowing how to contact experienced medical personnel by phone 24 h per day, 7 days per week
- having the constant presence of a relative or friend until the patient becomes familiar with the pump

For more details, a few good references include: *Understanding Insulin Pumps & Continuous Glucose Monitors* by H. Peter Chase, MD & Laurel Messer, RN, MPH, CDE, and the American Diabetes Association's *Putting Your Patients on the Pump* by Karen M. Bolderman RD, LDN, CDE. See Figure 3.4 for an example of the insulin effects of CSII therapy with rapid-acting insulin.

The initial programming of the pump is based on the total daily insulin dose of the previous regimen. Approximately 35–50% of the total dose is given as the basal rate, and the rest is divided among breakfast, lunch, dinner, and snacks. Ratios identified during MDI could be used or for insulin-to-carbohydrate ratio (divide 450 by the average total daily insulin dosage) and for insulin sensitivity factor (divide 1700—or 1500 if more insulin resistant—by the average total daily insulin dosage). The patient is generally started with a single basal rate over a 24-h period. Bedtime snacks are not given until the basal rate is correct overnight. The basal rate is adjusted every second or third day on the basis of the blood glucose levels at bedtime, mid-sleep, and on rising until the desired blood glucose target is obtained. Increments should be in the order of 10–15% or 0.1 units/h (or 0.025–0.05 units/h for young children). In the case of nocturnal hypoglycemia, basal rate should be lowered starting 2–3 h before the time of the hypoglycemic event. Patients exhibiting the dawn phenomenon may require increased basal rates in the early morning hours starting 2–3 h before waking and lasting 4–6 h. Children may have a reverse dawn phenomenon requiring higher basal rates between 10:00 P.M. and 2:00 A.M. Basal rates are adjusted during the day by delaying meals and withholding the bolus that would have accompanied the delayed

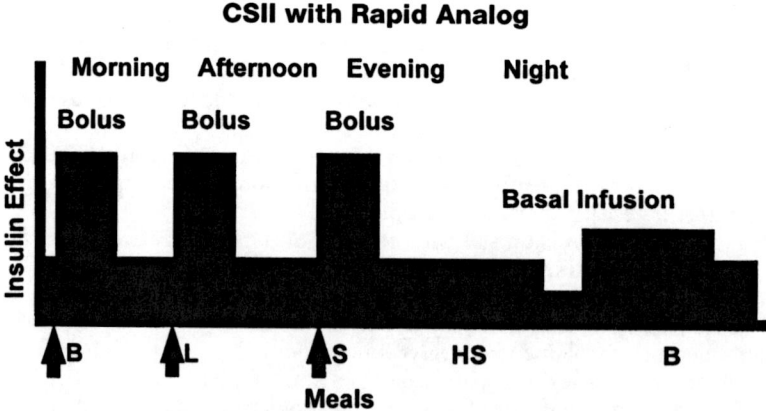

CSII with Rapid Analog

Figure 3.4 Schematic representation of idealized insulin effect provided by continuous subcutaneous insulin infusion (insulin pump) with rapid analog. B, breakfast; L, lunch; S, supper; HS, bedtime. *Arrow,* time of insulin bolus, at meals. Areas under heights of bars do not necessarily quantitatively reflect the relative doses. This schematic is just an example. The reduction of basal infusion could start earlier than shown here, possibly at HS.

meal, in order to assess drift of glucose. If glucose levels rise or fall >30 mg/dL (>1.7 mmol/L) during that time, typically observed over at least two days, then insulin needs to be adjusted appropriately. Daytime basal rates for those on rapid-acting analogs can often be determined by observing late postprandial glucose patterns (for example, pre-lunch and pre-dinner glucose levels, when the effects of the prior meal bolus are no longer in effect) or by skipping a meal and seeing the effect of basal rates alone.

Even when a patient's initial commitment persists, the use of pumps may be associated with various problems. These include local inflammation at catheter sites from infection or tape irritation, pump breakdown and/or malfunction, forgetting to refill reservoirs on time, or forgetting to give meal boluses. Appropriate education in troubleshooting hyperglycemia, hypoglycemia, and other problems must be provided. Many of the problems with the CSII of the past have been solved; there is less local irritation at insertion sites and less insulin precipitation, there are more programmable features to calculate bolus doses and duration of active insulin and more alerts, and pump therapy can be combined with CGM in some cases. As a result, pump therapy continues to increase in patients of all ages. Once initiated, most patients remain on CSII, and although there are no large-scale randomized trials, except for sensor-augmented pump studies, clinical reports and experience suggest that pump therapy patients (including toddlers and young children) have improved glycemic control, less hypoglycemia, and improved quality of life.

Continuous Glucose Monitoring Systems

The availability of continuous glucose monitoring (CGM) systems, which provide real-time sensor glucose values from a subcutaneously inserted electrochemical glucose sensor, has been a major advance for diabetes patients. Sensors are now showing improved accuracy and patients are reporting higher satisfaction with devices. Although not yet recommended to replace glucose meter measurements, it is clear that patients who frequently use continuous glucose monitoring are becoming increasingly reliant on their sensors to inform diabetes management decisions. More details about CGM can be found in the section titled Glucose Sensors (page 116).

Insulin pumps coupled with CGM and control algorithms are now able to automate some aspects of insulin delivery. For example, insulin delivery can be suspended automatically after a preset glycemic threshold has been reached, referred to as the 'threshold suspend' feature. This feature appears to be able to reduce time spent in hypoglycemia without increasing hyperglycemia. Predictive algorithms are being evaluated that will suspend insulin prior to reaching the threshold to prevent, not just reduce, hypoglycemia. These automated steps are part of ongoing efforts to automate insulin delivery based upon sensor glucose values.

Closed-Loop Insulin Delivery Systems

The concept of a closed-loop, automated insulin delivery system, with continuous glucose sensing and insulin delivery informed by a control algorithm without patient intervention, offers the potential to decrease the burden of daily diabetes management as well as modify the significant glycemic excursions associated with conventional therapy. Closed-loop technology represents a change in the treatment paradigm for diabetes as the transition is made from primarily self-management behaviors to automated insulin therapy (some systems are using dual hormone systems—insulin and glucagon), potentially relieving the burden and guilt of suboptimal glucose control.

The advances in this field have been rapid and clinical trials are currently underway worldwide testing several systems in various stages of development. Early studies demonstrated the feasibility of automated insulin modulation using subcutaneous insulin pumps and subcutaneous continuous glucose sensors. Further advances in both sensors and algorithms incrementally demonstrated improved protection against hypoglycemia, reduced variability, and decreased mean glucose levels in controlled, inpatient settings. Control-to-range strategies are intended to keep the glucose within a predetermined range with ranges being variable at different times of the day. Such controllers, combining both safety and range control modules, achieved almost 80% time in the range of 80–140 mg/dL in the overnight period in a study of 12 adults with type 1 diabetes. The performance of current systems is restricted by suboptimal sensor performance and the delayed onset and prolonged action of rapid-acting insulins, often beyond the time of meal absorption. These factors contribute to immediate postprandial hyperglycemia, and a delayed risk for postprandial hypoglycemia. Despite these limitations, the recently published studies of 24/7 closed-loop control for patients outside of the inpatient setting demonstrate that these systems can be safe and effective. The first-generation integrated, automated insulin delivery system that doses insulin based on continuous glucose sensor values was just approved by the FDA in September 2016. Early systems are expected to still rely heavily on patient input including premeal bolusing and frequent meter glucose testing. Input of timing of meals and exercise are both serious considerations for user inputs that would optimize performance of an otherwise closed-loop system, but there is not universal agreement about inclusion of these user inputs. Furthermore, studies are underway for dual hormonal systems that include the subcutaneous delivery of a glucagon infusion in addition to an insulin infusion.

ALTERNATIVE INSULIN DELIVERY SYSTEMS

Multiple alternative methods for delivering insulin have either been developed or are under development and investigation. These include pulmonary insulin delivered through inhalation, peritoneal insulin delivered via implantable pumps, and transdermal and buccal insulin delivery.

Pulmonary delivery of insulin in humans was initially reported in 1925, with further studies in the 1970s and 1980s confirming the feasibility of administering insulin by the aerosol route. In these studies, ~10–30% of the insulin inhaled was absorbed into the circulation and the aerosols appeared to be well tolerated. The first pulmonary insulin preparation (Exubera) was approved by the U.S. Food and Drug Administration (FDA) in January 2006, but was subsequently removed from the market by the manufacturer in late 2007 for financial/business reasons. In 2014, the FDA approved an inhaled, rapid-acting, dry powder formulation of recombinant human insulin, Technosphere insulin (Afrezza from Mannkind/Sanofi) for treatment of adults with type 1 or type 2 diabetes. Afrezza was approved by the FDA to cover prandial insulin requirements in nonsmoking adults with diabetes. The product is packaged in prefilled cartridges and delivered through a breath-powered inhalation device. The bioavailability of regular human insulin in Afrezza is approximately 25%.

Afrezza must be used in combination with basal/long-acting insulin in patients with type 1 diabetes. An unpublished pharmacokinetic study (summarized in the package insert) conducted in 12 patients with type 1 diabetes compared 8 units of Afrezza with the same dose of insulin lispro. Serum concentrations peaked earlier with inhaled insulin, but the onset of action was similar with both drugs. The maximum effect occurred about 50 min after administration of inhaled insulin and about 120 min after injection of insulin lispro. Inhaled insulin had a shorter duration of action than insulin lispro (~3 vs. ~4 h).

The intrasubject variability of inhaled insulin is comparable to subcutaneous regular insulin. Results of studies in patients with rhinovirus infection have been mixed, with most showing no substantial change in the pharmacokinetics of inhaled insulin. Results from studies of the use of inhaled pulmonary insulin have shown that they are as effective as subcutaneous insulin regimens in type 1 and type 2 diabetes patients. Quality of life and treatment satisfaction assessments have shown inhaled insulin therapy is preferred over subcutaneous insulin therapy by many patients. The most frequently reported adverse events are throat pain or irritation, cough, and hypoglycemia. Cough occurred in about 27% of patients who received inhaled insulin, and was the most common reason for discontinuing the drug. Mild changes in pulmonary function have been reported but have been felt to be reversible and of little clinical significance. Forced expiratory volume in 1 sec (FEV1) declined by 40 mL more in patients using inhaled insulin versus other diabetes medications within the first 3 months of therapy and persisted for 2 years. Therefore, it is recommended that pulmonary function be assessed before starting therapy, 6 months into therapy, and then annually. If FEV1 declines by >20% or the patient exhibits persistent wheezing, bronchospasm, breathing difficulties, or cough, then inhaled insulin should be stopped. Inhaled insulin is contraindicated in patients with chronic lung disease (asthma, COPD) because it increases the risk of bronchospasm, and it should not be used by patients who smoke or who stopped smoking <6 months previously.

Continuous peritoneal insulin infusions via programmable implantable insulin pumps, another alternative insulin delivery method, has been used for over 20 years, although only in research settings in the U.S. Intraperitoneal insulin is rapidly and predictably absorbed into the portal circulation, simulating physiologic insulin delivery and absorption. Such rapid and predictable absorption may avoid the peripheral hyperinsulinemia seen with subcutaneous insulin regimens and the theoretical risk of accelerated atherosclerosis. Clinical studies have proven implantable pump therapy to be safe and effective for achieving glycemic control (significant reductions in A1C, average glucose level, and glucose variability), decreasing the rate of severe hypoglycemia, and improving glucagon responses to hypoglycemia.

OPTIMIZING BLOOD GLUCOSE CONTROL

Physiologic insulin secretion in nondiabetic individuals involves both prandial and basal insulin secretion. Prandial insulin secretion is initiated by neural and gut factors, before there is a hyperglycemic stimulus to insulin release resulting from the meal ingestion. It is followed by a rapid return of insulin secretion to the baseline level. Basal insulin secretion occurs between meals and during the night to regulate amino acids and fatty acids in the fasting state and to prevent excessive fasting gluconeogenesis.

Proper diabetes management has the goal of approaching normal blood glucose levels without severe hypoglycemia. The ADA recommends a premeal blood glucose target of 80–130 mg/dL (4.4–7.2 mmol/L) and peak postprandial values of <180 mg/dL (<10.0 mmol/L). Safe middle-of-the-night values are in the range of 80–130 mg/dL (4.4–7.2 mmol/L). These targets are difficult to maintain safely except under very intensive programs, although use of CGM has been shown to reduce hyperglycemia by ~30%.

The implications of the Diabetes Control and Complications Trial (DCCT) findings are that optimal treatment should be offered to all patients. Such treatment has the goal of approaching normal blood glucose levels without severe hypoglycemia. This generally requires using multiple injections or insulin pump therapy with fairly frequent dose adjustments in response to treatment. Critical in determining success are the patient's and family's priorities, abilities, and willingness to adhere.

To achieve near-normal glycemic levels, it is advisable to use individualized calculations for adjusting the dose and timing of insulin and meals based on regularly monitored blood glucose levels or CGM. Dose adjustment algorithms also allow patients to adjust insulin doses in relation to amount and composition of food and exercise. The efficacy of insulin therapy is predicated on:

- reasonable and consistent adherence to carbohydrate counting
- adjustment of insulin based on SMBG
- appropriate dosing of insulin before the meal (in very young children, the dose may be given immediately after the meal or split with some pre-bolus and the rest delivered once the total amount consumed is known)
- a regular pattern of activity and willingness to make adjustments for unscheduled activities

Algorithms are used to correct for a given glucose value based on the sensitivity factor or to adjust insulin dosing in anticipation of any blood glucose–altering factors (e.g., increased carbohydrate intake, intercurrent stress, or changing physical activity).

Timing of Prandial Insulin

If using regular insulin, it is preferable to give the insulin injection 30–45 min before meals so that the peak corresponds to the postmeal glycemic peak, allowing for more optimal glucose disposal. If using a rapid-acting analog, the injections are given as much as 30 min before eating depending on the blood glucose level with consideration of timing in relation to any previous correction dose, and with consideration of blood glucose targets. In very young children or persons with nausea, for whom it is not possible to estimate meal intake before eating, rapid-acting insulin may be given immediately after the meal or split with some pre-bolus and the rest delivered once the total amount consumed is known.

Individuals with gastroparesis may need to move insulin boluses later to match meal delivery.

Insulin-to-Carbohydrate Ratios (Carb Ratios)

Patients with type 1 diabetes should be encouraged to learn carbohydrate counting and to calculate their insulin-to-carbohydrate (carb) ratio to enhance flexibility in their diet and improve postprandial glucose control. The carb ratio can vary, for example, between 1 unit insulin/5 g carbohydrate to 1 unit insulin/25 g carbohydrate. For young children, the carb ratio may be 0.25–0.5 units insulin/20–30 g carbohydrate. To determine the carb ratio, the patient can either *1)* eat a fixed amount of carbohydrates with a meal, adjust the premeal insulin to obtain adequate postmeal glucose control, and then determine the ratio, or *2)* start with an estimated ratio and adjust it based on the resulting patterns of postprandial glucose concentrations to obtain adequate postmeal control. The carb ratio can be determined initially using a statistically established formula with carb ratio estimated at 450 divided by the total daily dose (TDD) of insulin (though it is thought that young children may require a tighter carb ratio than older children and adults). For example, the initial estimate of carb ratio for a patient taking 25 units of insulin per day would be 18 (i.e., 1 unit of insulin per 18 g carbohydrate). Subsequently, the carb ratio can be adjusted by 2–5 g carbohydrate at a time based on analysis of postprandial glucose records. The carb ratio is usually the same at all meals but may be tighter in the morning because of insulin resistance at that time and looser at bedtime. The carb ratio can also change when there are changes in body weight or the total daily insulin dose, such as with change in physical activity or onset of puberty.

Correction Bolus

All patients on insulin should be provided with correction bolus calculations to correct out-of-range glucose values. To do this, the insulin sensitivity factor, or correction factor (CF), must be determined for each patient. The insulin CF is defined as the estimated number of mg/dL the blood glucose will drop over a 2- to 4-h period following administration of 1 unit rapid-acting insulin. Once this factor is determined, a corrective bolus or supplemental dose can be estimated and added to the normal premeal dose or can be given at other times to correct hyperglycemia.

The CF can be determined by using the "1700 rule," in which CF = 1700/TDD (young children may require a looser CF). For example, if a patient's TDD is 50 units insulin, the CF = 1700/50 = 35. In this case, 1 unit of insulin should lower the patient's blood glucose level by 35 mg/dL (2 mmol/L). The CF can be used to calculate an individual's supplemental or correction bolus dose, where:

Correction dose = (actual blood glucose [BG] – midtarget BG)/CF

For most people, midtarget blood glucose is 100 mg/dL (5.5 mmol/L). However, patients prone to hypoglycemia may have a higher target (120 mg/dL [6.7 mmol/L]), and pregnant patients may have a lower target (80 mg/dL [4.4 mmol/L]). The correction dose is added to the premeal dose to optimize postmeal glucose levels. When this is done, it is best to give the dose at least 10–30 min before the meal to start correcting hyperglycemia before eating. A patient's CF and correction dose are adjusted upon review of the SMBG records.

Glycemic Targets and Insulin Adjustments

Adjustments of the insulin doses are made on the basis of SMBG or CGM measurements and are aimed at achieving target blood glucose values. Target glucose values are individualized based on the patient's ability to detect hypoglycemia and his or her current state of health. In most cases, targets are the normal values of a person without diabetes. If a child or a person has a proven problem coping with hypoglycemia, the target may be set higher. If the patient is pregnant, the target is set toward normal values for a pregnant woman without diabetes to optimize fetal outcomes.

Adjustments of insulin should be made with care to avoid hypoglycemia and overinsulinization. Dose adjustments should generally not surpass 1–2 units (decreases or increases) and should be made only when patterns of out-of-range glucose levels occur at the same time of day and are not attributed to transient changes in activity, food intake, or erroneous insulin injection. Ideally, adjustments upward should be made every 2–3 days for short- or rapid-acting insulin and every 3–5 days for long-acting insulin until the desired blood glucose targets are achieved. Adjustments downward should be made the next day for unexplained hypoglycemia, especially if severe.

There are different ways to achieve treatment targets. One method is to change the basal insulin to normalize the morning blood glucose level while avoiding hypoglycemia at 1:00–3:00 A.M. Basal insulin during the day can best be adjusted when the patient delays or skips a meal and no food intake has occurred for a minimum of 4 h. Glucose levels should not fluctuate by more than 30 mg/dL in either direction. Bolus insulin is adjusted based on the postmeal glucose values if using rapid-acting analogs or the glucose values prior to the next meal if using regular insulin. Once blood glucose levels are normalized postmeal, after a known amount of carbohydrate for that meal, a carb ratio can be calculated for that mealtime. Correction bolus calculations are also adjusted if the glycemic response does not bring the glucose into the desired range. If the glycemic response consistently remains above target range, the insulin CF is lowered to allow more insulin to be delivered. If the glycemic response is too great and the glucose falls below target range, the insulin CF is increased.

Treatment options should be individualized according to meal plan, exercise, patient preferences, and lifestyle requirements. SMBG or CGM should be used frequently to profile glycemic values and to adjust therapy. Optimal type 1 therapy requires a high degree of knowledge, time, and commitment on the part of the patient, the family, and the diabetes management team. Insulin pump therapy requires even more rigorous adherence to SMBG or CGM and other aspects of management and careful coordination by a team of experienced professionals.

Barriers to Adherence

Even with initial commitment to intensified insulin therapy from the patient and diabetes management team, problems can arise. When the goals of the patient and the diabetes management team are not congruent, attempts at intensive insulin therapy are problematic. Patients may become frustrated by the normal variability of glucose levels in type 1 diabetes, despite their best efforts. Clinicians should be alert for signs such as "diabetes burnout," eating disorders, or depression.

COMMON PROBLEMS IN LONG-TERM THERAPY

Problems with insulin therapy may arise regardless of the insulin regimen, and they must be addressed. Detecting and eliminating patterns of hypoglycemia and hyperglycemia is a key part of caring for patients with diabetes. This is as true for the individual with diabetes of several years' duration as for the newly diagnosed patient.

Recurrent moderate or severe hypoglycemic reactions signal the need for evaluation of the insulin regimen, eating and exercise patterns, other diseases or autoimmune disorders (celiac, Addison's, thyroiditis), and other lifestyle factors (e.g., alcohol consumption). Exceptionally low A1C levels may identify patients at risk for moderate and/or severe hypoglycemia, but must be considered in the context of whether the A1C matches actual BG measurements. In this situation, clinical conditions that can artifactually reduce A1C, such as increased red blood cell turnover, must be excluded, and a confirmatory test such as fructosamine may be considered. Some patients have diminished symptoms of impending hypoglycemia (hypoglycemia-associated autonomic failure, or HAAF) and, thus, suffer from recurrent hypoglycemic reactions and/or hypoglycemic seizures. HAAF is more common with longer duration of diabetes. It also can be exacerbated by antecedent hypoglycemia and, conversely, partially reversed by stringent avoidance of hypoglycemia. In patients with HAAF, blood glucose targets must be increased, and insulin pump therapy and use of CGM should be considered. For patients with HAAF using CGM, the low alarm setting should be set at a higher level (i.e., 80–90 mg/dL) to mitigate the risk of severe hypoglycemia, and possibly allow recovery of counterregulatory response. All patients with diabetes should check their blood glucose prior to driving, but those with HAAF need to pay particular attention to this important safeguard and check their blood glucose every few hours during long car trips.

Fasting hyperglycemia may occur due to either over- or under-insulinization overnight. If glucose levels between 2:00 and 4:00 A.M. reveal nocturnal hypoglycemia, rebound hyperglycemia (Somogyi effect) may be operative, although blood glucose levels >200 mg/dL (>11.1 mmol/L) usually do not occur unless carbohydrate is given to treat hypoglycemia. In this case, a decrease in evening intermediate- or long-acting insulin or overnight basal rates on the pump is needed. However, if no nocturnal hypoglycemia can be documented, inadequate insulin in the early morning hours due to the dawn phenomenon and/or too little basal insulin at night may be causative. This should be addressed with either an increase in predinner or bedtime basal insulin or a change from a predinner injection to a bedtime injection schedule. If this fails, insulin pump therapy needs to be considered with appropriate titration of overnight basal rates.

Disordered eating and inconsistencies in food intake and/or activity, often associated with psychosocial factors, can be causes of unacceptable day-to-day glucose control and elevated A1C levels. Additional problems of insulin therapy, including changes in insulin absorption or sensitivity, surgery, and insulin allergy are discussed in subsequent parts of this chapter or in other chapters.

INSULIN ALLERGY

Allergic reactions to insulin are increasingly rare with the widespread use of human insulin. However, patients, particularly those with known atopic diseases, may exhibit local or systemic allergies to human insulin itself, protamine in NPH, or the low pH of glargine insulin.

Some allergic-type reactions may be transient or artifactual. Burning, itching, and hives at injection sites may result from improper injection technique (intradermal rather than subcutaneous injection or injection of cold insulin) or from localized allergic phenomena.

If symptoms do not resolve and the patient's injection technique is sound, a change from one brand or type of insulin to another may be in order. True anaphylaxis, although rare, occurs occasionally and should be treated according to well-established protocols (e.g., antihistamines, epinephrine, etc.). If changing insulin type does not result in improvement, antihistamines can be prescribed. If atopic phenomena continue or if systemic symptoms occur, consultation with an allergist or endocrinologist is recommended for alternative approaches, including insulin desensitization.

Local Reactions

Lipohypertrophy at the injection site is the most common local complication of insulin therapy. It is thought to occur as a result of insulin stimulation of fat cell growth; the exact incidence is unknown. Lipoatrophy, characterized by reduction of fat cells in size or number, is rare with human insulin. If it does occur, changing brands of insulin may help. If either lipohypertrophy or lipoatrophy occur, rotation of injection sites with avoidance of the affected sites is recommended.

Immunological Insulin Resistance

Immunological insulin resistance due to antibodies to insulin is exceedingly rare, particularly since the introduction of purified insulin and human insulin. If it is suspected in a patient with unexplained severe insulin resistance, i.e., >2 units/kg/day after correction of ketosis with intravenous insulin, insulin antibody titers should be obtained in a reliable research laboratory. If high, change in insulin brands and type of insulin should be considered. If problems persist, such patients should be seen by a consultant diabetologist experienced in the assessment and management of complex problems. Patients with insulin resistance due to high insulin antibodies sometimes improve with corticosteroid treatment or other immune suppression therapy. Apparent insulin resistance is much more likely to occur as the result of the patient's not taking insulin as prescribed or using insulin that has precipitated or aggregated from excessive shaking or heating.

SPECIAL CONSIDERATIONS

Exercise

Because physical activity offers numerous health benefits, it should be encouraged in every patient with diabetes. In anticipation of the glucose-lowering effects of exercise (e.g., 30–45 min of moderate to vigorous physical activity) it may be necessary to increase carbohydrate intake or decrease the insulin dose to avoid hypoglycemia during or after exercise. Exercise-related hypoglycemia results from increased glucose uptake and utilization by the exercising muscle. In the case of prolonged exercise (lasting >1–2 h), it is necessary to reduce the insulin dose because hypoglycemia can occur many hours after exercise. General guidelines for avoiding exercise-related hypoglycemia are given in Table 3.3. Recommended strategies for reducing an insulin dose to prevent exercise-related hypoglycemia include the following:

- decrease prebreakfast rapid- or short-acting insulin if exercising within 3 h of breakfast
- decrease prelunch rapid- or short-acting insulin and/or morning NPH for exercise occurring in the late morning or early afternoon

---

Table 3.3   General Guidelines for Avoiding Exercise-Induced Hypoglycemia in Insulin-Treated Patients

- Measure blood glucose before, during, and after exercise.
- Exercise may need to be preceded by extra carbohydrate depending on current glucose level and exercise intensity and duration (e.g., 15–30 g carbohydrate per 30 min exercise); insulin may need to be decreased after exercise.
- If exercise is planned, insulin dosages can be decreased before and after exercise according to the exercise intensity and duration as well as the personal experience of the individual with diabetes.
- Patients on pumps may suspend or temporarily decrease their basal rate beginning 30 min prior to exercise, and possibly extending to after completion of exercise.
- During exercise, fast-acting carbohydrate for hypoglycemia treatment should be readily available.
- After exercise, extra carbohydrate may be necessary and may be added to meals and snacks.
- Athletes and those who exercise for fitness need specific instructions and training on self-management skills for exercise.
- For athletes and those with delayed hypoglycemia during the night, bedtime snacks or reduction in basal insulin should be considered, and blood glucose should be checked through the night.

Source: Adapted from Berger M. Adjustment of insulin and oral agent therapy. In *Handbook of Exercise in Diabetes*. Ruderman N, Devlin JT, Schneider SH, Kriska A, Eds. Alexandria, VA, American Diabetes Association, 2002, p. 374.

- decrease predinner rapid- or short-acting insulin in anticipation of exercise occurring after dinner
- suspend (for a maximum of 2 h) or temporarily decrease basal insulin delivery with the pump during and after strenuous exercise

Management During Acute Illnesses

The increased secretion of counterregulatory hormones and decreased activity even in the face of reduced caloric intake or vomiting may increase insulin requirements during acute illnesses. Blood glucose and urine or blood ketone levels should be tested frequently (e.g., every 1–4 h or each time the patient urinates). The physician should be contacted immediately for advice if prior written guidelines are not known by the patient or family member. The following guidelines, based on whether the patient is able to take food or liquids by mouth, are useful for managing a patient during an illness.

An illness not accompanied by nausea or vomiting (e.g., minor infection or trauma requiring bed rest): If activity is normal, give the usual dose of basal insulin plus a correction bolus every 2–4 h as needed according to the blood glucose and ketone tests. If able to drink or eat, give, in addition to the correction bolus, the meal bolus insulin to cover the carbohydrate consumed.

An illness accompanied by nausea, vomiting, or marked anorexia: Blood glucose and urine or blood ketones should be measured as soon as possible and every 2–4 h until the illness or situation has resolved. If there are initial glucose excursions, repeat glucose measurements may need to be done hourly. The basal insulin dose must never be omitted because this could lead to ketoacidosis. If glucose is >240 mg/dL (>13.3 mmol/L) and ketones are large (blood ketones >3.0 mmol/L), the patient should give a correction bolus by syringe, call the health-care team, and consider emergency department care for probable diabetic ketoacidosis. If glucose is >240 mg/dL (>13.3 mmol/L) and ketones are moderate (blood ketones 0.6–3.0 mmol/L), the patient can take a correction bolus every 2–4 h and drink noncaloric fluids until the situation has resolved. If the patient is on CSII with hyperglycemia >240 mg/dL (>13.3 mmol/L) and moderate to large ketones (>0.6 mmol/L), the infusion set and tubing must be changed and the correction bolus given by subcutaneous injection. If glucose is <240 mg/dL (<13.3 mmol/L) and ketones are large, the patient can take a correction bolus or an insulin injection every 2–4 h and consume caloric fluids as tolerated until the situation is resolved. When in doubt or if the situation is not resolving, the patient should contact the health-care provider.

Vomiting that occurs after administration of the usual morning dose of insulin: Sips of sugar-containing fluids should be given every 20–30 min to maintain blood glucose levels between 100 and 180 mg/dL (5.67–10.0 mmol/L). If vomiting persists and blood glucose level falls to <100 mg/dL (<5.6 mmol/L), consider giving "mini-dose" of glucagon at 1 unit of mixed glucagon (0.01mg or 0.01 mL per unit) on the insulin syringe for every year of age, up to 15–20 units. This might be sufficient to resolve hypoglycemia and associated nausea/vomiting and allow for the ingestion of small amounts of sugar-containing fluids as above. If hypoglycemia persists, continuous mini glucagon doses will likely not be effective (used up glycogen stores) and the patient may require intravenous glucose therapy. A subcutaneous injection of remaining dosage of glucagon, or if not previously given "mini-dose" glucagon, or a full dose of glucagon based on age and weight should be given at home before departing if the patient lives some distance from the hospital.

Anytime the patient is sick and has blood glucose levels >240 mg/dL (>13.3 mmol/L) and moderate or large ketones (blood ketones >0.6 mmol/L), the diabetes care team should be advised immediately or the patient should be brought to the emergency room, because this could reflect impending ketoacidosis. Repeated vomiting lasting more than 4–6 h or accompanied by high fever, abdominal pain, severe headache, or drowsiness may require that the patient be evaluated by a health-care provider to ascertain whether he or she has a serious infection, appendicitis, meningitis, or other condition requiring antibiotics, surgery, or intensive medical care in a hospital setting.

Treatment of Diabetes in Newborns and Infants

Transient or permanent neonatal diabetes (NDM) occurs before 6 months of age, including in newborn infants. Neonatal diabetes is a rare monogenic form of diabetes occurring in 1 in 100,000–500,000 live births. Affected infants are insulin deficient leading to hyperglycemia, dehydration, and ketoacidosis; neonatal diabetes can be mistaken for the much more common type 1 diabetes, but type 1 diabetes usually does not occur before 6 months of age. In about half of the cases of neonatal diabetes, the condition is lifelong and is called permanent neonatal diabetes, and in the other half, it is transient and disappears during infancy, although it can reappear later in life. Over 20 identified genetic causes of NDM have been identified, but many of these are syndromic with clinical clues that can direct genetic testing.

Due to insulin deficiency, these babies usually suffer from severe intrauterine malnutrition and, therefore, are small for their gestational age. As a result of hypo-insulinemia and intrauterine growth failure, these infants must be treated with exogenous insulin and may require high doses of 1–2 units/kg/day. Insulin requirements are best established by starting a continuous intravenous insulin infusion at rates that provide at least 0.5 units/kg/day. Insulin treatment is simplified by using diluted insulins (e.g., a solution containing 10 units/ml instead of the standard 100 units/ml) so that inadvertent overdoses do not occur. It is very important to dilute the insulin with diluents received directly from the manufacturer. After birth, some infants fail to gain weight and grow as rapidly as expected; however, appropriate diabetes management improves and may normalize growth and development.

Heterozygous mutations of the genes KCNJ11 and ABCC8 encoding the two subunits of the ATP-sensitive potassium (KATP) channel account for approximately 50% of cases of permanent NDM. In most patients with KATP-related diabetes, oral sulfonylurea therapy permits insulin secretion through ATP-independent closure of overly active mutated channels. Therefore, transitioning to sulfonylurea therapy in these patients often results in improved glycemic control, quality of life, and decreased complications.

Type 1 diabetes can start in infancy, usually after 6 months of age. To differentiate type 1 diabetes from a monogenic form of neonatal diabetes, antibodies should be obtained as well as specific gene analyses. The treatment of type 1 diabetes in infancy is similar to that described for the infant with neonatal diabetes, but oral sulfonylureas should not be considered. Insulin requirements vary, and care of these patients should be supervised by an experienced specialist. The type of regimen used must be individualized depending on the ability to control hyperglycemia without an excess of hypoglycemia, since both may be particularly detrimental to the developing brain. Many infants are placed on CSII with dilute insulin, since this treatment might best facilitate decreasing extremes of glycemic variability.

CONCLUSION

Type 1 diabetes is characterized by a near-absolute deficiency in endogenous insulin secretion and resultant hyperglycemia. Thus, people with type 1 diabetes are dependent on insulin to survive. Insulin therapy should always be coupled with SMBG, monitoring of carbohydrate intake, and proper precautions for physical activity and illness. CGM should be considered as a method to improve glucose control. In this way, insulin therapy can be adjusted safely and effectively and individualized to age, lifestyle, eating habits, state of health, and physical activity. Effective insulin therapy helps the patient avoid extreme metabolic crises—such as severe hypoglycemia and ketoacidosis—achieve and maintain good glycemic control, and reduce the risk of diabetes complications.

BIBLIOGRAPHY

Agrawal P, Welsh JB, Kannard B, Askari S, Yan Q, Kaufman FR. Usage and effectiveness of the low glucose suspend feature of the Medtronic Paradigm Veo insulin pump. *J Diabetes Sci Technol* 2011;5:1137–1141

Ahern JA, Boland EA, Doane R, Ahern JJ, Rose P, Vincent M, Tamborlane WV. Insulin pump therapy in pediatrics: a therapeutic alternative to safely lower HbA1c levels across all age groups. *Pediatr Diabetes* 2002;3:10–15

American Diabetes Association. Standards of medical care in diabetes—2016. *Diabetes Care* 2016;39(Suppl. 1):S1–S112

American Diabetes Association. *Practical Insulin: A Handbook for Prescribers.* 4th ed. Alexandria, VA, American Diabetes Association, 2015

An inhaled insulin (Afrezza). *JAMA* 2015;313:2176–2177

Bergenstal RM. Glycemic variability and diabetes complications: does it matter? Simply put, there are better glycemic markers! *Diabetes Care* 2015;38:1615–1621

Bergenstal RM, Ahmann AJ, Bailey T, Beck RW, Bissen J, Buckingham B, Deeb L, Dolin RH, Garg SK, Goland R, Hirsch IB, Klonoff DC, Kruger DF, Matfin G, Mazze RS, Olson BA, Parkin C, Peters A, Powers MA, Rodriguez H, Southerland P, Strock ES, Tamborlane W, Wesley DM. Recommendations for standardizing glucose reporting and analysis to optimize clinical decision making in diabetes: The Ambulatory Glucose Profile (AGP). *Diabetes Technol Ther* 2013;15:198–211

Bode BW, Tamborlane WV, Davidson PC. Insulin pump therapy in the 21st century. Strategies for successful use in adults, adolescents, and children with diabetes. *Postgrad Med* 2002;111:69–77

Bolderman KM. *Putting Your Patients on the Pump*. 2nd ed. Alexandria, VA, American Diabetes Association, 2013

Bruttomesso D, Pianta A, Crazzola D, Scaldaferri E, Lora L, Guarneri G, Mongillo A, Gennaro R, Miola M, Moretti M, Confortin L, Beltramello GP, Pais M, Baritusso A, Casiglia E, Tienga A. Continuous subcutaneous insulin infusion (CSII) in the Veneto region: efficacy, acceptability and quality of life. *Diabet Med* 2002;19:628–634

Carmody D, Bell CD, Hwang JL, Dickens JT, Sima DI, Felipe DL, Zimmer CA, Davis AO, Kotlyarevska K, Naylor RN, Philipson LH, Greeley SA. Sulfonylurea treatment before genetic testing in neonatal diabetes: pros and cons. *J Clin Endocrinol Metab* 2014;99:E2709–E2714

Cefalu WT, Tamborlane WV. The artificial pancreas: are we there yet? *Diabetes Care* 2014;37:1182–1183

Cersosimo E, Jornsay D, Arce C, Rieff M, Feldman E, DeFronzo R. Improved clinical outcomes with intensive insulin pump therapy in type 1 diabetes (Abstract). *Diabetes* 2002;51(Suppl. 2):A128

Cryer PE. Mechanisms of hypoglycemia-associated autonomic failure in diabetes. *N Engl J Med* 2013;369:362–372

Cryer PE. Diverse causes of hypoglycemia-associated autonomic failure in diabetes. *N Engl J Med* 2004;350:2272–2279

Davidson PC, Hebblewhite HR, Bode BW, Richardson PL, Steed RD, Welch NS, Johnson J. Statistical estimates for CSII parameters: carbohydrate-to-insulin ratio (CIR); correction factor (CF); and basal insulin. *Diabetes Technol Ther* 2003;5:A28

Dean L, McIntyre JR; National Center for Biotechnology Information; National Library of Medicine; National Institutes of Health; National Institute of Diabetes and Digestive and Kidney Diseases. *The Genetic Landscape of Diabetes*. Bethesda, MD, National Center for Biotechnology Information (US), 2004. Available at: *http://www.ncbi.nlm.nih.gov/books/NBK1667*

DeSalvo DD, Buckingham B. Continuous glucose monitoring: current use and future direcions. *Curr Diab Rep* 2013;13:657–662

DeVries JH, Snoek FJ, Kostense PJ, Masurel N, Heine RJ; Dutch Insulin Pump Study Group. A randomized trial of continuous subcutaneous insulin infusion and intensive injection therapy in type 1 diabetes for patients with long-standing poor glycemic control. *Diabetes Care* 2002;25:2074–2080

Doyle FJ III, Huyett LM, Lee JB, Zisser HC, Dassau E. Closed-loop artificial pancreas systems: engineering the algorithms. *Diabetes Care* 2014;37:1191–1197

Dunn FL, Nathan DM, Scavini M, Selam JL, Wingrove TG. Long-term therapy of IDDM with an implantable insulin pump. The Implantable Insulin Pump Trial Study Group. *Diabetes Care* 1997;20:59–63

Garvey K, Wolfsdorf JI. The impact of technology on current diabetes management. *Pediatr Clin North Am* 2015;62:873–888

Greeley SA, Naylor RN, Philipson LH, Bell GI. Neonatal diabetes: an expanding list of genes allows for improved diagnosis and treatment. *Curr Diab Rep* 2011;11:519–532

Hanaire-Broutin H, Broussolie C, Jeandidier N, Renard E, Guerci B, Haardt MJ, Lassmann-Vague V. Feasibility of intraperitoneal insulin therapy with programmable implantable pumps in IDDM: a multicenter study: The EVA-DIAC Study Group (Evaluation dans le Diabète du Traitement par Implants Actifs). *Diabetes Care* 1995;18:388–392

Hattersley A, Bruining J, Shield J, Njølstad P, Donaghue K; International Society for Pediatric and Adolescent Diabetes. ISPAD clinical practice consensus guidelines 2006–2007: the diagnosis and management of monogenic diabetes in children. *Pediatr Diabetes* 2006;7:352–360

Heller S, Buse J, Fisher M, Garg S, Marre M, Merker L, Renard E, Russell-Jones D, Philotheou A, Francisco AM, Pei H, Bode B; BEGIN Basal-Bolus Type 1 Trial Investigators. Insulin degludec, an ultra-longacting basal insulin, versus insulin glargine in basal-bolus treatment with mealtime insulin aspart in type 1 diabetes (BEGIN basal-bolus type 1): a phase 3, randomized, open-label, treat-to-target non-inferiority trial. *Lancet* 2012;379:1489–1497

Henry RR, Mudaliar SRD, Howland WC III, Chu N, Kim D, An B, Reinhardt RR. Inhaled insulin using the AERx insulin Diabetes Management System in healthy and asthmatic subjects. *Diabetes Care* 2003;26:764–769

Jimenez C, Corcoran MH, Crawley JT, Guyton Hornsby W, Peer KS, Philbin RD, Riddell MC. National Athletic Trainers' Association position statement: management of the athlete with type 1 diabetes mellitus. *J Athl Train* 2007;42:536–545

Karges B, Boehm BO, Karges W. Early hypoglycaemia after accidental intramuscular injection of insulin glargine. *Diabet Med* 2005;22:1444–1445

King AB, Armstrong DU. Basal bolus dosing: a clinical experience. *Curr Diabetes Rev* 2005;1:215–220

Lepore G, Dodesini AR, Nosari I, Trevisan R. Both continuous subcutaneous insulin infusion and a multiple daily insulin injection regimen with glargine as basal insulin are equally better than traditional multiple daily insulin injection treatment. *Diabetes Care* 2003;26:1321–1322

Linkeschova R, Raoul M, Bott U, Berger M, Spraul M. Less severe hypoglycaemia, better metabolic control, and improved quality of life in type 1 diabetes mellitus with continuous subcutaneous insulin infusion (CSII) therapy: an observational study of 100 consecutive patients followed for a mean of 2 years. *Diabet Med* 2002;19:746–751

Litton J, Rice A, Friedman N, Oden J, Lee MM, Freemark M. Insulin pump therapy in toddlers and preschool children with type 1 diabetes mellitus. *J Pediatr* 2002;141:490–495

Ly TT, Nicholas JA, Retterath A, Lim EM, Davis EA, Jones TW. Effect of sensor-augmented insulin pump therapy and automated insulin suspension vs standard insulin pump therapy on hypoglycemia in patients with type 1 diabetes: a randomized clinical trial. *JAMA* 2013;310:1240–1247

Madiraju AK, Erion DM, Rahimi Y, et al. Metformin suppresses gluconeogenesis by inhibiting mitochondrial glycerophosphate dehydrogenase. *Nature* 2014;510:542–546

Phillip M, Battelino T, Rodriques H, Danne T, Kaufman F; European Society for Paediatric Endocrinology; Lawson Wilkins Pediatric Endocrine Society; International Society for Pediatric and Adolescent Diabetes; American Diabetes Association; European Association for the Study of Diabetes. Use of insulin pump therapy in the pediatric age group. Consensus statement from the European Society for Pediatric Endocrinology, the Lawson Wilkins Pediatric Endocrine Society, and the International Society for Pediatric and Adolescent Diabetes, endorsed by the American Diabetes Association and the European Association for the Study of Diabetes. *Diabetes Care* 2007;30:1653–1662

Pickup J, Matack M, Kerry S. Glycaemic control with continuous subcutaneous insulin infusion compared with intensive insulin injections in patients with type 1 diabetes: meta-analysis of randomized control trials. *BMJ* 2002;324:705

Pivovarov JA, Taplin CE, Riddell MC. Current perspectives on physical activity and exercise for youth with diabetes. *Pediatr Diabetes* 2015;16: 242–255

Rudolph JW, Hirsch IB. Assessment of therapy with continuous subcutaneous insulin infusion in an academic diabetes clinic. *Endocr Pract* 2002;8:401–405

Santiago JV, White N. Diabetes in childhood and adolescence. In *International Textbook of Diabetes Mellitus*. 2nd ed. Alberti KGMM, Zimmet P, DeFronzo RA, Eds. Chichester, U.K., Wiley, 1997, p. 1095–1122

Sinha VP, Choi SL, Soon DK, Mace KF, Yeo KP, Lim ST, Howey DC. Single-dose pharmacokinetics and glucodynamics of the novel, long-acting basal insulin LY2605541 in healthy subjects. *J Clin Pharmacol* 2014;54:792–799

Skyler JS, Cefalu WT, Kourides IA, Landschulz WH, Balagtas CC, Cheng SL, Gelfard RA. Efficacy of inhaled human insulin in type 1 diabetes mellitus: a randomized proof-of-concept study. *Lancet* 2001;357:331–335

Skyler JS. Insulin therapy in type 1 diabetes mellitus. In *Current Therapy of Diabetes Mellitus*. DeFronzo RA, Ed. St. Louis, MO, Mosby, 1998, p. 36–49

Wolfsdorf J (Ed.). *Intensive Diabetes Management*. 5th ed. Alexandria, VA, American Diabetes Association, 2012

Wolpert H (Ed.). *Smart Pumping for People with Diabetes: A Practical Approach to Mastering the Insulin Pump*. Alexandria, VA, American Diabetes Association, 2002

Type 1 diabetes manifests with near absolute insulin deficiency, and for over 90 years, insulin replacement therapy has been the only pharmacological treatment available for this disease. Despite considerable advances in the pharmacokinetics of injectable insulin and better insulin delivery systems, the majority of patients with type 1 diabetes are still unable to achieve and maintain optimal glycemic control. The T1D Exchange Clinic Registry, involving at least 75 U.S.-based pediatric and adult endocrinology practices, recently reported an overall average hemoglobin A1C of 8.4%, with <30% of patients meeting the ADA-defined A1C goal.

Among the clinical barriers that hinder the attainment of glycemic goals with insulin therapy alone are the increased risk of hypoglycemia, postprandial hyperglycemia, excessive glucose fluctuations throughout the day, and undesired weight gain. Non-insulin adjunctive therapy complements intensive insulin therapy by addressing physiologic disturbances that result from endogenous β-cell destruction, offering potential for helping patients reach their glycemic targets and preventing diabetes-related complications (see Table 3.4). The aim of adjunct therapy is to complement, rather than replace, intensive inulin therapy. This section will highlight this area of promising research that may impact the clinical care of individuals with type 1 diabetes in the near future. It should be noted that most clinical trials in this area have been small and short-term in design.

TYPES OF ADJUNCTIVE THERAPY

Amylin

It has been recognized that pancreatic β-cells secrete another glucoregulatory hormone, amylin, which is normally co-secreted with insulin in response to meals. Consequently, the autoimmune-mediated destruction of pancreatic β-cells in type 1 diabetes results in a near absolute deficiency not only of insulin, but also of amylin.

Amylin is a 37–amino acid neuroendocrine hormone that binds with high affinity to certain areas of the brain and complements the effects of insulin in postprandial glucose control. Specifically, while insulin is the major hormone in the regulation of glucose disposal (efflux) out of the circulation, amylin regulates the inflow of glucose into the circulation after meals. This is achieved by suppression of glucagon secretion and regulation of gastric emptying. In addition, amylin has been shown to reduce food intake and body weight in laboratory animals, suggesting that it may also act as a physiological satiety signal.

The findings that amylin is normally co-secreted with insulin, that it complements the effect of insulin, and that it is deficient in type 1 diabetes led to the hypothesis that amylin replacement may convey additional benefits to patients with type 1 diabetes when added to existing insulin regimens. Human amylin itself is not optimal for clinical use because of its insolubility and tendency to self-aggregate; thus, a soluble, nonaggregating equipotent amylin analog, pramlintide, was developed.

Pramlintide is an adjunct to insulin therapy in people with type 1 or type 2 diabetes who use mealtime insulin therapy and have failed to achieve desired

Table 3.4 Non-insulin Adjunct Therapies in Type 1 Diabetes

Drug	Actions	Potential benefits in type 1
Metformin	Inhibits hepatic gluconeogenesis Improves insulin-mediated glucose utilization in peripheral tissues (i.e., muscle and liver) Reduces intestinal glucose absorption Reduces fatty acid oxidation Reduction of LDL and VLDL Reduction of pro-coagulant factors	Improved postprandial and fasting glucose profile Improved overall glycemic effect Insulin-sparing effect Weight reduction Improved cardiovascular outcomes
Amylin analogs	Regulation of postprandial glucagon release Inhibits hepatic gluconeogenesis Reduces gastric emptying Central effect of satiety	Improved postprandial glucose profile Improved overall glycemic effect Weight reduction
GLP-1 agonists in C-peptide positive and C-peptide negative	Augments insulin secretion Regulation of postprandial glucagon release Delays gastric emptying Central effect of satiety	Inhibition of β-cell apoptosis Halt progression and reversal of disease Insulin-sparing effect Improved postprandial glucose profile Reduction in glycemic variability Improved overall glycemic effect Weight reduction
DPP-4 inhibitors	Inhibits endogenous GLP-1 breakdown	Improved postprandial glucose profile Improved overall glycemic effect Insulin-sparing effect
Pioglitazone	Improved glucose delivery to the periphery through action on peroxisome proliferator-activated receptor-γ 1, 2 and α Decreases gluconeogenesis	Reduces insulin resistance Improved overall glycemic effect
Alpha-glucosidase inhibitors	Inhibits digestion of disaccharide to monosaccharide	Improved postprandial glucose profile Improved overall glycemic effect Insulin-sparing effect
Sodium glucose co-transporter-2 (SGLT2) inhibitors	Reduces renal glucose absorption in proximal renal tubules	Improved overall glycemic effect Weight reduction

Source: Reprinted with permission from George P, McCrimmon RJ. Potential role of non-insulin adjunct therapy in type 1 diabetes. *Diabet Med* 2013;30:179–188. Published by John Wiley and Sons. ©2012 The Authors. Diabetes Medicine ©2012 Diabetes UK.

glucose control despite optimal insulin therapy. Like insulin, pramlintide is given via subcutaneous injection. In short-term studies (days or weeks) of patients with type 1 diabetes, addition of pramlintide to insulin injections before meals reduced postprandial glucose excursions by at least 75%, regardless of whether pramlintide was used with regular insulin or a rapid-acting insulin analog. Adjunctive treatment with pramlintide reduced excessive glucose fluctuations over the course of the day, as demonstrated in a 4-week study with a continuous glucose monitoring device in an intensively treated type 1 diabetes patient. Of note, these effects were achieved with pramlintide doses (30 and 60 µg) that yield a plasma pramlintide profile similar to the normal postprandial amylin response in healthy subjects, indicating that the improvement in postprandial glucose control is achieved via physiological replacement of the absent amylin action. Additional studies in patients with type 1 diabetes have shown that the improvement in postprandial glucose control with pramlintide is attributable to both a correction of postprandial glucagon hypersecretion, thereby controlling excessive glucose output from the liver, and a slowing of gastric emptying, thereby controlling glucose inflow from the gut. These pramlintide effects are entirely consistent with the known physiological functions of amylin.

In studies of 6–12 months duration in patients with type 1 diabetes, addition of pramlintide to preexisting insulin regimens led to a significant A1C reduction of ~0.3–0.5% compared to placebo, and a doubling of the proportion of patients achieving recommended glycemic targets (A1C <7%). In a longer-term (29 weeks) safety and efficacy study evaluating dose escalation of pramlintide with mealtime insulin reduction, followed by insulin optimization, pramlintide was shown to drecrease postprandial glucose excursions and weight, with a decreased prandial insulin dose and without severe hypoglycemia. More insulin modification and glucose monitoring may be needed when more active, ill, etc. as would be expected even if not on amylin.

Pramlintide was the first pharmacological agent other than insulin to show improved long-term glycemic control in patients with type 1 diabetes. It is important to note that the glycemic improvement with pramlintide was not accompanied by the long-term increases in body weight or severe hypoglycemia typically seen when glycemic control is improved by increasing the dose of insulin. On the contrary, compared to placebo, pramlintide treatment was associated with a relative decrease in insulin use and reduction in body weight that was most pronounced (~1.5–3 kg) in overweight and obese patients (lean patients did not have unwarranted weight loss). Pramlintide treatment was generally well tolerated; the most common adverse event was mild nausea, which typically occurred during the first few weeks of therapy and dissipated over time.

Amylin replacement with pramlintide elicits a combination of clinical benefits that addresses some of the unresolved challenges with insulin therapy in type 1 diabetes. Adjunctive therapy with pramlintide is useful for those patients with type 1 diabetes in whom there are excessive unpredictable glucose fluctuations, postprandial hyperglycemia, undesired weight gain, or repeated episodes of insulin-induced hypoglycemia that hinder the achievement of glycemic targets. The clinical benefits of pramlintide are achieved by replacing the action of a second, naturally occurring β-cell hormone that is deficient in type 1 diabetes. By better matching the rate of glucose inflow to the rate of insulin-mediated glucose disposal, pramlintide improves glucose control via a unique mechanism of action that is distinct from, and complementary to, the action of insulin and its analogs.

GLP-1 Agonists

Glucagon-like peptide-1 (GLP-1) is an incretin that is normally secreted in response to nutrient ingestion to enhance insulin secretion, delay gastric emptying, suppress glucagon, and induce satiety. Injectable GLP-1 agonists such as liraglutide, exenatide, albiglutide, and dulaglutide are commonly used in type 2 diabetes, and have been demonstrated to improve fasting and postprandial blood glucose and A1C while promoting weight loss. Few studies have focused on GLP-1 agonist treatment in type 1 diabetes.

In a study investigating the effect of 4 weeks of treatment with liraglutide on inulin dose and glycemic control in patients with type 1 diabetes, insulin dose decreased significantly with improved or unaltered glycemic control. The treatment effect was greater in patients with residual β-cell function, and almost all patients lost weight. In a longer duration, open-label, pilot study involving 8 patients with type 1 diabetes on intensive insulin therapy plus liraglutide for 24 weeks, mean fasting and weekly glucose concentrations, glycemic excursions, and insulin doses significantly decreased. Additionally, mean A1C decreased significantly from 6.5% at baseline to 6.1% after 24 weeks of therapy, and weight decreased by 4.5 ± 1.5 kg. In a study involving 14 adults with long-standing type 1 diabetes, 6 months of high-dose exenatide therapy reduced postprandial blood glucose but was associated with higher fasting glucose concentrations without net changes in hemoglobin A1C. In adolescents with type 1 diabetes, there is evidence that exenatide therapy reduces postprandial hyperglycemia even with concurrent reduction in insulin doses.

Although there are few studies of GLP-1 agonists as adjunctive therapy in type 1 diabetes, there is clearly potential for therapeutic benefit including improved glycemic control, lower insulin doses, and weight loss. Longer-duration clinical trials are currently underway to assess the potential benefit of GLP-1 agonists in inhibiting β-cell apoptosis and promoting β-cell regeneration.

SGLT2 Inhibitors

Sodium-glucose cotransporter-2 (SGLT2) inhibitors are highly selective, orally active agents that reduce renal glucose absorption in the proximal renal tubules. SGLT2 inhibitors have been shown in type 2 diabetes to reduce hemoglobin A1C by as much as 1% with accompanying decrease in insulin dose and weight loss. The potential risks of SGLT2 inhibition include hypoglycemia, hypokalemia, hypotension (especially in patients using diuretics), syncope, and *Candida albicans* vaginitis in the female and balanitis in the uncircumcised male. The insulin-independent glucosuric mode of action led to the hypothesis that SGLT2 inhibitors may offer therapeutic benefits as an adjunct to intensive insulin therapy in type 1 diabetes.

In a short-term pilot study assessing the safety and efficacy of the SGLT2 inhibitor dapagliflozin in combination with insulin in type 1 diabetes, there were suggested dose-related reductions in average blood glucose, glycemic variability (mean amplitude of glycemic excursion), and insulin doses with no unexpected short-term safety concerns. A proof of concept study showed that the SGLT2 inhibitor empagliflozin when added to insulin therapy improved glycemic control in type 1 diabetes with concurrent reductions in insulin dose, body weight, and frequency of hypoglycemia. Improvements in blood pressure, renal hyperfiltration, and arterial stiffness have also been reported to occur with empagliflozin as adjunctive therapy in type 1 diabetes.

Sotagliflozin is a novel, orally delivered dual inhibitor of SGLT1 and SGLT2 designed to reduce glucose absorption in the gastrointestinal tract via SGLT1 inhibition in addition to renal glucose reabsorption via SGLT2 inhibition. In a small, short-term safety study, sotagliflozin as adjunctive therapy to insulin in type 1 diabetes resulted in improved glycemic control (hemoglobin A1C reduction of 0.55% in just 29 days of treatment) with associated reduction of bolus insulin (32.1% reduction from baseline) and weight loss (1.7 kg in 29 days), and no increased hypoglycemia compared to placebo.

Off-label use of SGLT2 inhibitors as adjunctive therapy in type 1 diabetes is increasing. Recently, the concern that SGLT2 inhibitors may predispose patients to ketoacidosis has been raised, and in May 2015 the U.S. Food and Drug Administration (FDA) issued a warning to that end. A recent case report described 7 individuals with type 1 diabetes on SGLT2 inhibitors who experienced euglycemic diabetic ketoacidosis (DKA). The loss of hyperglycemia as a marker of DKA with SGLT2 inhibitors was attributed to their insulin-independent glucose clearance, hyperglucagonemia, and volume depletion. Risk factors for euglycemic ketoacidosis associated with SGLT2 inhibitor therapy include the use of very low doses of insulin or withholding of insulin, and little to no food intake. Therefore, it should be cautioned that patients with type 1 diabetes on SGLT2 inhibitor therapy who experience nausea, vomiting, malaise, or develop a metabolic acidosis should be promptly evaluated for serum or urine ketones even if glucose levels are normal. Further study on the safety and efficacy of SGLT2 inhibitors is clearly needed.

Metformin

Studies show that a significant proportion of individuals with type 1 diabetes are overweight or obese, often with associated insulin resistance and worsening glycemic control. In a U.S. study of 507 youths (age 8–16 years) with type 1 diabetes, 33% were overweight or obese. Some studies point to a beneficial effect of metformin used adjunctively with insulin in these patients.

Metformin is an inexpensive and well-established oral glucose-lowering agent commonly used as first-line therapy for type 2 diabetes. A principal mode of metformin action is activation of the energy-regulating enzyme AMP-activated protein kinase, principally in muscle and liver, with associated decreased hepatic glucose production. Metformin therapy in type 2 diabetes is associated with decreased fasting glucose, hemoglobin A1C reduction, weight stabilization/loss, and decreased triglyceride, VLDL, and LDL levels.

Recently, in a multicenter (26 pediatric endocrinology clinics), double-blinded, placebo-controlled randomized clinical trial, involving 140 overweight adolescents with type 1 diabetes, the addition of metformin to insulin did not improve glycemic control after 6 months. Of multiple secondary endpoints, findings favored metformin only for insulin dose and measures of adiposity; conversely, metformin resulted in an increased risk for gastrointestinal adverse events. Otherwise, evidence on the effects of metformin in type 1 diabetes is limited. In a review of 9 other studies of patients with type 1 diabetes there were varying results, but, overall, use of metformin was associated with reduced insulin dose requirements (5.7–10.1 units/day), reduced hemoglobin A1C (0.6–0.9%), weight loss (1.7–6.0 kg), and decreased total cholesterol (0.3–0.41 mmol/l).

Metformin has generally been well tolerated, although with an increase in gastrointestinal side effects and increased episodes of mild hypoglycemic events. It remains unclear whether these effects are sustained beyond 1 year and whether there are benefits for cardiovascular and other key clinical outcomes.

DPP-4 Inhibitors

Sitagliptin, a dipeptidyl peptidase-IV (DPP-4) inhibitor approved for type 2 diabetes, increases endogenous GLP-1 levels by inhibiting its rapid metabolism through the DPP-4 enzyme. There are limited published data available on DPP-4 use in type 1 diabetes. In an 8-week, double-blind, crossover trial of patients with type 1 diabetes receiving adjunctive sitagliptin versus placebo, hemoglobin A1C was reduced by 0.27±0.11% after just 8 weeks, and total daily insulin decreased by 13.8%, but there was no significant weight loss. In a study assessing the effect of sitagliptin on glucagon and other counterregulatory hormones in response to hypoglycemia on 16 adult males with type 1 diabetes, sitagliptin treatment significantly increased active levels of GLP-1, but no significant differences were observed for glucagon or adrenergic counterregulatory responses. Further investigation with larger cohorts to assess clinical efficacy of DPP-4 inhibitor use as adjunctive therapy in type 1 diabetes is needed.

Alpha-Glucosidase Inhibitors

Miglitol is an alpha-glucosidase inhibitor used primarily in treating type 2 diabetes that targets postprandial hyperglycemia via inhibition of digestion of carbohydrates (such as disaccharides, oligosaccharides, and polysaccharides) into monosaccharides, particularly in the upper small intestine. There are limited data on their use as adjunctive therapy in type 1 diabetes. In a small, open-label study analyzing the effect of preprandial miglitol in combination with intensive insulin therapy over 12 weeks, there were significant decreases in hemoglobin A1C by 0.5%, preprandial hypoglycemic episodes, insulin doses (~2.4 units/day), and body mass index (BMI). No substantial change in appetite, nausea, bloating sensation, constipation, or diarrhea was reported. Interestingly, the authors also reported an increase in GLP-1 levels at 2 h with a mixed-meal tolerance test.

Thiazolidinediones

Pioglitazone is a thiazolidinedione approved for use in type 2 diabetes that works by increasing insulin sensitivity by activating peroxisome proliferator-activated receptors. In a double-blinded, placebo-controlled study analyzing the effect of pioglitazone as adjunctive therapy for 6 months in postpubertal lean individuals (BMI 18–25 kg/m^2) with type 1 diabetes, pioglitazone was modestly effective in improving postprandial glucose levels and hemoglobin A1C (0.22±0.29%) without alteration in body weight, insulin requirement, or lipid parameters. Of concern, however, are reports that pioglitazone may accelerate the disease course of type 1 diabetes. One study reported a more rapid decrease in C-peptide to undetectable levels with oral glucose tolerance test indicating loss of insulin secretion in subjects with type 1 diabetes receiving adjunctive pioglitazone.

Bromocriptine

Bromocriptine, a dopamine agonist, was recently approved for glucose-lowering in type 2 diabetes but not type 1 diabetes; however its use has not become widespread. Studies are ongoing to determine whether this agent may also be effective in type 1 diabetes.

CONCLUSION

Even with the remarkable advances in diabetes care over the last century or so since insulin was first used to treat diabetes, our ability to safely achieve glycemic targets in type 1 diabetes remains very limited. The loss of insulin secretion, dysfunctional glucagon secretion, and limitations in pharmacokinetics of injected insulin all contribute to this issue. Non-insulin adjunctive therapy may play an important therapeutic role in the management of type 1 diabetes. Although data are currently limited, adjunctive therapy appears to be beneficial in reducing postprandial glucose excursions, improving A1C, and reducing body weight, the net effect of which may lead to a reduction in micro- and macrovascular complications of diabetes. In order for these therapies to be considered for routine clinical practice, well-designed, randomized, placebo-controlled trials are needed to clearly demonstrate safety and efficacy.

BIBLIOGRAPHY

American Diabetes Association. Standards of medical care in diabetes—2016. *Diabetes Care* 2016;39(Suppl. 1):S1–S112

Baron AD, Kim D, Weyer C. Novel peptides under development for the treatment of type 1 and type 2 diabetes. *Curr Drug Targets Immune Endocr Metabol Disord* 2002;2:63–82

Baskaran C, Volkening LK, Diaz M, Laffel LM. A decade of temporal trends in overweight/obesity in youth with type 1 diabetes after the Diabetes Control and Complications Trial. *Pediatr Diabetes* 2015;16:263–270

Bhat R, Bhansal A, Bhadada S, Sialy R. Effect of pioglitazone therapy in lean type 1 diabetes mellitus. *Diabetes Res Clin Pract* 2007;78:349–354

Buse JB, Weyer C, Maggs DG. Amylin replacement with pramlintide in type 1 and type 2 diabetes: a physiological approach to overcome barriers with insulin therapy. *Clinical Diabetes* 2002;20:137–144

Chereney DZ, Perkins BA, Soleymanlou N, et al. Renal hemodynamic effect of sodium-glucose cotransporter 2 inhibition in patients with type 1 diabetes mellitus. *Circulation* 2014;129:587–597

Chereney DZ, Perkins BA, Soleymanlou N, et al. The effect of empaglifozin on arterial stiffness and heart rate variability in subjects with uncomplicated type 1 diabetes mellitus. *Cardiovasc Diabetol* 2014;13:28

DeFronzo RA. Bromocriptine: a sympatholytic, D2-dopamine agonist for the treatment of type 2 diabetes. *Diabetes Care* 2011;34:789–794

Edelman S, Garg S, Frias J, Maggs D, Wang Y, Zhang B, Strobel S, Lutz K, Kolterman O. A double-blind, placebo-controlled trial assessing pramlintide treatment in the setting of intensive insulin therapy in type 1 diabetes. *Diabetes Care* 2006;29:2189–2195

Edelman SV, Weyer C. Unresolved challenges with insulin therapy in type 1 and type 2 diabetes: potential benefit of replacing amylin, a second β-cell hormone. *Diabetes Technol Ther* 2002;4:175–189

Ellis SL, Moser EG, Snell-Bergeon JK, Rodionova AS, Hazenfield RM, Garg SK. Effect of sitagliptin on glucose control in adult patients with type 1 diabetes: a pilot, double-blind, randomized, cross-over trial. *Diabet Med* 2011;28:1176–1181

George P, McCrimmon RJ. Potential role of non-insulin adjunct therapy in type 1 diabetes. *Diabet Med* 2013;30:179–188

Gottlieb A, Velte M, Fineman M, Kolterman O. Pramlintide as an adjunct to insulin therapy improved glycemic and weight control in people with type 1 diabetes during treatment for 52 weeks (Abstract). *Diabetes* 2000;49(Suppl. 1):A109

Henry RR, Rosentock J, Edelman S, Mudaliar S, Chalamandaris AG, Kasichayanula S, Bogle A, Iqbal N, List J, Griffen SC. Exploring the potential of the SGLT2 inhibitor dapaglifozin in type 1 diabetes: a randomized, double-blind, placebo-controlled pilot study. *Diabetes Care* 2015;38:412–419

Kielgast U, Krarup T, Holst JJ, Madsbad S. Four weeks of treatment with liraglutide reduces insulin dose without loss of glycemic control in type 1 diabetic patients with and without residual beta-cell function. *Diabetes Care* 2011;34:1463–1468

Levetan C, Want LL, Weyer C, Strobel SA, Crean J, Wang Y, Maggs DG, Kolterman OG, Chandran M, Mudaliar SR, Henry RR. Impact of pramlintide on glucose fluctuations and postprandial glucose, glucagon, and triglyceride excursions among patients with type 1 diabetes intensively treated with insulin pumps. *Diabetes Care* 2003;26:1–8

Libman IM, Miller KM, DiMeglio LA, et al. Effect of metformin added to insulin on glycemic control among overweight/obese adolescents with type 1 diabetes: a randomized clinical trial. *JAMA* 2015;314:2241–2250

Miller MM, Foster NC, Beck RW, Bergenstal RM, DuBose SN, DiMeglio LA, Maahs DM, Tamborlane WV; T1D Exchange Clinic Network. Current state of type 1 diabetes treatment in the U.S.: updated data from the T1D Exchange clinic registry. *Diabetes Care* 2015;38:971–978

Nagai E, Katsuno T, Miyagawa JI, Konishi K, Miuchi M, Ochi F, Kusunoki Y, Tokuda M, Murai K, Hamaguchi T, Namba M. Effects of miglitol in combination with intensive insulin therapy on blood glucose control with special reference to incretin responses in type 1 diabetes mellitus. *Endocr J* 2011;58:869–877

Nyholm B, Brock B, Ørskov L, Schmitz O. Amylin receptor agonists: a novel pharmacological approach in the management of insulin-treated diabetes mellitus. *Expert Opin Investig Drugs* 2001;10:1–12

Perkins BA, Cherney DZI, Partridge H, et al. Sodium-glucose cotransporter 2 inhibition and glycemic control in type 1 diabetes: results of an 8-week open-label proof-of-concept trial. *Diabetes Care* 2014;37:1480–1483

Peters AL, Buschur EO, Buse JB, Cohan P, Diner JC, Hirsch IB. Euglycemic diabetic ketoacidosis: a potential complication of treatment with sodium-glucose cotransporter 2 inhibition. *Diabetes Care* 2015;38:1687–1693

Raman VS, Mason KJ, Rodriguez LM, Hassan K, Yu X, Bomgaars L, Heptulla RA. The role of adjunctive exenatide therapy in pediatric type 1 diabetes. *Diabetes Care* 2010;33:1294–1296

Sands AT, Zambrowicz BP, Rosenstock J, Lapuerta P, Bode BW, Garg SK, Buse JB, Banks P, Heptulla R, Rendell M, Cefalu WT, Strumph P. Sotagliflozin, a dual SGLT1 and SGLT2 inhibitor, as adjunct therapy to insulin in type 1 diabetes. *Diabetes Care* 2015;38:1181–1188

Sarkar G, Alattar M, Brown RJ, Quon MJ, Harlan DM, Rother KI. Exenatide treatment for 6 months improves insulin sensitivity in adults with type 1 diabetes. *Diabetes Care* 2014;37:666–670

Shimada A, Shigihar T, Okubo Y, Katsuki T, Yamada Y, Oikawa Y. Pioglitazone may accelerate disease course of slowly progressive type 1 diabetes. *Diabetes Metab Res Rev* 2011;27:951–953

Varanasi A, Bellini N, Rawal D, Vora M, Makdissi A, Dhindsa S, Chaudhuri A, Dandona P. Liraglutide as additional treatment for type 1 diabetes. *Eur J Endocrinol* 2011;165:77–84

Vella S, Bluetow L, Royle P, Livingstone S, Colhoun HM, Petrie JR. The use of metformin in type 1 diabetes: a systematic review of efficacy. *Diabetologia* 2010;53:809–820

Weyer C, Maggs DG, Kim D, Crean J, Wang Y, Burrell T, Fineman M, Kornstein J, Schwartz S, Guiterrez M, Kolterman OG. Mealtime amylin replacement with pramlintide markedly improves postprandial glucose excursions when added to regular insulin or insulin lispro in patients with type 1 diabetes: a dose-timing study. *Diabetologia* 2002;45(Suppl. 2):A240

Weyer C, Maggs DG, Young AA, Kolterman OG. Amylin replacement with pramlintide as an adjunct to insulin therapy in type 1 and type 2 diabetes mellitus: a physiological approach toward improved metabolic control. *Curr Pharm Des* 2001;7:1353–1373

Whitehouse F, Kruger DF, Fineman M, Shen L, Ruggles JA, Maggs DG, Weyer C, Kolterman OG. A randomized study and open-label extension evaluating the long-term efficacy of pramlintide as an adjunct to insulin therapy in type 1 diabetes. *Diabetes Care* 2002;25:724–730

Zambrowicz B, Freiman J, Brown PM, et al. LX4211, a dual SGLT1/SGLT2 inhibitor, improved glycemic control in patients with type 2 diabetes in a randomized, placebo-controlled trial. *Clin Pharmacol Ther* 2012;92:158–169

MONITORING

Monitoring, performed by patients, families, and diabetes management teams, is an integral feature of diabetes care. Specifically, results of blood or interstitial glucose monitoring are useful in preventing hyperglycemia and hypoglycemia, reducing glycemic excursions, and adjusting insulin, other medications such as pramlintide, diet, and exercise so that target blood glucose levels are achieved. Additionally, testing for urine or blood ketones provides an early warning sign of impending ketoacidosis.

PATIENT-PERFORMED MONITORING

Patients can manage their diabetes effectively and safely only if they are able to perform self-monitoring of blood glucose (SMBG). In certain circumstances (infants, young children, hospitalized or incapacitated patients), monitoring may be performed by family members, school personnel, child care providers, and health-care providers.

SMBG is a direct method of testing glucose that allows patients to determine their glucose levels anywhere (at home, school, or work) and to adjust therapy on the basis of accurate and timely results. To perform SMBG, a drop of blood is obtained from a fingertip or alternative site by use of a sharp lancet, usually with the aid of an automatic spring-loaded puncturing device. The capillary blood is then applied to a chemically impregnated or electrochemical strip, and after a specified time, the result is quantitated and displayed on the meter. With most meters, the results, as well as additional data (date, time, and, in some cases, additional data entered by the patient, such as whether the reading is pre- or postprandial), are stored in memory for later analysis.

Alternative-site testing is available with some meters that need only a small amount of blood. Such testing, usually performed on the forearm but also possible at other sites (heel of hand, thigh), is reliable and correlates well with finger-stick testing in the premeal or fasting state, but can have up to a 15- to 30-min lag if testing is done when glucose levels are changing rapidly (postmeal or with hypoglycemia). Therefore, it is recommended that patients be aware of this lag and not make decisions based on alternative testing at these times, but rather test the fingertip.

Many commercially available strips and meters have been evaluated in clinical studies, and are relatively reliable and reasonably accurate, though there are some concerns that with competitive bidding accuracy and reliability may be at risk. Lists of SMBG products can be found in the *Consumer Guide*, published annually in the January issue of *Diabetes Forecast*, the American Diabetes Association's magazine. With appropriate education, most patients can perform the testing technique successfully. However, office return demonstrations of the patient's skills and the use of quality control techniques at home are essential. Patients should be encouraged to bring their meters to every office visit to assess their accuracy and, if possible, to download the memory. Downloads have logbook displays of values above and below target, mean values, pie charts, graphs, etc. Inaccurate measurements can be obtained due to faulty meters, wrong coding of strips, unclean or wet hands, or use of control solutions instead of blood for testing. Using inaccurate measurements to make treatment adjustments can be more dangerous than having no measurements at all.

Frequency of SMBG

The frequency and timing of glucose monitoring should be dictated by the particular needs and goals of the patient. If the goal is to obtain near-normal glucose levels and prevent hyperglycemia, hypoglycemia, and extremes of glycemic excursions, then most patients with type 1 diabetes should test 6–10 (or more) times daily—although individual needs may vary. A database study (Type 1 Diabetes Exchange) of almost 27,000 children and adolescents with type 1 diabetes showed that, after adjustment for multiple confounders, increased daily frequency of SMBG was significantly associated with lower A1C (~0.2% per additional test). Additional testing after meals may be needed periodically or regularly to adjust prandial insulin doses. Testing before, during, and/or after exercise can help the patient avoid serious hypoglycemia (see Exercise, page 150). Adding a test periodically in the middle of the night is particularly important for patients who aim for near-normal blood glucose levels, those with unexplained fasting hyperglycemia, and for any patient during illness or after intense physical activity. Patients should vary testing times to learn about their blood glucose patterns over the entire day. Patients who are ill (Table 2.10), pregnant, or whose usual schedule has changed require more frequent monitoring.

Glycemic Variability

A1C does not provide a measure of glycemic variability or hypoglycemia. It is thought that high glycemic variability is a risk factor for vascular complications, besides genetic and environmental risks, and should be a primary treatment target. However, the ideal glycemic variability value as well as the effect, as measured within or between days, on the risk of developing diabetic complications is uncertain. There are many ways to analyze glycemic variability, including standard deviation (SD), coefficient of variation (CV), interquartile range (IQR), mean amplitude of glucose excursion (MAGE), M-value, mean of daily difference (MODD), continuous overall net glycemic action (CONGA), and others; however, most clinicians focus on SD, CV, and IQR.

Adjusting Insulin Dose

SMBG results are crucial in making appropriate insulin adjustments to optimize glycemic control, prevent hypoglycemia, and avoid hyperglycemic crisis. Insulin dose adjustments are covered earlier in this chapter under the section Glycemic Targets and Insulin Adjustments (page 94). SMBG results are also used at mealtimes to calculate a correction bolus in addition to the meal bolus needed to cover that meal. Thus, most patients should be encouraged to monitor a minimum of 4 times a day (before meals and at bedtime),, with additional monitoring at other times (during the night, during hypoglycemia, exercise, and illness, and after meals) to ensure safe and effective therapy. Since there is evidence that more monitoring improves glucose levels, it is not uncommon to see patients monitoring 8–10 or more times per 24 h, either routinely or occasionally.

Pregnant women need to perform SMBG more frequently (8–10, or more, times daily) to adjust insulin doses to obtain stringent glycemic targets and to avoid hypoglycemia. As with other elements of diabetes management, the prescription for glucose monitoring must be individualized.

The value of SMBG is not limited to adjustments in insulin dose. Patients with suspected nocturnal hypoglycemia can use SMBG to check their blood glucose levels at 3:00 A.M. SMBG is a valuable educational tool to help the patient differentiate between symptoms truly arising from hypoglycemia or hyperglycemia and those from other causes.

Common Causes of Error

Despite the relative simplicity of SMBG, the information is not free of errors. Many of the previous problems with SMBG have been resolved with test strips that do not require wiping, meters with built-in timers, meters with memory, and strips that do not require coding. The most common problems now with SMBG, independent of specific methodologies, include the use of an inadequate drop of blood on the strip, wet or dirty hands, wrong use of the control solution instead of blood, or a poorly calibrated meter. These problems stress the need to provide proper patient education and training in SMBG. Finally, some patients report their results inaccurately, perhaps to please their spouses, parents, or diabetes management team with the right results. The use of meters that automatically store glucose results in an electronic memory may simplify the recording, reporting, and analysis of SMBG; these results should be downloaded before or during office visits. Faxing data, or transmitting through emails or internet cloud with proper precautions to protect patient privacy, saves considerable amounts of time and enhances compliance to SMBG and intensive diabetes management.

Successful SMBG

If the goal of SMBG is to improve glycemic control, the diabetes management team should ensure that the patient:

- reviews results of glycemic patterns with the diabetes management team
- responds to the results by making appropriate changes in the insulin regimen
- receives the necessary psychosocial support and technical guidance
- monitors as frequently as recommended
- reads and reports tests accurately
- uses additional SMBG during intercurrent illnesses, exercise, traveling, and when the routine is not followed

To support successful glycemic control, there should be mutual efforts to maintain education, motivation, and adherence. Furthermore, it is essential for the diabetes management team to provide feedback by monitoring progress with A1C (eAG) tests every 3 months.

GLUCOSE SENSORS

Continuous interstitial glucose sensing is an adjunct to SMBG that provides additional data to optimize glycemic control and alarms to help prevent hypoglycemic and hyperglycemic crises. Several different systems have been approved in the U.S. by the FDA, and others are in development. The devices that are available are calibrated by fingerstick SMBG measurements and then sense glucose in the interstitial fluid using glucose oxidase enzymatic methodology. Interstitial fluid has been shown to correlate well with blood glucose, and the glucose concentration in the interstitial fluid has been shown to reflect glucose concentrations and glucose dynamics in the brain. However, there is a physiological lag between the interstitial fluid and the blood. This lag is usually <5 min in the fasting or premeal state but can be up to 15–30 min in the postprandial state. As a result of this lag time and other factors, these devices are currently recommended for use as an adjunct to, not a replacement for, SMBG. The glucose trends and alarms/alerts, rather than the absolute glucose values, obtained from these devices are used to make therapy changes to optimize glucose control. For immediate therapy decisions, such as deciding on premeal insulin doses or treatment of hypoglycemia, patients should use the SMBG results. Most continuous glucose sensors can be worn for 3–7 days.

The original continuous glucose monitoring (CGM) system was used like a Holter-style monitor system and measured glucose continuously in interstitial fluid for up to 72 h. The data was not displayed to the patient in real time, but was used by a physician or member of the diabetes team for retrospective monitoring and interpretation of the readings. To use this system, an electrochemical sensor was inserted by an insertion device into the subcutaneous tissue (usually the abdomen, buttocks, or back) and worn for up to 72 h. The sensor used in the original systems measured glucose every 10 sec and provided an average glucose every 5 min for up to 288 readings per day. These readings were collected and stored in a monitor connected by a cable to the sensor. Calibration by fingerstick blood glucose measurements was done at least three times per day with entry of the value into the monitor. Patients were also instructed to keep a food diary and enter event markers for specific behaviors such as eating, insulin administration, exercise, and hypoglycemia symptoms. After wearing the device, the sensor was removed and the monitor was downloaded into a computer for further analysis and evaluation by the health-care provider and the patient.

Retrospective (also called professional or blinded) CGM devices used now employ the same sensor that is used with real-time CGM, and instead of transmitting the interstitial glucose values to a monitor, the information is stored and downloaded to a computer program at the end of the sensor wear (3–7 days depending on sensor life). During the use of retrospective CGM, the patient must calibrate the sensor with SMBG and use SMBG to manage their diabetes. Patients are also instructed to keep a food diary and enter event markers for specific behaviors such as eating, insulin administration, exercise, and hypoglycemia symptoms. These systems are used one time or at repeated intervals to obtain continuous glucose monitoring information when the patient is not ready to wear a real-time device. The 288 glucose values per day can be used to determine the presence of hypoglycemia (particularly at night), the dawn phenomenon, and postprandial hyperglycemia. It is of particular value in those suspected of having hypoglycemia unawareness and can be used at the time of a change in the diabetes regimen, such as when switching from MDI to CSII. Retrospective CGM can also be used to help patients understand the effect of certain lifestyle choices, such as glycemic patterns associated with exercise or the ingestion of specific foods.

The uploaded data is displayed on a number of pages including a logbook that displays values above and below glycemic targets, individual tracings by day, mean glucose by day and time of day, pie charts, and area and percent above and below targets. Retrospective CGM is also used in research protocols to compare the glycemic outcomes between the groups being evaluated in the research study.

Data from the landmark Juvenile Diabetes Research Foundation Continuous Glucose Monitoring (JDRF-CGM) trial demonstrated that in adults with an A1C >7%, the use of continuous glucose monitoring was associated with a 0.5% reduction in A1C and that 83% of adults used sensors for at least 6 days a week. In children and young adults, aged 8–24 years, however, sensor use was not associated with an overall reduction in A1C, although in a subset of participants who used sensors for at least 6 days a week, a reduction of 0.5% in A1C was also seen.

Despite the use of continuous glucose monitoring, data from the JDRF-CGM trial still demonstrated a high incidence of prolonged nocturnal hypoglycemia. This is not surprising given the evidence that patients sleep through 71% of alarms and that adolescents with type 1 diabetes have a high acoustic arousal threshold from sleep. During the overnight period, the presence of continuous glucose monitoring alone is unlikely to prevent prolonged nocturnal hypoglycemia.

Real-Time Continuous Glucose Monitoring System

Continuous glucose monitoring systems are meant to be worn chronically or intermittently by the same patient and provide real-time as well as stored glucose data (which can be uploaded through a computer program for retrospective analysis). The system consists of a sensor, a monitor, and a transmitting device, which sends the signal from the sensor to the monitor in real time. When CGM is integrated with an insulin pump, referred to as sensor-augmented pump therapy, the pump itself is used as the monitor and the stored glucose and pump data can be uploaded together. Real-time CGM systems have alarms to alert for high and low glucose levels or a rapid change in glucose value, and predictive alarms to warn of impending hypoglycemia and hyperglycemia.

Although originally there were only short-term and not rigorously controlled studies on CGM, there has been an increasing number of longer-term studies (a 6–12-month study phase with up to a 12–18-month continuation phase) in adults and children showing that CGM is associated with reduced glycemic variability (less time spent in the hyperglycemic and hypoglycemic ranges) and improved glycemic control. In subjects with A1C < 7%, CGM usage has been shown to assist in maintaining target A1C levels while limiting the risk of hypoglycemia. These studies have also shown that the greater the sensor usage, the more the reduction in A1C levels. A recent meta-analysis of 6 randomized, controlled trials involving 449 patients showed that CGM was associated with significant reduction in A1C. Those with the highest baseline A1C and those who used sensors the most had the greatest reduction in A1C. The devices and sensors are expensive and may not be covered by third-party payors. However, the devices are increasingly being prescribed, especially for children and adults with severe hypoglycemia. In 2008, the American Diabetes Association recommendation (level E, based on expert opinion) was that such systems may be a useful supplemental tool to

SMBG for selected patients with type 1 diabetes who have demonstrated that they can use these devices.

Advances continue to be made with next-generation glucose oxidase sensors being more accurate, smaller, more comfortable, and of longer duration. Research continues not only with this methodology, but with other methods to measure glucose in the interstitial fluid as well as in other parts of the body. The ultimate goal is to develop CGM methodologies that will replace SMBG and be reliable enough for the artificial pancreas.

KETONE TESTING

The ketone bodies acetoacetate (AcAc), acetone, and β-hydroxybutyric acid (β-HBA) are catabolic products of free fatty acids. Determinations of ketones in the urine and blood are widely used as adjuncts for both the diagnosis and ongoing monitoring of diabetic ketoacidosis (DKA). Measurements of ketone bodies can be routinely performed both in the office/hospital setting and by patients at home.

Urine ketone testing remains the most commonly used method to detect impending ketosis at home. Most urine methods use reagent strips containing nitroprusside that form a colorimetric reaction on contact with AcAc (and in some strips, acetone), resulting in a purple color. Care should be taken not to use out-of-date strips. The strips are manually read as measuring negative, small, moderate, or large ketones. Urine methodologies do not measure β-HBA and are thus not useful in monitoring the response to DKA treatment, because AcAc and acetone may increase as β-HBA falls during successful treatment of DKA.

Testing for ketonuria should be a regular feature of sick-day instructions and should be done every time blood glucose levels are consistently >240 mg/dL (>13.3 mmol/L), patient is on SGLT2 inhibitors, or patient is symptomatic. The presence of persistent moderate or large amounts of ketones in the urine suggests the possibility of impending or established DKA and should prompt patients to adjust insulin as recommended or seek assistance by calling their health-care provider. Note that positive urine ketone readings are found in up to 30% of first morning urine specimens from pregnant woman (with and without diabetes), during starvation, and after hypoglycemia.

Blood ketone testing is also available for home and office/hospital use. Most blood methods measure β-HBA, which is the predominant ketone in DKA. Reference intervals for β-HBA differ among the assay methods, but concentrations <0.5 mmol/L are considered normal, 0.6–1.5 mmol/L indicate the potential for DKA, and >1.5 mmol/L indicate high risk for DKA or that DKA is already present (at which point, the β-HBA is typically much higher than 1.5 mmol/L).

Specific measurements of β-HBA in blood can be used by both the patient and health-care provider for the diagnosis and monitoring of DKA. Testing for blood ketones is not mandatory for either the patient or the health-care provider because the patient can use urine testing to troubleshoot hyperglycemia and the health-care provider can use measurements of serum CO_2, anion gap, and pH to diagnose and monitor DKA treatment. However, blood ketone testing is much more specific than urine testing and much quicker and easier than these hospital laboratory methods, and thus has a role in the prevention, diagnosis, and management of DKA.

PHYSICIAN-PERFORMED MONITORING

Because blood glucose levels can fluctuate widely in type 1 diabetes, sporadic testing in the physician's office is not sufficient as the sole means of monitoring. Intermittent testing does not reliably predict glucose levels at other times or the level of chronic glycemic control. Laboratory glucose determinations by a calibrated meter or approved instrument can be performed, if needed, to validate the accuracy of patient-performed monitoring and meter accuracy.

Glycated Hemoglobin (A1C Test)

The introduction of the A1C assay has revolutionized the ability to follow glucose control over time. When hemoglobin and other proteins are exposed to glucose, the glucose becomes attached to the protein in a slow, nonenzymatic, and concentration-dependent fashion. A1C is a weighted average of blood glucose levels during the life of the red blood cells (~3 months). Therefore, glycemic control within the month prior to A1C testing contributes more to the A1C value than glycemic control between 1 and 3 months prior to A1C testing.

This measurement is performed on a single tube of blood or with a fingerstick capillary sample, and when correctly performed by a reliable laboratory or certified kit, the test is unaffected by acute changes in blood glucose; therefore, the test can be performed at any time during the day.

The Diabetes Control and Complications Trial (DCCT) established the major role of glycemic control in the development and progression of microvascular complications in type 1 diabetes. Although glycemic control can be assessed directly by analyzing multiple blood glucose levels over time, A1C is strongly associated with the mean of the blood glucose values and is easier to obtain. However, factors other than just mean blood glucose have been shown to affect A1C; these include biological variation for glycation and glucose variability or instability. The contribution of glycemic variability or instability to A1C in studies derived from DCCT data appears to be minor. This suggests that glucose variability, particularly the instability of postprandial values, may influence outcome through other pathways, such as oxidative stress.

Assay methods. Many different types of glycohemoglobin assay methods were available in the past, differing considerably with respect to the glycated components measured, interferences, and nondiabetic range. Glycated hemoglobin A1C has become the preferred standard for assessing glycemic control and, in 1996, the National Glycohemoglobin Standardization Program (NGSP) was formed to standardize the A1C test to DCCT values. Since then, A1C measurements in North America have been almost universally standardized to the DCCT assay range.

In recent years, the International Federation of Clinical Chemistry (IFCC) developed a new standard for A1C that results in a measurement of concentration (mmol A1C/mol HbA) rather than percent and a reference range that is different than the DCCT standard. Although small studies had already suggested it to be the case for type 1 populations, a recent multicenter study in subjects with type 1 diabetes, type 2 diabetes, and no diabetes; of multiple ethnic groups, and on multiple types of diabetes therapies confirmed that there is a close association of

A1C with the mean blood glucose over the prior 2–3 months across the entire study population.

Hemoglobin variants have the potential to cause falsely low or high A1C readings, especially with older assays. A list of assays and whether or not they are accurate in patients with hemoglobin variants can be found on the NGSP website (visit www.ngsp.org/interf.asp). Additionally, patient comorbidities affecting red blood cell turnover (hemolytic anemias, chronic kidney disease) will make interpretation of the test difficult.

Utility. A properly performed A1C test provides the best available index of chronic glucose levels. Other glycated protein molecules can be measured for this purpose (e.g., glycated albumin or fructosamine), especially in patients with abnormalities of red blood cell turnover, but their role in clinical practice is less well established.

A1C testing is invaluable in identifying patients who have relatively high, average, or near-normal levels of chronic glucose control. Discrepancies between the A1C level and the results of SMBG may indicate that the latter is either inaccurately performed or fabricated, or that the patient has an interfering hemoglobinopathy or disorder of red blood cell turnover.

The measurement of A1C allows physician and patient to set objective goals for therapy and to measure the efficacy of changes in therapy. The usual frequency for performing this assay in type 1 diabetes should be four times per year.

A1C testing at the time of the patient's visit with immediate results is available via several NGSP-certified instruments. Such testing allows the patient and physician to discuss the results at that visit and make immediate changes in treatment, if needed, to optimize glycemic control. Such point-of-care testing has resulted in a drop of 0.5–1% in the A1C value. A1C testing by home NGSP-certified kits is also commercially available, but the value of such testing remains to be determined.

A1C can also be used to make the diagnosis of diabetes in adults, and likely in children although this has not been confirmed. A value ≥6.5% is sufficient to suggest diabetes, while a value of ≥5.7–6.4% suggests prediabetes.

The GlycoMark blood glucose test measures monosaccharide 1,5-anhydroglucitol in the blood, which is a specific index of elevated postmeal glucose levels and short-term glycemic control. This test has proven useful in pharmaceutical research, as well as in patient care, when methods are being employed that specifically target glucose instability after meals.

OTHER MONITORING

In addition to monitoring for glycemia and A1C, patients need ongoing monitoring of fasting lipid profiles, urine albumin excretion, and kidney function, as further described in the Complications chapter (page 243) and in the American Diabetes Association's Standards of Medical Care in Diabetes. Thyroid-stimulating hormone (TSH) testing is recommended periodically for all patients with type 1 diabetes. Screening for celiac disease or other autoimmune diseases may be indicated in patients with signs or symptoms.

CONCLUSION

The appropriate application of SMBG techniques provides the patient with type 1 diabetes the opportunity to adjust therapy safely and effectively. The type and frequency of monitoring must be individualized and will be dictated primarily by the patient's lifestyle and the intensity of insulin therapy. A1C testing provides an objective index of long-term glucose levels and can be used to determine efficacy of treatment.

BIBLIOGRAPHY

American Diabetes Association. Standards of medical care in diabetes—2016. *Diabetes Care* 2016;39(Suppl. 1):S1–S112

American Diabetes Association. Tests of glycemia in diabetes (Position Statement). *Diabetes Care* 2004;27(Suppl. 1):S91–S93

Bergenstal RM. Glycemic variability and diabetes complications: does it matter? Simply put, there are better glycemic markers! *Diabetes Care* 2015;38:1615–1621

Bergenstal RM, Ahmann AJ, Bailey T, Beck RW, Bissen J, Buckingham B, Deeb L, Dolin RH, Garg SK, Goland R, Hirsch IB, Klonoff DC, Kruger DF, Matfin G, Mazze RS, Olson BA, Parkin C, Peters A, Powers MA, Rodriguez H, Southerland P, Strock ES, Tamborlane W, Wesley DM. Recommendations for standardizing glucose reporting and analysis to optimize clinical decision making in diabetes: the ambulatory glucose profile (AGP). *Diabetes Technol Ther* 2013;15:198–211

Bergenstal RM, Tamborlane WV, Ahmann A, Buse JB, Dailey G, Davis SN, Joyce C, Perkins BA, Welsh JB, Willi SM, Wood MA; STAR 3 Study Group. Sensor-augmented pump therapy for A1C reduction (STAR 3) study. *Diabetes Care* 2011;34:2403–2405

Bergenstal RM, Tamborlane WV, Ahmann A, Buse JB, Dailey G, Davis SN, Joyce C, Perkins BA, Welsh JB, Willi SM, Wood MA; STAR 3 Study Group. Effectiveness of sensor-augmented insulin-pump therapy in type 1 diabetes. *N Engl J Med* 2010;363:311–320

Bode BW, Sabbah H, Davidson PC. What's ahead in glucose monitoring? *Postgrad Med* 2001;109:41–44

Boland E, Monsod T, Delucia M, Brandt CA, Fernando S, Tamborlane WV. Limitations of conventional methods of self-monitoring of blood glucose: lessons learned from three days of continuous glucose sensing in pediatric patients with type 1 diabetes. *Diabetes Care* 2001;24:1858–1862

Chase HP, Kim LM, Owen SL, MacKenzie TA, Klingensmith GJ, Murtfeldt R, Garg SK. Continuous subcutaneous glucose monitoring in children with type 1 diabetes. *Pediatrics* 2001;107:222–226

Cheyne EH, Cavan DA, Kerr D. Performance of a continuous glucose monitoring system during controlled hypoglycaemia in healthy volunteers. *Diabetes Technol Ther* 2002;4:607–613

Diabetes Research in Children Network (DirecNet) Study Group; Buckingham B, Beck RW, Tamborlane WV, Xing D, Kollman C, Fiallo-Scharer R, Mauras N, Ruedy KJ, Tansey M, Weinzimer SA, Wysocki T. Continuous glucose monitoring in children with type 1. *J Pediatr* 2007;151:388–393

Garb S, Zisser H, Schwartz S, Bailey T, Kaplan R, Ellis S, Jovanovic L. Improvement in glycemic excursions with a transcutaneous, real-time continuous glucose sensor: a randomized controlled trial. *Diabetes Care* 2006;29:44–50

Garg SK, Schwartz S, Edelman SV. Improved glucose excursions using an implantable real-time continuous glucose sensor in adults with type 1 diabetes. *Diabetes Care* 2004;27:734–738

Jungheim K, Koschinsky T. Risky delay of hypoglycemia detection by glucose monitoring at the arm. *Diabetes Care* 2001;24:1303–1306

Juvenile Diabetes Research Foundation Continuous Glucose Monitoring Study Group; Tamborlane WV, Beck RW, Bode BW, et al. Continuous glucose monitoring and intensive treatment of type 1 diabetes. *N Engl J Med* 2008;359:1464–1476

Kerr D, Cheyne EH, Weiss M, Ryder J, Cavan DA. Accuracy of MiniMed continuous glucose monitoring system during hypoglycaemia. *Diabetology* 2001;44(Suppl. 1):A239

Klonoff DC, Buckingham B, Christiansen JS, Montori VM, Tamborlane WV, Vigerskky RA, Wolpert H; Endocrine Society. Continuous glucose monitoring: an Endocrine Society Clinical Practice Guideline. *J Clin Endocrinol Metab* 2011;96:2968–2979

McCarter RJ, Hempe JM, Chalew SA. Mean blood glucose and biological variation have greater influence on HbA1C levels than glucose instability: an analysis of data from the Diabetes Control and Complications Trial. *Diabetes Care* 2006;29:352–355

Miller KM, Beck RW, Bergenstal RM, et al.; T1D Exchange Clinic Network. Evidence of a strong association between frequency of self-monitoring of blood glucose and hemoglobin A1c levels in T1D Exchange Clinic Registry participants. *Diabetes Care* 2013;36:2009–2014

Nielsen JK, Djurhuus CB, Gravholt CH, Carus AC, Granild-Jensen J, Orskov H, Christiansen JS. Continuous glucose monitoring in interstitial subcutaneous adipose tissue and skeletal muscle reflects excursions in cerebral cortex. *Diabetes* 2005;54:1635–1639

Pickup JC, Freeman SC, Sutton AJ. Glycaemic control in type 1 diabetes during real-time continuous glucose monitoring compared with self monitoring of blood glucose: meta-analysis of randomized controlled trials using individual patient data. *BMJ* 2011;343:d3805

Sacks DB, Bruns DE, Goldstein DE, Maclaren NK, McDonald JM, Parrott M. Guidelines and recommendations for laboratory analysis in the diagnosis and management of diabetes mellitus. *Clin Chem* 2002;48:436–472

Schiaffini R, Ciampalini P, Fierabracci A, Spera S, Borrelli P, Bottazzo G, Crinò A. The continuous glucose monitoring system (CGM) in type 1 diabetic children is the way to reduce hypoglycemic risk. *Diabetes Metab Res Rev* 2002;18:324–329

NUTRITION

The effectiveness of medical nutrition therapy (MNT) in the medical management of type 1 diabetes is well established. MNT includes a comprehensive assessment of the patient's nutritional status, diabetes and health status, weight for height or BMI, lifestyle, support systems, and willingness and ability to make changes or initiate new behaviors. MNT is implemented in a nutrition care plan based on individual goals negotiated with the patient, and monitoring and evaluation of goal-directed activities. Success and satisfaction are measured by goal achievement and improved metabolic and other health outcomes.

Managing eating is one of the most challenging aspects of diabetes self-management and requires knowledge, time, effort, and commitment from those involved. Although there are many other variables besides food that affect blood glucose levels, physicians and other diabetes management team members often attribute poor glycemic control to a lack of dietary adherence. In the best-case scenario, all team members are knowledgeable about nutrition therapy and supportive of the person with diabetes who is struggling to make lifestyle changes. Because of the complexity of nutrition issues, it is recommended that a registered dietitian, knowledgeable and skilled in implementing diabetes MNT, be the team member providing individualized MNT, which is recommended for all people with type 1 diabetes. Also, all patients with type 1 diabetes should be referred to a registered dietitian when diagnosed (sometimes in an initial series of three to four encounters), then routinely consult with a registered dietitian as part of the continuing medical care of their diabetes. Follow-up may be appropriate every 3–6 months for children and every 6–12 months for adults.

NUTRITION RECOMMENDATIONS

The American Diabetes Association has published the evidence-based position statement Nutrition Therapy Recommendations for the Management of Adults With Diabetes as a stand-alone document and as part of the 2014 Standards of Medical Care (see references). These recommendations attempt to translate research data and clinically applicable evidence into nutrition care. The Food and Nutrition Board in the Health and Medicine Division of the National Academies of Sciences, Engineering, and Medicine has published dietary reference values for the intake of macronutrients. This report covers dietary reference intakes (DRIs) for energy, carbohydrates, fiber, fat, fatty acids, cholesterol, protein, and amino acids. Competing with the science-based recommendations are media and commercially generated nutrition recommendations based on misinformation, opinion, and a desire to sell a product or program. The target audience for these questionable products and practices is often individuals with chronic diseases lured by the promise of a quick or easy solution.

Diabetes management team members must not only be knowledgeable about science- or evidence-based recommendations, but must also be aware of the latest health or nutrition fads or products in the marketplace. When applying scientific principles and recommendations, team members will continue to focus on the patient's individual circumstances and preferences. The patient is the central team member, and the one who most actively manages his or her diabetes with the exception of young children with diabetes, in which case the parent(s) or guardian(s) play key roles in successful management of diabetes.

The Nutrition Prescription

An individualized nutrition prescription based on nutrition assessment and treatment goals has replaced the historical one-size-fits-all "American Diabetes Association diet," which was a formulated prescription of calorie intake and macronutrient composition. The primary goals of diabetes MNT are:

- to promote and support healthful eating patterns, emphasizing a variety of nutrient-dense foods in appropriate portion sizes, in order to improve overall health and specifically to:
  - attain individualized glycemic, blood pressure, and lipid goals
  - achieve and maintain body weight goals
  - delay or prevent complications of diabetes
- to address individual nutrition needs based on personal and cultural preferences, health literacy and numeracy, access to healthful food choices, willingness and ability to make behavioral changes, and barriers to change
- to maintain the pleasure of eating by providing non-judgmental messages about food choices
- to provide the individual with diabetes with practical tools for developing healthful eating patterns rather than focusing on individual macronutrients, micronutrients, or single foods

Additional MNT goals for specific situations include:

- for youth with type 1 diabetes, pregnant and lactating women, and older adults, to meet the nutritional needs of these unique times in the life cycle
- for all type 1 diabetes patients, to provide self-management training for safe conduct of exercise, including the prevention and treatment of hypoglycemia, and diabetes treatment during acute illness

Nutrition recommendations advise that macronutrient composition and distribution be individualized based on an assessment of patient's current eating patterns, preferences, and metabolic goals to achieve desired metabolic outcomes, since evidence suggests that there is no single ideal percentage of calories from carbohydrate, protein, and fat for all people with diabetes (Table 3.5).

NUTRITION THERAPY FOR TYPE 1 DIABETES

Nutritional management of type 1 diabetes requires paying careful attention to the glycemic effect of foods in order to contain postprandial blood glucose excursions, maximize the effectiveness of exogenous insulin, and minimize hypoglycemia. MNT also must provide for optimal growth and development of the individual and reduce nutrition-related health risks. Although individuals with diabetes have the same nutritional needs as individuals without diabetes, the amount and type of food and coordination with insulin delivery directly affect blood glucose levels. In regards to specific eating patterns for the management of diabetes (Mediterranean, Dietary Approaches to Stop Hypertension [DASH], Low Carb, Low Fat, and Vegetarian/Vegan), please refer to the American Diabetes Associa-

Table 3.5 Nutrition Recommendations: Historical Perspective

| Year | Distribution of Calories | | |
	Carbohydrate (%)	Protein (%)	Fat (%)
Before 1921		Starvation diets	
1921	20	10	70
1950	40	20	40
1971	45	20	35
1986	50–60	10–20	30
1994	A	10–20	A, B
2002	A, C	15–20*	A, B, C, D
2008	A	15–20	A, E
2014	A	A	A, D

A, based on nutrition assessment; B, <10% saturated fat; C, carbohydrate and monounsaturated fatty acids together = 60–70% energy intake; D, avoid trans fatty acids and encourage monounsaturated fats; E, saturated fat < 7%.
*If renal function is normal.

tion Nutrition Therapy Recommendations for Management of Adults with Diabetes (see Bibliography), although these 5 specific eating patterns are really geared more toward adults with type 2 diabetes.

Insulin Regimens

Individuals on multiple daily injections (MDI) of insulin or CSII therapy (i.e., insulin pumps), should adjust their premeal short- or rapid-acting insulin based on the total amount of carbohydrate in their meals. Those receiving fixed daily insulin doses should emphasize consistency of daily carbohydrate content at meals and snacks. Along with the type of insulin regimen, the nutrition care plan addresses caloric requirements, macro- and micronutrient intake, the glycemic effect of foods and meal patterns, lifestyle, exercise, overall health status, and patient goals.

Caloric Requirements

Caloric requirements should be prescribed for people with type 1 diabetes in order to achieve and maintain reasonable body weight in all patients and normal linear growth in children. Note that reasonable weight is defined as the weight an individual and health-care provider acknowledge as achievable and maintainable, both short term and long term. This may not be the same as the traditionally defined desirable or ideal body weight. In addition to weight, body mass index (BMI; weight in kg/height in meters squared) may also be measured with the goal of having a healthy BMI, out of the obese and overweight range. Daily caloric requirements vary depending on age, gender, body size, and activity patterns. Additional calories are needed to promote growth during childhood, adolescence, pregnancy, and lactation and for catabolic illnesses.

Estimated Energy Requirement (EER) is defined by the Food and Nutrition Board (of the Health and Medicine Division of the National Academies of Sciences, Engineering, and Medicine) as "the dietary energy intake that is predicted to maintain energy balance in a healthy individual of a defined age, gender, weight, height, and level of physical activity consistent with good health." The Food and Nutrition Board has published several tables of EER for adults based on BMI and four physical activity levels: sedentary, low active, active, and very active. The board also published gender- and age-based EER tables for infants, children, and adolescents. These tables are available on the Internet from the National Academies Press website (see Resources for Professionals or visit www.nap.edu/catalog/10490/dietary-reference-intakes-for-energy-carbohydrate-fiber-fat-fatty-acids-cholesterol-protein-and-amino-acids-macronutrients). Several other methods for estimating caloric requirements are available, including the Harris-Benedict or World Health Organization equations, which compute calories for basal or resting energy expenditure (REE) and then add activity calories to the basal requirement. Simple methods for routine use are outlined in Table 3.6. Accurate records of food intake offer another means for estimating energy requirements and provide useful information on food preferences and eating patterns. Adjustments in caloric intake will need to be made to promote growth, weight gain, weight loss, or weight maintenance. In addition to meeting energy requirements, the caloric prescription promotes a consistency in daily food intake that is helpful in managing type 1 diabetes.

Macronutrients

In general, recommendations for the macronutrient composition of the meal plan for people with diabetes correspond to guidelines for healthy eating for all

Table 3.6 Estimating Adult Daily Energy Needs

Basal calories	20–25 kcal/kg desirable body wt 25–35 kcal/kg for catabolic illness	
Add calories for activity	If sedentary If moderately active If strenuously active	30% more calories 50% more calories 100% more calories
Adjustments	Add 500 kcal/day to gain 1 lb/week Subtract 500 kcal/day to lose 1 lb/week Pregnancy: add 340 kcal/day during 2nd trimester, 452 kcal/day during 3rd trimester* Lactation: add 330 kcal/day during 1st 6 months, 400 kcal/day during 2nd 6 months*	

Source: Margaret Powers, Issues in prescribing calories. In *Handbook of Diabetes Medical Nutrition Therapy 2nd Edition*, 1996: Jones & Bartlett Learning, Burlington, MA. www. jblearning.com. Reprinted with permission.

*See Food and Nutrition Board Institute of Medicine: *Dietary Reference Intakes for Energy, Carbohydrate, Fiber, Fat, Fatty Acids, Cholesterol, Protein, and Amino Acids (Macronutrients)*. Washington, DC, National Academies Press, 2005.

Americans. The composition and distribution will be guided by the individual's needs and preferences, keeping total calorie and metabolic goals in mind.

Carbohydrate

The primary role of carbohydrate (sugars and starches) is to provide energy to cells in the body. The recommended daily allowance (RDA) for carbohydrate is set at 130 g/day for adults and children and is based on the average minimum amount of glucose utilized by the brain. Individuals with type 1 diabetes should be offered education using the carbohydrate counting meal planning approach, which has been shown to improve glycemic control in several clinical studies. Individuals using fixed insulin doses because of self-care limitations, health literacy, and/or health numeracy concerns should be counseled to have consistent timing and amount of carbohydrate intake to optimize glycemic control and minimize hypoglycemia. Education regarding a simple diabetes meal planning approach that includes portion control and healthful food choices can be quite effective.

Carbohydrate Classification

The focus for type 1 diabetes care is on the total amount of carbohydrate in the foods that are eaten, so the appropriate amount of insulin can be given. People with type 1 diabetes, however, should also be aware of the category of carbohydrates in foods, which includes sugars (monosaccharides, disaccharides, and polyols) and polysaccharides (starches and nonstarch polysaccharides [fiber]) (Table 3.7). Insulin doses may need to be adjusted based on the amount of sugars or polysaccharides in a meal. The terms "complex carbohydrates" and "simple sugars" are no longer used. Intrinsic sugars are sugars that are present within the cell walls of plants (naturally occurring), whereas extrinsic sugars are those that are typically added to foods. Added sugars are defined as sugars and syrups that are added to foods during production and do not include naturally occurring sugars such as lactose in milk or fructose in fruits. Foods and beverages with a high added sugar content include soft drinks, cookies, cakes, pastries, and candy. These foods and beverages have lower micronutrient (vitamins and minerals) densities compared to those that are major sources of naturally occurring sugars. Current U.S. food labels do not distinguish between sugars naturally present in foods and

Table 3.7 Classification of Carbohydrates

Class	Subgroup	Components
Sugars	Monosaccharides	Glucose, galactose, fructose
	Disaccharides	Sucrose, lactose
	Polyols	Sorbitol, mannitol, xylitol
Polysaccharides	Starch	Amylose, amylopectin, modified starches
	Nonstarch polysaccharides (fiber)	Cellulose, hemicellulose, pectins, hydrocolloids

added sugars, but labels may in the future. Historically, sugars, particularly sucrose, were restricted in diets for individuals with diabetes. However, studies show that this restriction is not warranted metabolically. The U.S. Department of Agriculture (USDA; ChooseMyPlate.gov) guidelines allow for added sugars as part of discretionary calories once food is consumed from nutrient-dense food groups. Generally speaking, this would be <10% of calories for most calorie levels. Carbohydrates providing vitamins, minerals, and fibers should receive first priority in food choices over foods high in added sugars and low in nutrient density. Beverages high in sugar, like soda and juice, should be avoided because current insulin analogs are not rapid enough to keep blood glucose in target range when consumed.

Healthy carbohydrates. Foods containing carbohydrate from whole grains, fruits, vegetables, legumes, dry beans, and fat-free or low-fat milk are important sources of vitamins, minerals, phytochemicals, and fiber and are preferred choices for carbohydrate-containing foods. Healthy eating programs such as ChooseMyPlate.gov from the USDA, Fruits & Veggies—More Matters (previously 5 a Day) program, and the DASH diet encourage increased intake of fruits and vegetables, whole grains, and low-fat milk.

Glycemic effect of carbohydrate. The American Diabetes Association's position states that the total amount of carbohydrate in meals and snacks is usually the primary determinant of postprandial response, but the type of carbohydrate may also affect this response. A key strategy in achieving glycemic control is monitoring carbohydrate, whether by carbohydrate counting, choices/exchanges, or experienced-based estimation. The use of the glycemic index and load may provide a modest additional benefit over that observed when total carbohydrate is considered alone, and is a tool to fine tune blood glucose control.

Individuals using MDI or CSII therapy should adjust premeal insulin doses based on the total carbohydrate content of the meal. Those on fixed doses of insulin should be consistent with their carbohydrate intake pattern with respect to both time and amount. There is widespread interest and controversy surrounding the concepts of glycemic index and glycemic load. See Figure 3.5 and Figure 3.6 for definitions.

Glycemic index. Glycemic index (GI) is a concept and meal-planning approach based on published tables ranking carbohydrate foods according to glycemic response (Figure 3.5). The tables propose that, per gram of carbohydrate, foods with a high GI produce a higher peak in postprandial blood glucose and a greater overall glucose response during the first 2–3 h after consumption than do foods with a low GI. The International Tables of Glycemic Index and Glycemic Load Values: 2008 contains 2,480 individual food items. Study subjects included "healthy" volunteers and 20% of table entries are from subject with diabetes or impaired glucose metabolism.

The concept of GI seemed straightforward when it was first introduced as a research tool in the 1980s, but the use of GI in preventing and treating disease has created much controversy. Proponents of GI support its role in treating and preventing chronic diseases, including diabetes, obesity, coronary heart disease, and cancer. Critics of GI point out flaws in epidemiologic studies cited in support of GI as a public health tool. Additional concerns are related to the utility of the tables as a tool for nutritional management. Within each food category, there is

"The glycemic index is a classification proposed to quantify the relative blood glucose response to carbohydrate-containing foods. It is defined as the area under the curve for the increase in blood glucose after the ingestion of a set amount of carbohydrate in an individual food (e.g., 50 g) in the 2-h postingestion period as compared with ingestion of the same amount of carbohydrate from a reference food (white bread or glucose) tested in the same individual under the same conditions using the initial blood glucose concentration as a baseline."

Figure 3.5 Glycemic Index: Food and Nutrition Board definition.

"Thus, the GL of a typical serving of food is the product of the amount of available carbohydrate in that serving and the GI of the food." The GL values in the tables were calculated "by multiplying the amount of carbohydrate contained in a specified serving size of the food by the GI value of that food (with the use of glucose as the reference food), which was then divided by 100." Because portion sizes vary from country to country, researchers and health professionals are advised to calculate their own GL data by using appropriate serving sizes and carbohydrate composition data.

Figure 3.6 Glycemic load (GL): International Table of Glycemic Index and Glycemic Load Values: 2002 definition.

wide variability; values can vary as much as fivefold, depending on the food form, study setting, and other factors. In earlier studies, cooked carrots received a GI rating of 92 ± 20, whereas in more recent studies, they are rated at 32 ± 5. Many factors affect the glycemic response, including variation in the food and its preparation and the circumstances under which it is ingested (Table 3.8). Additionally, variability within and between subjects is large.

Table 3.8 Factors Affecting the Rate of Digestibility and Glycemic Response

Factors inherent in a food	Grain, particle size Amylose-amylopectin (starch) ratio Fiber content Enzyme inhibitors Physical interaction with fat or protein within a food Degree of ripeness in fruit
Factors related to preparation	State of hydration Raw vs. cooked Amount of food processing
Factors related to consumption	Addition of protein, fat, other foods Acidity of a meal Preceding meal Time of day Palatability Duration of the meal Rate of gastric emptying

Glycemic load. The portion sizes for many of the foods studied for GI were not realistic or usual. To obtain 50 g carbohydrate from carrots, almost 5 cups of cooked carrots would need to be ingested. The concept of glycemic load (GL) was introduced to take into account the amount of carbohydrate in a usual serving of a particular food. The GL is calculated using the average GI of the particular food, multiplied by the grams of carbohydrate available in a typical serving of that food (Figure 3.6). GL has been calculated for the foods listed in the International Tables. Concerns about GL are based on the use of imprecise values multiplied to give yet another imprecise number. To use GI, or GL, as a meal-planning tool, one would select foods with low or medium GI versus those with a high GI or, if consuming high-GI foods, also select low-GI foods for balance. The assumption is that the higher the GI or GL, the greater the expected elevation in blood glucose and insulin requirements.

Using GI for meal planning. The American Diabetes Association position is that GI adds another level of complexity to meal planning without scientific evidence to recommend its use as a primary strategy. As for all Americans, individuals with diabetes should be encouraged to replace refined carbohydrates and added sugars with whole grains, legumes, vegetables, and fruits. The consumption of sugar-sweetened beverages and "low-fat" or "nonfat" products with high amounts of refined grains and added sugars should be discouraged.

In general, there is little difference in glycemic control and CVD risk factors between low-GI and high-GI diets or other diets. A slight improvement in glycemia may result from a lower-GI diet; however, confounding by higher fiber content must be accounted for in some of these studies.

Resistant starch. There are no published long-term studies proving benefit from use of resistant starch in subjects with diabetes.

Nutritive Sweeteners

Sucrose. Sucrose restriction in a diet for diabetes cannot be justified on the basis of its glycemic effect. Sucrose can be included in diets of people with diabetes by making appropriate substitutions for other carbohydrate sources to maintain consistent carbohydrate intake. If the sucrose-containing food is added as an extra, it can be covered with additional short- or rapid-acting insulin. However, patients should consider the potential for a decrease in nutrient value and an increase in fat intake and calories that often accompanies sucrose-containing foods.

Fructose. Fructose consumed as "free fructose" (i.e., naturally occurring in foods such as fruit) may result in better glycemic control compared with isocaloric intake of sucrose or starch. People with diabetes should limit or avoid intake of caloric sweeteners including high fructose corn syrup to reduce the risk of weight gain and worsening cardiometabolic risk profile.

Natural sweeteners. Fruit juice, honey, molasses, corn syrup, and other natural sweeteners require the same considerations as sucrose. They contribute 4 cal/g and need to be counted as carbohydrate in meal planning.

Sugar alcohols. Sugar alcohols (e.g., sorbitol) and hydrogenated starch hydrolysates have less of a glycemic effect than sucrose and yield about 2 cal/g on average. Some individuals report gastric discomfort after eating foods sweetened with these products, and consumption of large quantities can cause diarrhea.

Nonnutritive Sweeteners

Nonnutritive sweeteners currently approved for use in the U.S. include ace-sulfame potassium, aspartame, neotame, advantame, saccharin, and sucralose (ste-via is not FDA approved yet). The FDA determines an acceptable daily intake (ADI) for products it approves that is defined as a safe amount for daily consumption over a lifetime. The ADI includes a 100-fold safety factor and greatly exceeds average consumption levels. All FDA-approved sweeteners can be used by individuals with diabetes, including pregnant women. However, moderation is often recommended. Please refer to the USDA's Nutritive and Nonnutritive Sweetener Resources page (https://fnic.nal.usda.gov/food-composition/nutritive-and-non-nutritive-sweetener-resources) for more information.

Fiber

Dietary fiber appears to benefit overall bowel health, including prevention and treatment of constipation and possible prevention of colon cancer. Soluble fiber in large amounts has been shown to be effective in reducing total and LDL cholesterol levels in subjects with and without diabetes. The beneficial effect of soluble dietary fiber on glycemic control, although intuitively attractive, is difficult to substantiate. An overall benefit to blood glucose control from dietary fiber has not been established, and it may require large amounts (>50 g fiber) to achieve a significant effect. The Food and Nutrition Board in the Health and Medicine Division of the National Academies of Sciences, Engineering and Medicine, for the first time, has indicated an adequate intake (AI) for fiber (see Table 3.9). In the American Diabetes Association and Academy of Nutrition and Dietetics' booklet *Choose Your Foods: Food Lists for Diabetes*, the starch, vegetable, fruit, and plant-based protein lists identify foods that provide more than 3 g of dietary fiber per serving.

Protein

Daily requirements. The RDA for protein is 0.8 g/kg/day of high-quality protein for adults, which corresponds to ~10% of calories. This is lower than the usual protein intake of 15–20% of calories consumed by adults in the general U.S. population. The long-term effects of diets with 20% of energy as protein on renal function have not been determined. Protein requirements for children range from 1.5 g/kg/day for infants to 0.85 g/kg/day for adolescent males through 18

Table 3.9   Adequate Intake for Total Fiber

	Men	Women
Adults aged <50 years	38 g	25 g
Adults aged ≥50 years	30 g	21 g

Source: Adapted from Food and Nutrition Board Institute of Medicine: *Dietary Reference Intakes for Energy, Carbohydrate, Fiber, Fat, Fatty Acids, Cholesterol, Protein, and Amino Acids* (Macronutrients). Washington, DC, National Academies Press, 2005.

years of age. Some patients who are interested in strength training and muscle development are advised by trainers, coaches, and others to take large amounts of protein or amino acids, often in powdered form, to build muscle. When patients indicate an interest in strength training activities, diabetes clinicians must be prepared to discuss with them safe amounts of protein intake for their individual kidney function status.

Protein and diabetic kidney disease. There is no evidence to suggest that protein intake needs to be limited if renal function is normal. However, in patients with diabetic kidney disease (albuminuria and/or reduced estimated glomerular filtration rate (eGFR), dietary protein should be maintained at 0.8 g/kg/day and should make up ≤20% of total calorie intake per day to slow the rate of decline in renal function, since protein intake >1.3 g/kg/day and >20% of total daily calories has been associated with worsening of albuminuria, more rapid loss of kidney function, and cardiovascular disease (CVD) mortality.

Protein and insulin requirements. Meal doses of insulin are normally calculated based on the carbohydrate content of the meal, with the assumption that the basal insulin will cover the attenuated glycemic effects of the protein in the meal. Those eating large amounts of protein during meals may need an individualized insulin dosing plan and may require additional insulin 3–5 h following the meal. Individuals using CSII may use extended delivery of meal bolus insulin for this type of meal. A dual-wave or extended bolus can deliver part of the meal bolus before the meal and the remainder over 2–4 h following the meal. The amount of insulin to administer for grams of protein consumed should be discussed with a diabetes health-care provider familiar with this concept. Use of continuous glucose monitors can help with determining how large protein meals affect blood glucose levels. If eating a regular diet, the benefits of adjusting insulin doses based on the grams of protein eaten will be limited.

Fat

The 80–85% of daily calories not allocated to dietary protein are distributed between carbohydrate and fat sources. Saturated fat and trans unsaturated fatty acids (trans fats) are highly atherogenic and have a greater impact on serum cholesterol than dietary cholesterol. Because diabetes is an independent risk factor for cardiovascular disease, the American Diabetes Association recommends restricting saturated fat intake to <7% of calories and avoiding trans fats. Dietary cholesterol intake should be <200 mg/day. Content of the diet from monounsaturated and polyunsaturated fats should be individualized, and type of fat should be emphasized more than quantity.

Foods that contain omega-3 fatty acids have cardioprotective effects; the American Diabetes Association recommends that people with diabetes (as is recommended for the general population as well) eat 2–3 servings per week of foods providing omega-3 polyunsaturated fat, such as fish, walnuts, and flaxseed, as well as including plant stanols/sterols in their diets.

Alcohol

Most adults with type 1 diabetes may drink alcohol in moderation if they so choose. Exceptions include individuals whose blood glucose is out of control, those with elevated blood triglycerides, and pregnant women. Daily alcohol intake should be limited to one drink for women and two drinks for men. One drink is 12 oz beer, 5 oz wine, or 1.5 oz 80-proof distilled spirits. Each drink contains 15 g alcohol.

In addition to the precautions regarding alcohol use that apply to the general public, people with type 1 diabetes risk alcohol-induced hypoglycemia for up to 24 h after ingestion, especially if meals are skipped or delayed or they drink during fasting. Therefore, alcoholic beverages should be ingested with food. If the patient is overweight and consumes alcohol on a regular basis, adjustments to the meal plan to account for calories from alcohol (7 cal/g) without increasing risk for hypoglycemia should be considered. A reduction in fat (9 cal/g) intake is preferable to a reduction in carbohydrate intake, because of the hypoglycemia implications, to offset calories consumed in an alcoholic beverage.

Micronutrients

Sodium and hypertension. People differ greatly in their sensitivity to sodium and its effect on blood pressure. The recommendation for individuals with diabetes—with or without hypertension—is a reduced sodium intake of ≤2,300 mg/day. The American Heart Association recommends an even lower sodium intake of <1,500 mg/day for patients with hypertension or diabetes. The DASH diet (Dietary Approaches to Stop Hypertension) may also be helpful in reducing blood pressure in individuals with hypertension. For individuals with symptomatic heart failure, reducing sodium to ≤2,000 mg/day is usually recommended to prevent heart failure exacerbations. Sodium intake can be minimized by reducing the use of table salt, processed and convenience foods, starchy carbohydrates from grains, and fast foods. *Choose Your Foods: Food Lists for Diabetes* highlights foods with a sodium content >480 mg/serving. The Nutrition Facts panel on food labels provides useful information by indicating, for a single serving, the amount of sodium in milligrams and the percent of the daily value (the % of 2,400 mg). A consumer may wish to reconsider use of a food containing >25% of the daily value of sodium.

Potassium. Individuals taking diuretics may experience a loss of potassium sufficient to warrant supplementation. Potassium restriction may be required if hyperkalemia occurs in patients such as those with renal insufficiency, those taking angiotensin-converting enzyme inhibitors, or angiotensin II receptor blockers, etc.

Magnesium. Magnesium deficiency can be easily detected and treated. The deficiency may occur as a result of poorly controlled diabetes and the accompanying urinary loss.

Calcium. The Food and Nutrition Board of the Health and Medicine Division of the National Academies of Science, Engineering, and Medicine has established Dietary Reference Intakes (DRIs) for calcium based on age (Table 3.10). The values are mostly the same for males and females. Because of enhanced absorption of calcium during pregnancy and lactation, calcium requirements are similar to the nonpregnant and nonlactating state and are based on age.

Vitamin and mineral supplementation. At this time, there is no clear evidence that vitamin and mineral requirements of individuals with type 1 diabetes are different from those of other healthy people. If a nutrition assessment reveals a deficiency, individuals should be counseled on how to adjust food intake to meet these needs. If they are unable to do so, supplements should be recommended. When caloric intake is ≤1,200 cal/day, use of a multivitamin and mineral supple-

Table 3.10 Dietary Reference Intakes for Calcium

Age	Adequate intake (mg/day)
0–6 months	200
7–12 months	260
Age	**Recommended dietary allowance (mg/day)**
1–3 years	700
4–8 years	1,000
9–18 years	1,300
19–50 years	1,000
Females 51–70 years	1,200
Males 51–70 years	1,000
>70 years	1,200

Source: Adapted/Reprinted with Permission from *Dietary Reference Intakes for Calcium and Vitamin D,* 2010, by the National Academy of Sciences, Courtesy of the National Academies Press, Washington, D.C.

ment should be advised. There may be safety concerns regarding the long-term use of antioxidant supplements such as vitamins E and C and carotene. Several conditions may create a deficiency in one or more micronutrients that would warrant supplementation. These include poor diabetes control, celiac disease (fat soluble vitamins), use of diuretics, critical care environments, medications that alter micronutrient metabolism, strict vegetarian diets (especially vegan diets), nutritional intakes that do not meet established RDAs or AIs, pregnancy, and lactation. Pregnancy increases requirements for folate and iron.

Herbal and botanical supplements. Many people who balk at taking prescription or over-the-counter medications view herbal and botanical products as a safe and natural alternative or adjunct to their diabetes management plan. Very few randomized, clinical trials have examined the safety and efficacy of these products, especially for people with diabetes. Herbal and botanical supplements, sports supplements, vitamins, minerals, and other specialty products represent a multi-billion-dollar industry in the U.S. The Dietary Supplement Health and Education Act of 1994 (DSHEA) changed the regulation of dietary supplements and associated label claims. DSHEA places the burden of proof of unsafe or adulterated products or of false or misleading labeling on the FDA rather than on the manufacturer. However, DSHEA restricts the FDA in regulation of these products. The Federal Trade Commission regulates the advertising of dietary supplements and has taken action against sponsors of false and misleading information. Until proven otherwise, consumers have no assurance that a product contains what the label says it does or that it is free from harmful contaminants. Some herbal preparations have been found to surreptitiously contain pharmaceutical agents that produce hypoglycemia. Health-care providers should ask whether their patients are using these products, as many patients do not voluntarily share this information. While providing individualized, science-based information, it is also important to be sensitive to the patient's decisions to use products that might be considered questionable. The

FDA Center for Food Safety & Applied Nutrition and the National Institutes of Health Office of Dietary Supplements can provide reliable information about many of these products (see Resources for Professionals, page 148).

ADDITIONAL NUTRITION CONSIDERATIONS

Sick-Day Management

Individuals with type 1 diabetes must be educated to manage brief periods when they cannot ingest solid foods. They must understand the need to continue insulin therapy and carbohydrate consumption. Fruit juices and sugar-containing soda, sports drinks, popsicles, or gelatin can replace the usual carbohydrate in the meal plan. Frequent intermittent intake of small amounts of these foods and beverages helps to provide fluids and energy and helps to avoid hypoglycemia. Individuals should also be taught the value of ingesting fluids containing sodium and potassium (e.g., vegetable and fruit juices and broths) to help replace electrolytes lost from diarrhea and vomiting. The usual meal plan should be reintroduced gradually (see Table 2.10, page 56).

Growth Years

For infants, children, and adolescents, height and weight data can be plotted on standardized growth grids. The caloric prescription for children with diabetes should include adequate calories for growth and development. Poor diabetes control during the growth years can contribute to failure to attain height potential. During these years, it is helpful to schedule visits with the dietitian every 3–6 months to adjust calories and other nutrients and to account for changes in food preferences and habits. Parents of infants and young children with diabetes may need frequent nutrition counseling to deal with the eating challenges common to children that present particular difficulty when coupled with type 1 diabetes.

Pregnancy

The USDA's ChooseMyPlate.gov provides nutrition guidelines for pregnant women. Additional calorie intake is not needed in the first trimester, but calorie requirements should increase by 340 kcal/day during the second trimester and 450 kcal/day during the third trimester. The RDA for protein during pregnancy is 1.1 g/kg, or approximately an additional 25 g/day of protein. The 1990 National Academy of Sciences recommendations for optimum weight gain for pregnant women are based on prepregnancy BMI (Table 3.11). These guidelines anticipate delivery of babies weighing 3–4 kg at term. The 1998 Food and Nutrition Board publication, *Dietary Reference Intakes for Thiamin, Riboflavin, Niacin, Vitamin B6, Folate, Vitamin B12, Pantothenic Acid, Biotin, and Choline*, recommends that, to reduce the risk of neural tube defects for women capable of becoming pregnant, 400 µg folic acid should be taken daily from fortified foods, supplements, or both in addition to consuming folate from a varied diet. Therefore, prescribing a multivitamin plus up to 400 µg/day folate from preconception through the first trimester is recommended. The RDA for iron during pregnancy is 27 mg/day. Assessment of nutritional status and dietary intake should guide prescription of supplements. Because of the additional metabolic stress of diabe-

Table 3.11 Recommendations for Total and Rate of Weight Gain during Pregnancy, by Prepregnancy BMI

Prepregnancy BMI	Total weight gain		Rates of weight gain 2nd and 3rd trimester	
	Range in kg	Range in lb	Mean (range) in kg/week	Mean (range) in lb/week
Underweight (<18.5 kg/m²)	12.5–18	28–40	0.51 (0.44–0.58)	1 (1–1.3)
Normal weight (18.5–24.9 kg/m²)	11.5–16	25–35	0.42 (0.35–0.50)	1 (0.8–1)
Overweight (25.0–29.9 kg/m²)	7–11.5	15–25	0.28 (0.23–0.33)	0.6 (0.5–0.7)
Obese (≥30.0 kg/m²)	5–9	11–20	0.22 (0.17–0.27)	0.5 (0.4–0.6)

Source: Committee to Reexamine IOM Pregnancy Weight Guidelines, Institute of Medicine National Research Council. *Weight Gain During Pregnancy: Reexamining the Guidelines.* Rasmussen KM, Yaktine AL, Eds. Washington, D.C., National Academies Press, 2009. Reprinted with permission from the National Academies Press, Copyright 2009, National Academy of Sciences.

tes on pregnancy, nutritional guidelines need to be individualized for each pregnant diabetes patient to promote optimal blood glucose levels and appropriate maternal and fetal weight gain.

A plan of three meals and three to four snacks will help patients minimize blood glucose excursions and facilitate tight glycemic control. If there is morning ketosis with normal blood glucose levels, the amount of food in the prebedtime snack can be increased or a snack at 3:00 A.M. can be considered. In the first trimester, hyperemesis may be a problem. A very liberal meal plan allowing the patient to eat whatever is tolerated can be helpful. Insulin dosage should be adjusted to allow for minimum food intake at critical points during the day.

Lactation

The protein RDA for lactation is an additional 25 g/day above prepregnancy requirements. Additional EER for lactation is based on a milk energy output of 330 kcal/day in the first 6 months and 400 kcal/day in the second 6 months. Many women with diabetes report wide swings in blood glucose levels while they are breast-feeding, which may be related to the amount of milk produced and the frequency of feedings. Continuing the pregnancy meal pattern of three meals and three to four snacks per day may help prevent hypoglycemia and decrease the need for additional insulin to cover the extra calories.

Obesity Management

People with type 1 diabetes may gain excessive weight for several reasons, including:

■ overinsulinization

- frequent and inappropriate treatment of insulin reactions
- efforts to avoid insulin reactions with the use of extra food
- failure to decrease caloric intake to compensate for decreased urinary caloric loss with improved glucose control
- general overemphasis on food intake

Individuals and parents of children with diabetes should be advised about the consequences of obesity on general health. Individuals with diabetes who are attempting to lose weight should avoid fad diets that promote inappropriate food combinations or omissions and rapid weight loss, because dehydration, fluid and electrolyte imbalances, and starvation ketosis may result. Weight-loss programs for individuals with type 1 diabetes must include advice about insulin dose adjustment, careful monitoring of diabetes control, and realistic weight-loss goals.

The American Diabetes Association advises that either low-carbohydrate, low-fat, or Mediterranean-style calorie-restricted diets may be effective for short-term weight loss (up to 2 years—the duration of comparative studies). If patients are following a low-carbohydrate diet, clinicians should monitor lipid profiles, because these diets can raise LDL cholesterol. Because low-carbohydrate diets may be high in protein, those with diabetic kidney disease should be counseled about appropriate protein intake, and renal function should be monitored. Patients using carb ratios can adjust their prandial insulin downward to account for the lower carbohydrate intake. Patients who lose weight from either type of diet are likely to need changes in their carb ratio due to the effects of weight loss on insulin sensitivity.

To enable the overweight or obese patient with type 1 diabetes to alter his or her eating, motivational interviewing can be employed to initiate behavior change. Motivational interviewing is a patient-centered method for enhancing intrinsic motivation to change by exploring and resolving ambivalence; however, the basic tenet is that the patient must be ready to change, and that desire must emanate from within, and not be thrust upon the patient by a member of the health-care team.

Long-term maintenance of weight loss is a challenge. Strategies for successful weight management are emerging from the National Weight Control Registry (NWCR), a prospective study of individuals age ≥18 years who have successfully maintained a 30-lb weight loss for a minimum of 1 year. The NWCR, a collaborative effort between the University of Colorado School of Medicine and Brown University, currently includes over 5,000 individuals and offers the opportunity to study the eating and exercise habits of successful weight-loss maintainers (visit www.nwcr. ws). The average registrant was overweight as a child (66%), has a family history of obesity, and has a lifetime average gain and loss of 271 lb. Half followed a formal weight-loss program. Additional characteristics of the average registrant include:

- a resting metabolic rate equal to the rate of a nondieting counterpart in the same weight range
- has lost 66 lb and kept it off for 5.5 years
- takes in an average of 1,400 calories/day (macronutrient composition is 49% carbohydrate, 22% protein, and 29% fat)
- exercises, on average, about 1 h per day
- walks for exercise
- eats breakfast every day

NWCR registrants indicate that weight-loss maintenance becomes easier over time. Additional strategies used by these registrants include keeping many healthy foods in the house (87%), keeping records of food intake or exercise (43%), and buying books or magazines related to nutrition or exercise (74%).

Disordered Eating

An increasing number of children, adolescents, and adults in the general population appear to be affected with anorexia nervosa, bulimia, or a combination of the two. Disordered eating in type 1 diabetes is more common than previously thought. A meta-analysis evaluating the prevalence of eating disorders in type 1 diabetes in 748 and 1,587 female subjects with and without diabetes, respectively, showed the prevalence of anorexia nervosa was not different between controls and subjects with type 1 diabetes. However, the prevalence of bulimia nervosa and bulimia plus anorexia combined was significantly higher in patients with diabetes. Type 1 diabetes complicated by an eating disorder is very difficult to manage because of erratic eating patterns and purging behaviors such as vomiting, laxative abuse, or excessive exercise. A purging behavior unique to type 1 diabetes is self-induced glycosuria (also called diabulemia), achieved by insulin omission. These destructive behaviors can lead to recurrent diabetic ketoacidosis and early development of long-term complications. Risk factors for disordered eating in girls and women with type 1 diabetes include higher BMI, increased body weight and shape dissatisfaction, low self-esteem and depression, and dietary restraint. Recognition and treatment are critical, along with referral to experienced medical, psychological, and nutrition counselors (see Resources for Patient Education, page 147).

THE PROCESS OF MEDICAL NUTRITION THERAPY

The process of MNT begins with a comprehensive assessment of the patient's diabetes status and nutritional status. Following the assessment, the intervention includes collaboration on setting the metabolic and self-care goals determined by the patient and dietitian to be priorities and creating a plan for action. Achievement of goals will be monitored by ongoing communication between the patient and dietitian. Follow-up visits will provide opportunities to evaluate progress, identify barriers to success, solve problems, and make necessary changes in the plan of care. Although the dietitian is the primary provider of MNT, this component of diabetes management must be integrated into the care provided by all members of the core team. Coordination of this effort is supported by concise and accurate documentation, communication among team members, and consistency of diabetes and nutrition messages provided to the patient.

Assessment

A comprehensive nutrition assessment (Table 3.12) contains components of the medical evaluation and the education assessment for overall diabetes education needs. Recognizing that the other members of the patient's diabetes care team need similar information should encourage communication among clini-

Table 3.12   Comprehensive Nutrition Assessment

Clinical Data
- Height, weight, BMI
- Body frame
- Reasonable weight
- Blood pressure

- Family history
- Blood glucose and lipids
- A1C
- Abnormal laboratory findings

Nutrition History
- Usual food intake
- Attitudes toward nutrition and health
- Previous nutrition education and outcomes

- Cultural food practices
- Physical activity
- Allergies and intolerances

Nutrient Intake
- Overall nutritional adequacy
- Caloric intake
- Nutrient distribution

- Types of carbohydrate, protein, and fat eaten
- Use of vitamins, minerals, and herbal and botanical products

Social History
- Daily schedule
- Family relationships
- Friends—social support
- Finances and living environment

- Education—learning style
- Literacy and numeracy
- Self-efficacy

Diabetes and Health Status
- Duration of diabetes
- Insulin regimen
- Hypoglycemia treatment and history
- Diabetes knowledge and skills

- History and current status of complications
- Other medications
- Smoking
- Alcohol

cians, collaboration on treatment goals, and consistency of messages provided to the patient.

Setting Goals

Specific goals for MNT are identified through the nutrition assessment. These goals must correspond with the overall treatment goals for the individual and must agree with the patient's personal goals for therapy. Goal-setting is often a negotiation process involving clinicians and the patient. Goals should be realistic and specific.

Nutrition Care Plan

The meal plan for type 1 diabetes is directed by the insulin deficiency that characterizes the condition. Food intake and insulin regimens must be coordinated to accommodate the patient's food preferences and lifestyle while achieving goal glucose levels as closely as is safely possible. Fortunately, SMBG, basal-bolus insulin regimens, CSII, and CGM support this coordination effort. Specific strategies for the nutritional management of type 1 diabetes include:

- integrating insulin therapy with an individual's food and physical activity preferences
- basing the food plan on assessment of appetite, preferred foods, and usual eating and exercise habits
- using information from SMBG, CGM, insulin, food, and physical activity records and uploads to make adjustments in food intake or insulin dose to achieve target glucose levels
- modifying caloric and nutrient composition of the food plan as appropriate to achieve metabolic and weight goals and for different stages of the life cycle

The individualized self-management plan should also reflect the patient's lifestyle, exercise patterns, and resources. Important considerations include:

- daily schedule (weekday and weekend), travel to and from work or school, schedule during work/school, recreational and social activities
- individual's and family's eating patterns, including usual time and size of meals, where meals are eaten, who meals are eaten with, food preferences, social habits, and cultural customs
- availability of food at home, school, or work; and food budget
- facilities and equipment for preparation and storage of food

Evaluation

The effectiveness of the nutrition treatment plan is evaluated by outcomes specifically related to the goals of therapy. Outcomes would include metabolic and behavior change measures.

Practice Guidelines for MNT of Type 1 Diabetes

Practice guidelines offer a systematic approach to disease management designed to increase assurance that desired outcomes will be achieved. Nutrition practice guidelines for type 1 and type 2 diabetes were developed using criteria set forth by the former Institute of Medicine (now the Health and Medicine Division of the National Academies of Sciences, Engineering, and Medicine). In field tests of the nutrition practice guidelines for type 1 diabetes, practice guideline patients achieved greater reduction in A1C than usual care patients. These guidelines are available from the Academy of Nutrition and Dietetics (see Resources for Patient Education, page 147).

PRACTICAL APPROACHES TO NUTRITION COUNSELING

Pattern Management

SMBG, CGM, insulin, food, and physical activity records and uploads provide patients and clinicians an evaluation mechanism that can be used to closely examine the effectiveness of the treatment regimen and to make adjustments to improve glycemic control. Finding and interpreting blood glucose patterns leads to possible changes in either the amount or timing of insulin, food, or physical activity.

Carbohydrate Counting for Intensive Insulin Therapy

Carbohydrate counting is a meal planning approach that focuses on carbohydrate as the primary nutrient affecting postprandial glycemic response. Carbohydrate counting can be used at basic or advanced levels depending on the interest and skills of the individual.

Basic carbohydrate counting. Carbohydrate counting can be used at a basic level by patients whose goals include consistency of carbohydrate intake to support improved glycemic control. Patients first learn to estimate how much carbohydrate is in their meals and snacks by becoming familiar with reference amounts of foods similar to the food lists in the American Diabetes Association's resource *Choose Your Foods: Food Lists for Diabetes* or other published carbohydrate food lists. Other skills include reading food labels accurately for carbohydrate values and estimating carbohydrate amounts in combination foods, such as pizza, and in restaurant meals or meals prepared by others. A person must be willing to spend time and effort learning and practicing measuring and weighing foods, reading food labels, and using reference books to develop the skills necessary to accurately estimate carbohydrate amounts in the portions usually eaten. These skills require moderate levels of literacy and numeracy. Some institutions teach certain patients to carb count by servings or choices/exchanges, each serving having a fixed number of grams. Nutrient databases are available on the Internet, as software for loading into personal computers, or as applications for smartphones.

Advanced carbohydrate counting. Individuals on intensive insulin therapy, either basal-bolus regimens or CSII, can learn to match their premeal insulin to their carbohydrate foods using an individualized insulin-to-carbohydrate ratio. Patients striving for tight glucose control while trying to maintain flexibility in meals and snacks are candidates for using this counting method.

The insulin-to-carbohydrate ratio is determined for individuals based on records of SMBG, CGM, insulin doses, food intake, and physical activity. The ratio is based on the amount of short- or rapid-acting insulin needed to cover a specific amount of carbohydrate in order to achieve postprandial glucose targets. For example, if a patient uses 1 unit rapid-acting insulin for every 10 g carbohydrate eaten to achieve a specific blood glucose target 2 h postprandially, this person has an insulin-to-carbohydrate ratio of 1:10 (i.e., 1 unit insulin covers 10 g carbohydrate). To adjust insulin for varying amounts of carbohydrate, divide the total grams of carbohydrate to be consumed by the insulin-to-carbohydrate ratio. For example, with an insulin-to-carbohydrate ration of 1:10, a meal with 100 g carbohydrate would require 10 units of premeal insulin (100 g divided by 10 = 10 units insulin). Some formulas for initially calculating insulin-to-carbohydrate ratio include weight and total daily insulin dose as part of the equation (e.g., 450 divided by total daily dose; see Optimizing Blood Glucose Control, page 91).

An absolute prerequisite for insulin-to-carbohydrate ratio use is that the patient must already be extremely well versed in carbohydrate counting. The insulin-to-carbohydrate ratio's effectiveness depends on the patient's ability to accurately estimate carbohydrate amounts that can be covered by insulin. Miscalculation of consumed carbohydrate will result in taking too much or too little insulin. Time, effort, and practice are needed to become proficient enough in carbohydrate counting to use it safely and effectively in insulin dose calculation and adjustment.

Individuals using insulin-to-carbohydrate ratios also need to consider other factors that affect glycemic response and be aware that they may need to adjust timing of insulin delivery as well as amount of insulin for specific situations. For example, high-fat meals can delay stomach emptying and may require delivery of a divided dose of insulin, where part of the dose is taken before and part after the meal. CSII allows delivery of extended boluses that help to accommodate this type of insulin delivery.

Nutrition Self-Management Tools

Meal planning tools, such as the print resources *Count Your Carbs: Getting Started, Match Your Insulin to Your Carbs*, and *Choose Your Foods: Food Lists for Diabetes* or its simplified version, *Eating Healthy With Diabetes: An Easy Reading Guide* (see Resources for Patient Education on page 147) can be used to guide patients in implementing their nutrition management plan. These tools are available from the American Diabetes Association and the Academy of Nutrition and Dietetics. These associations also offer nutrition education materials related to several ethnic and regional food practices. The American Diabetes Association has published a variety of cookbooks and meal planning books (visit www. shopdiabetes.org), and also has carb counting and nutrition resources for patients available on its website, www.diabetes.org. A meal planning resource should be selected that is appropriate for the patient's lifestyle, reading level, culture, and intensity of diabetes management.

Staged Nutrition Counseling

Eating habits are not easy to change. For the person with type 1 diabetes, the need to balance food intake and activity, the potential for hypoglycemia, and the psychological stress of managing a chronic disease make changing food habits even more difficult. Nutrition counseling should be provided in stages to allow the patient time to absorb information, try out self-management skills, and test the nutrition plan in daily living. Staged nutrition counseling also provides an opportunity to evaluate the effectiveness of the treatment plan and to make modifications to improve diabetes control. Staged nutrition counseling can be effective when timely, such as developing a diabetes nutrition plan right before a holiday or social event. MNT is a lifetime treatment of diabetes. Therefore, nutrition counseling must be included in the ongoing care of the patient with type 1 diabetes.

CONCLUSION

Diabetes MNT is more than mere calculation of a caloric prescription with appropriate macronutrient composition and distribution of foods into meals and snacks. It is a complex process that requires commitment on the part of clinicians and the patient to design an individualized nutrition self-management plan. The effectiveness of MNT is evaluated by success in achieving nutrition-related goals. MNT cannot be limited to the time of diagnosis, but must continue through life with adjustments made for growth and development; changes in lifestyle, diabetes status, and health status; and advances in the field of diabetes nutritional care.

BIBLIOGRAPHY

American Diabetes Association. Standards of medical care in diabetes—2016. *Diabetes Care* 2016;39(Suppl. 1):S25–S27

American Diabetes Association. Foundations of care: education, nutrition, physical activity, smoking cessation, psychosocial care, and immunization. *Diabetes Care* 2015;38(Suppl. 1):S20–S30

American Diabetes Association; Bantle JP, Wylie-Rosett J, Albright AL, Apovian CM, Clark NG, Franz MJ, Hoogwerf BJ, Lichtenstein AH, Mayer-Davis E, Mooradian AD, Wheeler ML. Nutrition recommendations and interventions for diabetes (Position Statement). *Diabetes Care* 2008;31(Suppl. 1):S61–S78

Atkinson F, Foster-Powell K, Brand-Miller JC. International table of glycemic index and glycemic load values: 2008. *Diabetes Care* 2008;31:2281–2283

Committee on Nutritional Status During Pregnancy and Lactation; Institute of Medicine. *Nutrition During Pregnancy Part I: Weight Gain.* Washington, DC, National Academy Press, 1990

Dietary Supplement Health and Education Act of 1994, Public Law 103–417 (S.784) (1994) (codified at 42 USC 287C–11)

Evert AB, Boucher JL, Cypress M, Dunbar SA, Franz MJ, Mayer-Davis EJ, Neumiller JJ, Nwankwo R, Verdi CL, Urbanski P, Yancy WS. Nutrition therapy recommendations for the management of adults with diabetes. *Diabetes Care* 2014;37(Suppl. 1):S120–S143

Evert AB, Boucher JL, Cypress M, et al. Nutrition therapy recommendations for the management of adults with diabetes. *Diabetes Care* 2013;36:3821–3842

Food and Nutrition Board Institute of Medicine. *Dietary Reference Intakes for Calcium and Vitamin D.* Washington, DC, National Academies Press, 2010

Food and Nutrition Board Institute of Medicine. *Dietary Reference Intakes for Energy, Carbohydrate, Fiber, Fat, Fatty Acids, Cholesterol, Protein, and Amino Acids (Macronutrients).* Washington, DC, National Academies Press, 2005

Food and Nutrition Board Institute of Medicine: *Dietary Reference Intakes for Vitamin A, Vitamin K, Arsenic, Boron, Chromium, Copper, Iodine, Iron, Manganese, Molybdenum, Nickel, Silicon, Vanadium, and Zinc.* Washington, DC, National Academy Press, 2002

Food and Nutrition Board Institute of Medicine. *Dietary Reference Intakes for Thiamin, Riboflavin, Niacin, Vitamin B6, Folate, Vitamin B12, Pantothenic Acid, Biotin, and Choline.* Washington, DC, National Academy Press, 1998

Franz MJ, Bantle JP, Beebe CA, Brunzell JD, Chiasson JL, Garg A, Holzmeister LA, Hoogwerf B, Mayer-Davis E, Mooradian AD, Purnell JQ, Wheeler M.

Evidence-based nutrition principles and recommendations for the treatment and prevention of diabetes and related complications (Technical Review). *Diabetes Care* 2002;25:148–198

Goebel-Fabbri AE. Disturbed eating behaviors and eating disorders in type 1 diabetes: clinical significance and treatment recommendations. *Curr Diab Rep* 2009;9:133–139

Jenkins DJA, Kendall CWC, Augustin LSA, Franceschi S, Hamidi M, Marchie A, Jenkins AL, Axelsen M. Glycemic index: overview of implications in health and disease. *Am J Clin Nutr* 2002;76(Suppl.):266S–273S

Joint National Committee on the Prevention, Detection, Evaluation, and Treatment of High Blood Pressure. *Seventh Report of the Joint National Committee on the Prevention, Detection, Evaluation, and Treatment of High Blood Pressure.* Washington, DC, National Institutes of Health National Heart Lung and Blood Institute, 2004

Joyce M. Issues in prescribing calories. In *Handbook of Diabetes Medical Nutrition Therapy.* 2nd ed. Powers MA, Ed. Gaithersburg, MD, Aspen Publishers, 1996, p. 364–375

Klem ML, Wing RR, Lang W, McGuire MT, Hill JO. Does weight loss maintenance become easier over time? *Obesity Res* 2000;8:438–444

Mannucci E, Rotella F, Ricca V, Moretti S, Placidi GF, Rotella CM. Eating disorders in patients with type 1 diabetes: a meta-analysis. *J Endocrinol Invest* 2005;28:417–419

Marsh K, Barclay A, Colagiuri S, Brand-Miller J. Glycemic index and glycemic load of carbohydrates in the diabetes diet. *Curr Diab Rep* 2011;11:120–127

Miller WR, Rollnick S. *Motivational Interviewing: Preparing People for Change.* 2nd ed. New York, Guilford Press, 2002

National Institutes of Health. *National Cancer Institute: 5-a-Day for Better Health Program Monograph.* Washington, DC, National Institutes of Health, 2002

Pastors JG, Franz MJ, Warshaw H, Daly A, Arnold MS. How effective is medical nutrition therapy in diabetes care? *J Am Diet Assoc* 2003;103:827–831

Pastors JG, Warshaw H, Daly A, Franz M, Kulkarni K. The evidence for the effectiveness of medical nutrition therapy in diabetes management. *Diabetes Care* 2002;25:608–613

Peters AL, Davidson MB. Protein and fat effects on glucose response and insulin requirements in subjects with insulin-dependent diabetes mellitus. *Am J Clin Nutr* 1993;58:555–560

Pi-Sunyer FX. Glycemic index and disease. *Am J Clin Nutr* 2002;76(Suppl.):290S–298S

Polonsky WH. Identifying and treating eating disorders in persons with diabetes. In *Handbook of Diabetes Medical Nutrition Therapy.* Powers MA, Ed. Gaithersburg, MD, Aspen Publishers, 1996, p. 585–601

Report of a Joint FAO/WHO Expert Consultation. *Carbohydrates in Human Nutrition*. Rome, Italy, Food and Agriculture Organization of the United Nations and World Health Organization, 1998

Sacks FM, Appel LJ, Moore TJ, Obarzanek E, Vollmer WM, Svetkey LP, Bray GA. Dietary approaches to prevent hypertension: a review of the Dietary Approaches to Stop Hypertension (DASH) study. *Clin Cardiol* 22(Suppl. 7):III6–III10, 1999

Thomas D, Elliott EJ. Low glycaemic index, or low glycaemic load, diets for diabetes mellitus (review). *The Cochrane Collaboration*. John Wiley and Sons 2009, 3:1–31, or *Cochrane Database of Systematic Reviews* 2009;1:CD006296. DOI: 10.1002/14651858,CD006296.pub2

Toeller M, Buyken A, Heitkamp G, Bramswig S, Mann J, Milne R, Gries FA, Keen H; the EURODIAB IDDM Complications Study. Protein intake and urinary albumin excretion rates in the EURODIAB IDDM Complications Study. *Diabetologia* 1997;40:1219–1226

Wheeler ML, Dunbar SA, Jaacks LM, Karmally W, Mayer-Davis EJ, Wylie-Rosett J, Yancy WS. Macronutrients, food groups, and eating patterns in the management of diabetes: a systematic review of the literature, 2010. *Diabetes Care* 2012;35:434–445

RESOURCES FOR PATIENT EDUCATION

Academy of Nutrition and Dietetics, American Diabetes Association. *Choose Your Foods: Food Lists for Diabetes*. Alexandria, VA, American Diabetes Association, and Chicago, Academy of Nutrition and Dietetics, 2014

Academy of Nutrition and Dietetics, American Diabetes Association. *Choose Your Foods: Plan Your Meals*. Alexandria, VA, American Diabetes Association, and Chicago, Academy of Nutrition and Dietetics, 2014

Academy of Nutrition and Dietetics, American Diabetes Association. *Count Your Carbs: Getting Started*. Alexandria, VA, American Diabetes Association, and Chicago, Academy of Nutrition and Dietetics, 2014

Academy of Nutrition and Dietetics, American Diabetes Association. *Diabetes Care and Education Practice Group of the American Dietetic Association: Ethnic and Regional Food Practices: A Series*. Alexandria, VA, American Diabetes Association, and Chicago, Academy of Nutrition and Dietetics, various publication dates

Academy of Nutrition and Dietetics, American Diabetes Association. *Eating Healthy with Diabetes: An Easy Reading Guide*. Alexandria, VA, American Diabetes Association, and Chicago, Academy of Nutrition and Dietetics, 2014

Academy of Nutrition and Dietetics, American Diabetes Association. *Healthy Food Choices*. Alexandria, VA, American Diabetes Association, and Chicago, Academy of Nutrition and Dietetics, 2014

Academy of Nutrition and Dietetics, American Diabetes Association. *Match Your Insulin to Your Carbs.* Alexandria, VA, American Diabetes Association, and Chicago, Academy of Nutrition and Dietetics, 2014

Holzmeister LA. *Diabetes Carbohydrate & Fat Gram Guide.* 4th ed. Alexandria, VA, American Diabetes Association, 2010

McCarren M. *Carb Counting Made Easy for People with Diabetes.* Alexandria, VA, American Diabetes Association, 2002

Warshaw HS. *Diabetes Meal Planning Made Easy.* 4th ed. Alexandria, VA, American Diabetes Association, 2010

Warshaw HS, Kulkarni K. *Complete Guide to Carb Counting.* 3rd ed. Alexandria, VA, American Diabetes Association, 2011

Warshaw HS, Webb R. *Diabetes Food and Nutrition Bible.* Alexandria, VA, American Diabetes Association, 2001

RESOURCES FOR PROFESSIONALS

American Dietetic Association. *Nutrition Practice Guidelines for Type 1 and Type 2 Diabetes Mellitus.* Chicago, American Dietetic Association, 1998

Diabetes Care and Education Dietetic Practice Group of the American Dietetic Association. *The American Dietetic Association Guide to Diabetes Medical Nutrition Therapy and Diabetes Education.* Ross TA, Boucher JL, O'Connell BS, Eds. Chicago, American Dietetic Association, 2005

Evert AB, Boucher JL, Cypress M, Dunbar SA, Franz MJ, Mayer-Davis EJ, Neumiller JJ, Nwankwo R, Verdi CL, Urbanski P, Yancy WS. Nutrition therapy recommendations for the management of adults with diabetes. *Diabetes Care* 2014;37(Suppl. 1):S120–S143

Fragakis AS. *The Health Professional's Guide to Popular Dietary Supplements.* Chicago, American Dietetic Association, 2000

Franz MJ, Evert A (Eds.). *American Diabetes Association Guide to Nutrition Therapy for Diabetes.* 2nd ed. Alexandria, VA, American Diabetes Association, 2012

National Academies Press website for online review of publications on dietary reference intakes for macronutrients and micronutrients: www.nap.edu

NIH Office of Dietary Supplements website (with IBIDS-International Bibliographic Information on Dietary Supplements, which contains over 690,000 scientific citations and abstracts about dietary supplements). Available from http://ods.od.nih.gov/

Pastors J (Ed.). *Diabetes Nutrition Q & A for Health Professionals: 101 Essential Questions Answered by Experts.* Alexandria, VA, American Diabetes Association, 2003

Powers M (Ed.). *Handbook of Diabetes Medical Nutrition Therapy.* Gaithersburg, MD, Aspen Publishers, 1996

Shane-McWhorter L. *Complementary and Alternative Medicine (CAM) Supplement Use in People with Diabetes: A Clinician's Guide.* Alexandria, VA, American Diabetes Association, 2007

U.S. Food and Drug Administration, Center for Food Safety and Applied Nutrition Dietary Supplements website. http://www.fda.gov/food/dietarysupplements/default.htm

Warshaw HS, Bolderman KM. *Practical Carbohydrate Counting: A How-to-Teach Guide for Health Professionals.* 2nd ed. Alexandria, VA, American Diabetes Association, 2008

EXERCISE

In addition to insulin and medical nutrition therapy, physical activity and exercise play a key role in diabetes management. Important health benefits of physical activity for individuals with diabetes include a reduction in cardiovascular risk factors, increased sensitivity to insulin, better ability to maintain a healthy weight and level of body fat, and a heightened sense of well-being. Given these health benefits, regular physical activity should be considered an integral part of the treatment plan for individuals with type 1 diabetes.

Because exercise can significantly affect blood glucose levels, it must be carefully integrated into the diabetes management regimen. When individuals with type 1 diabetes are given appropriate guidance and support and attain good self-management skills, they can achieve optimal glycemic control, exercise safely, and achieve desired levels of exercise performance. Children and adolescents can participate fully in gym classes, team sports, and other activities and can have at least 60 min of moderate to vigorous physical activity a day. In the absence of contraindications, all adults should accumulate at least 150 min per week of moderate-intensity aerobic physical activity at 50–70% of maximum heart rate, spread over at least 3 days/week, with no more than 2 consecutive days without exercise to improve health and reduce the risk of chronic disease. All individuals, including those with diabetes, should be encouraged to reduce time spent in sedentary activity and to break up extended time periods (>90 min) spent sitting. Adults with type 1 diabetes should be encouraged to achieve at least this level of daily activity. Individuals with physical limitations should be encouraged to maintain an active lifestyle and offered guidance about safe and appropriate exercise options that will enable them to do so.

Success with any physical activity program is greatly enhanced when exercise goals are appropriately established. Goals must be individualized based on the patient's interests, likes and dislikes, unique lifestyle and psychosocial variables, age, general health, level of physical fitness, and prior exercise experience.

GLYCEMIC RESPONSE TO EXERCISE

Exercise requires rapid mobilization and redistribution of metabolic fuels to ensure an adequate energy supply for working muscles. For individuals who do not have diabetes, this complex process is coordinated via neural and hormonal responses that increase production of glucose and free fatty acids (FFA) and facilitate uptake and utilization of these fuels by working muscles (Table 3.13). Insulin levels fall while counterregulatory hormones rise, so that increased glucose utilization by exercising muscles is matched precisely by increased glucose production by the liver. For individuals with type 1 diabetes, the metabolic adjustments that maintain fuel homeostasis during and after exercise are lacking. The result can be a mismatch between hepatic glucose production and muscle glucose utilization, and significant deviation from normal glycemia. The glycemic response to exercise can be variable and is influenced by multiple factors. These include:

- overall metabolic control
- circulating insulin level

- plasma glucose at the start of exercise
- timing of exercise in relation to food intake
- glycogen stores
- level of training and fitness
- intensity, duration, time, and type of exercise

Plasma insulin level is a primary determinant of the glycemic response to exercise. In individuals who do not have diabetes, the circulating insulin level normally falls at the onset of light or moderate-intensity exercise. In those with type 1 diabetes, this response is absent, and insulin adjustments need to be made in anticipation of exercise. If circulating insulin levels are too high, a state of relative hyperinsulinemia results, which leads to enhanced muscle glucose uptake, inhibited hepatic glucose production, and potentiation of hypoglycemia. In contrast, if circulating insulin levels are too low, as evidenced by pre-exercise hyperglycemia and poor metabolic control, an inadequate level of insulin combined with the heightened counterregulatory hormone release associated with exercise can lead to a marked increase in glucose production and FFA mobilization from the liver. When availability of these substrates exceeds muscle uptake, a further worsening of hyperglycemia and ketosis may result.

Table 3.13 Metabolic Response to Light and Moderate Exercise: Normal vs. Type 1 Diabetes

Normal response	Response in type 1 diabetes
Insulin level decreases - ↑ glucose release from liver - ↑ FFA mobilization - restricts use of glucose by nonexercising skeletal muscle	Insulin level fails to change at the onset of exercise - insulin excess: muscle glucose uptake exceeds liver glucose production - insulin deficiency: liver glucose production exceeds muscle uptake; FFA release and ketone body formation increase - adequate insulin level: liver glucose output matches muscle glucose uptake
Counterregulatory hormones increase - ↑ hepatic glucose production and release - ↑ muscle glycogenolysis - adipose tissue lipolysis	Counterregulatory hormones generally increase, although response may be blunted in some individuals
Glucose uptake and utilization by working muscle increases	Glucose uptake and utilization by working muscle may or may not increase depending on insulin availability
Precise integration of glucose production and utilization and stable blood glucose levels	Potential mismatch between glucose production and utilization and variable blood glucose levels

POTENTIAL BENEFITS OF EXERCISE

Because individuals with type 1 diabetes are at high risk for the development of cardiovascular disease, exercise, through its ability to improve multiple cardiovascular risk factors, offers important health benefits. Regular exercise can improve the lipoprotein profile by lowering VLDL cholesterol and triglycerides and by increasing HDL cholesterol. It can also reduce blood pressure, decrease adiposity, improve cardiac work capacity, decrease platelet adhesiveness, and lower the adrenergic response to stress.

Beyond cardiovascular benefits, participation in regular exercise assists with weight loss and is essential for long-term success with maintaining a healthy weight. It enhances the sense of well-being and reduces feelings of stress and anxiety. It improves muscle strength and agility, reduces bone loss, and prevents the loss of functional capacity that can occur with aging.

Although exercise increases insulin sensitivity and can lower the requirement for insulin, it has not consistently been shown to lead to improvements in glycemic control in individuals with type 1 diabetes as measured by A1C. However, when exercising individuals learn to self-adjust their management plan to accommodate physical activity through careful meal planning, frequent SMBG and record keeping, and correct application of insulin-adjustment strategies, they can achieve excellent glycemic control and A1C levels.

POTENTIAL RISKS OF EXERCISE

Although exercise offers many health benefits, it also carries potential risks for those with type 1 diabetes. Both acute complications, hyper- and hypoglycemia, and long-term microvascular and macrovascular complications may be exacerbated by physical activity, especially if an exercise option is contraindicated given existing complications or physical limitations or is incorrectly performed.

Hyperglycemia and Hypoglycemia

Because exercise potentiates the effects of insulin, hypoglycemia may occur during, immediately after, or many hours after a period of physical activity. Hypoglycemia poses a risk to individuals who perform unusually long-duration or strenuous exercise or to those who exercise sporadically without adjusting their usual insulin dose or meal plan. In contrast, hyperglycemia can occur if preexercise metabolic control is poor or if exercise is performed at a very high-intensity, anaerobic level (>80% of VO_{2max}).

Individual glycemic response patterns can differ markedly with exercise. SMBG, use of continuous glucose sensing, careful record keeping, and recognition of glucose patterns with activity are important skills that can enable individuals with type 1 diabetes to understand unique glycemic responses to exercise, enhance their ability to make self-management decisions that support optimal glycemic control and exercise safety, and enhance performance. Frequent SMBG helps with anticipation of the onset of hypo- or hyperglycemia and enables individuals to make decisions about taking corrective actions before either complication becomes severe. When data from monitoring are carefully recorded and analyzed, they can provide a valuable basis for making decisions about adjustments in management for subsequent exercise sessions. In the future, it may be possible to use computer-based algorithms and sensor-augmented pumps with threshold or predictive low glucose suspend features to help avoid aberrations of glycemia during and after exercise.

Microvascular and Macrovascular Complications

Although regular participation in physical activity tends to reduce cardiovascular risk factors, the risk of arrhythmias, myocardial ischemia or infarction, and cardiac arrest is transiently elevated during exercise. Because individuals with type 1 diabetes are at high risk for cardiovascular disease, careful evaluation to assess risk for preexisting disease is advisable before an exercise program is initiated, especially in previously sedentary adults with long duration of diabetes. For those with known or suspected disease, a moderate, safe level of exercise that will minimize risk of negative cardiac events should be prescribed.

Screening for microvascular diabetes complications before initiation of exercise is also advisable. Worsening of complications is possible (Table 3.14) if exercise is not carefully prescribed. Exercise can aggravate preexisting joint disease or lead to musculoskeletal injuries.

REDUCING EXERCISE RISKS

Potential exercise risks can be reduced if a thorough medical evaluation that includes screening for microvascular, macrovascular, and neurologic complications of diabetes precedes initiation of exercise. Based on findings of this evaluation, an individualized physical activity program should be carefully planned and supported by an appropriate level of supervision to minimize exercise risks and promote progressive gains in health and fitness. Exercise should be prescribed with caution in individuals with previous poor metabolic control (including severe hyperglycemia and ketonuria, frequent hypoglycemia or hypoglycemia

---

Table 3.14   Potential Risks of Exercise with Microvascular Diabetes Complications

Microvascular complication	Potential exercise risk
Proliferative retinopathy	Retinal detachment, vitreous or retinal hemorrhage, blood pressure elevation
Peripheral neuropathy	Loss of protective sensation, soft tissue injury, foot ulcers, injury to bones and joints, infection
Autonomic neuropathy	Reduced heart rate and blood pressure response to exercise, silent ischemia, orthostatic hypotension, impaired counterregulatory response to exercise, hypoglycemia unawareness, impaired body temperature regulation, dehydration, reduced exercise tolerance
Diabetic kidney disease	Marked blood pressure elevations with high intensity, which may lead to transient increases in proteinuria/ albuminuria

unawareness), cardiovascular disease, neuropathy, proliferative retinopathy, or diabetic kidney disease (Table 3.15). Individuals with these complications should be offered guidance about safe exercise options as well as activities that should be avoided (Table 3.16). Patients should also be assessed for conditions that might contraindicate certain types of exercise or predispose to injury, such as uncontrolled hypertension, autonomic neuropathy, peripheral neuropathy, a history of foot lesions, and untreated proliferative retinopathy. Exercise regimens should be customized for the individual. Some individuals may benefit from initially participating in a supervised exercise program. Performance of frequent SMBG before, during, and after exercise should be encouraged.

Table 3.15   Pre-exercise Testing Indications for Exercise Program Greater Than Brisk Walking

- Age >40 years
- Age >35 years and
  - Type 1 or type 2 diabetes of >10 years duration
  - Hypertension
  - Cigarette smoking
  - Dyslipidemia
  - Proliferative or preproliferative retinopathy
  - Diabetic kidney disease, including albumin levels 30–299 mg/dL/24 h

- Any of the following, regardless of age:
  - Known or suspected coronary artery disease, cerebrovascular disease, and/or peripheral vascular disease
  - Autonomic neuropathy
  - Renal failure
  - Uncontrolled hypertension
  - Peripheral neuropathy
  - History of foot lesions

Table 3.16   Exercise Options with Diabetes Complications

Diabetes complications	Best exercise options	Inadvisable exercise options
Proliferative retinopathy	Low-impact activities like walking, swimming, low-impact aerobics, stationary cycling	Pounding, jarring, or "head-low" activities, high-impact sports, heavy lifting, breath-holding and Valsalva-like maneuvers
Insensitive feet/peripheral vascular insufficiency	Non-weight-bearing activities like cycling, swimming, arm chair exercises, light weight lifting, yoga, tai chi	Repetitive weight-bearing or high-impact activities like prolonged walking or jogging
Diabetic kidney disease	Light to moderate daily activities, low-intensity aerobic activity, light weight lifting	Heavy lifting or intensive exercise that results in blood pressure increase
Hypertension	Dynamic exercises that primarily use large, lower-extremity muscle groups	Heavy lifting and Valsalva-like maneuvers

Participation in a cardiac rehabilitation program may benefit individuals with known cardiovascular disease. For these individuals, the exercise prescription should be based on results of a graded exercise test. Special precautions and monitoring are warranted for those who have hypertension or thyroid disease and for anyone who is taking cardiac or blood pressure medications that can mask hypoglycemia, alter heart rate response to exercise, or influence cardiac work capacity (e.g., β-blockers).

EXERCISE PRESCRIPTION

Before initiating exercise, all individuals should be given specific guidance about appropriate exercise options, exercise goal-setting, methods for self-monitoring exercise performance, strategies for maintaining optimal glycemic control, and exercise safety precautions (Table 3.17).

Table 3.17   Exercise Safety Guidelines

General

- Carry a medical identification card and wear an identification bracelet, necklace, or tag that alerts others that the individual has diabetes
- Exercise with an informed partner
- Measure pre-exercise blood glucose level and if at risk for hyperglycemia or hypoglycemia, take the following action:
  - If <100 mg/dL: eat a carbohydrate-containing snack before exercising
  - If >250 mg/dL: test for ketones and troubleshoot reason for hyperglycemia; if ketones are present, delay exercising until ketones are negative
- Frequently consume fluids before, during, and after exercise to prevent dehydration
- Wear footwear and clothing that is appropriate for the activity you plan to do and for the exercise climate
- Make changes in exercise regimen, intensity, and timing slowly. Do not vary exercise dramatically from one day to the next
- Avoid exercising in extreme heat, humidity, or cold

To Prevent Hypoglycemia

- Perform SMBG periodically during prolonged exercise; monitor more frequently postexercise
- Have immediate access to a source of readily absorbable carbohydrate (such as glucose tablets) to treat hypoglycemia
- Consume carbohydrate every 30–45 min during prolonged bouts of exercise, particularly with moderate to strenuous exercise
- Be alert for signs of hypoglycemia during and several hours after an exercise session
- Administer insulin away from working limbs if exercise is to be initiated within 30 min of an insulin injection
- Consider reducing the dose of insulin that will be acting during a period of exercise (e.g., reduce premeal bolus for the preceding meal OR reduce or suspend basal rate if using an insulin pump)

The purpose of an exercise prescription is to offer specific exercise recommendations that will safely and successfully guide an individual toward achieving a level of physical activity that will improve health, fitness, functional capacity, and quality of life. Individualization is the key to the success of any exercise program. Unique lifestyle variables, likes and dislikes regarding exercise options, stage of readiness to make necessary lifestyle changes, age, prior exercise experience, and level of fitness should all be considered.

Recommendations regarding frequency, intensity, duration, and type of exercise should similarly be individualized. The most precise exercise prescriptions are based on exercise testing that determines heart rate and blood pressure response to exercise and aerobic capacity ($VO_{2\,max}$).

An aerobic conditioning program is desirable for most individuals with diabetes. In addition, all people can benefit from informally increasing daily lifestyle activities (e.g., walking and climbing stairs). The very unfit person may benefit from beginning with a lifestyle activity program before progressing to structured, aerobic exercise.

Whenever possible, an exercise contract that guides an individual toward achieving exercise goals should be established. Goals should be established collaboratively with input from the exercising individual. The person's progress toward achieving goals should regularly be assessed and the exercise plan adjusted as needed. Specific recommendations that are established with active involvement and input from the individual with diabetes are most likely to lead to successful exercise outcomes.

AEROBIC TRAINING

Individuals who are interested and physically able should be encouraged to participate in aerobic activity. Aerobic training, which uses large muscle groups repetitively and continuously for an extended time, promotes optimal improvements in cardiorespiratory fitness, body composition, functional capacity, and overall health when it is consistently done at a level that accrues an energy expenditure of 1,000–2,000 calories per week. Generally, aerobic activity should be performed:

- 20–60 min per session, although benefits have been demonstrated for three or more 10-min bouts per day
- 150 min/week
- at an intensity of 55–79% of maximum heart rate (40–74% of maximal oxygen uptake reserve [VO_2R] or heart rate reserve [HRR]), or a rating of perceived exertion (RPE) of 12-13-14 "somewhat hard" level of effort; a lower intensity of 55–65% of maximum heart rate (40–50% of VO_2R or HRR) and RPE of 12 is appropriate for those who are unfit (Table 3.18)

Participation in aerobic exercise is safest and most effective if individuals monitor exercise intensity to ensure that they are working in an appropriate "target zone" or level of effort. Three methods that can be used to monitor exercise intensity are heart rate or pulse count monitoring, RPE, and the "talk test" (Table 3.18). Individuals with known coronary artery disease should be informed about symptoms of myocardial ischemia. Exercise-related chest pain or discom-

Table 3.18 Methods of Determining and Monitoring Exercise Intensity with Exercise

Target heart rate	Rating of perceived exertion	"Talk test"
Monitor 10-s pulse count by palpating carotid or radial pulse or use heart rate monitor	Determine perception of effort required or level of difficulty associated with exercising at a given workload	Access ability to talk or carry on a conversation while exercising as an indicator of staying within/not exceeding an aerobic training level
Target heart rate: 55–79% of HR_{max} or 40–74% VO_2R or HRR*	Target: rating of perceived exertion of 12-13-14 "somewhat hard" level of effort	Target: maintaining ability to talk during an exercise session; avoid extreme shortness of breath

*HR_{max} = 220 – age (or maximal heart rate achieved on exercise stress test).
VO_2R = VO_{2max} – resting VO_2 (maximal oxygen uptake reserve; can be calculated if VO_{2max} is measured during exercise stress test). HRR = HR_{max} – HR_{rest}) + HR_{rest} (heart rate reserve; formula accounts for true resting as well as maximal heart rate).

fort, excessive shortness of breath, lightheadedness, or nausea are all indicators that an individual should immediately stop an activity. Any discomfort or worrisome symptoms associated with exercise should be reported to the individual's physician.

Each session of aerobic exercise should include a 5- to 10-min warm-up and a 5- to 10-min cooldown period. The warm-up should include light general muscle movement, e.g., slow walking or stationary cycling, followed by stretching. The warm-up should be followed by the more vigorous aerobic training period during which the exercise "target zone" should be achieved. At the end of an exercise session, the cooldown period should include light general muscle movement and stretching. Calisthenics or other light resistance activities can be incorporated into the cooldown. The heart rate should approach a resting level (<100 beats/min) before the cooldown is completed.

When prescribing exercise, it is important to start each individual at a level that can reasonably be achieved. This may require that an individual who is very deconditioned begin by doing short, 5- to 10-min exercise sessions two to three times per day. The duration of each session can gradually be increased as the person becomes more fit. As the duration of each exercise session increases, the number of daily sessions can be reduced. It is important not to overlook the considerable health benefits that can be gained even if exercise is performed at an intensity below an optimal target range for improving cardiorespiratory fitness. Promoting all types of physical activity, even forms that require only a low-to-moderate level of effort, is important. For individuals who dislike vigorous exercise, a physical activity program that focuses on weekly energy expenditure rather than on intensity of exercise may support improved adherence and better exercise outcomes.

RESISTANCE TRAINING

Resistance exercises such as weight lifting or calisthenics can improve body composition, increase muscle strength and endurance, improve flexibility, increase insulin sensitivity and glucose tolerance, and decrease cardiovascular risk factors. Individuals who are interested in resistance exercise should be carefully screened for diabetes complications, especially proliferative retinopathy, so that a program can be safely adapted to minimize risk of aggravating existing complications. All individuals should be taught proper technique at the onset of a training program to minimize the risk of injury.

If a diabetes clinician does not feel knowledgeable enough about principles of exercise to prescribe and supervise an aerobic and/or resistance training exercise program, a referral should be made. Hospital-based cardiac rehabilitation or wellness programs, YMCA programs, and programs offered through college and university physical education departments can be excellent and appropriate options for exercise referral. A well-qualified exercise physiologist or exercise specialist who has clinical experience and is knowledgeable about diabetes can also be a valuable resource.

STRATEGIES FOR MAINTAINING OPTIMAL GLYCEMIC CONTROL WITH EXERCISE

Based on results of SMBG, CGM, record keeping, uploads, and identification of exercise-related blood glucose patterns, individuals with type 1 diabetes can learn to make adjustments in their diabetes management plan to maintain optimal glycemic control with exercise. Adjustments can be made to the meal plan, insulin dosage, or both in combination. Diligence with glucose monitoring either by SMBG or CGM (before, during, and after exercise), careful record keeping, and uploading data to retrospectively determine glucose response patterns are crucial for success in making sound exercise-related adjustment decisions.

Adjusting Carbohydrate Intake

The decision to adjust carbohydrate intake for exercise should be based on a number of factors. These include pre-exercise blood glucose level, planned exercise intensity and duration, the time of day of the planned activity and time in relation to previous food intake, the individual's level of training, and previous glycemic response to exercise. Additional carbohydrate may be necessary to prevent hypoglycemia, treat hypoglycemia if it occurs, or fuel muscles and delay fatigue during periods of prolonged activity.

When an activity session is of short duration or is unplanned, consuming additional carbohydrate is useful. For moderate activity lasting <30 min, insulin adjustment is rarely necessary, but a small snack that provides ~15 g carbohydrate may be needed. Consuming additional carbohydrate is certainly indicated if the pre-exercise blood glucose is <100 mg/dL (<5.6 mmol/L). Evidence is lacking regarding the optimal blood glucose range before planned exercise, although 100–200 mg/dL is a reasonable range in the absence of clinical research data. During periods of prolonged or intense exercise when energy expenditure is high, additional carbohydrate is often necessary. Intake of 15 g carbohydrate every 30–60 min of activity is a general, safe starting guideline. Extra carbohydrate may also be needed in the postexercise period when insulin sensitivity is increased and glycogen storage is enhanced. Intake of additional carbohydrate at this time can reduce the risk of hypoglycemia and enhance glycogen storage. For individuals who exercise in the late afternoon or evening, it is particularly important to be alert to the possibility of nocturnal hypoglycemia and adjust the evening snack as needed to prevent its occurrence.

The rigid recommendation to consume extra carbohydrate based only on the planned intensity and duration of exercise and without regard to the glycemic level at the start of exercise, previous metabolic response to exercise, and insulin therapy is no longer appropriate. Such an approach can easily neutralize the beneficial blood glucose–lowering effect and energy deficit that results from exercise. The amount of carbohydrate required to prevent hypoglycemia and optimize exercise performance must be determined on an individual basis and can vary with each exercise situation.

Adjusting Insulin

The increasing use of intensive insulin therapy has provided individuals with type 1 diabetes with great flexibility and the ability to make precise insulin adjustments for various activities. In certain exercise situations, it may be necessary to reduce the insulin dosage to prevent hypoglycemia.

A reduction in insulin dosage is often necessary when a vigorous exercise session lasts greater than or equal to 30 min. The specific adjustment that will be needed depends on the insulin dosage, the timing of exercise in relation to insulin "peak" action time, and the planned intensity and duration of an activity. For a moderate amount of exercise, a modest reduction (~20–30%) in the insulin component that is most active during the period of exercise may be sufficient to prevent hypoglycemia. However, for very prolonged, vigorous exercise such as distance running, cross-country skiing, cycling, or backpacking, a large decrease in the total daily insulin dosage (by as much as 50–80%) may be needed to prevent hypoglycemia. In this case, both short- or rapid- and longer-acting insulin may need to be decreased proportionally. The DirecNet study in children using CSII showed that during strenuous activity in children, basal insulin delivery via insulin pump should be discontinued to avoid hypoglycemia. Care should be taken to avoid discontinuation of insulin delivery for long periods of time. In addition, DirecNet has shown that after 1 h of exercise in the afternoon, children experience significantly more hypoglycemia during the ensuing night compared to sedentary days. The nadir glucose was between midnight and 2:00 A.M. after an afternoon exercise session between 4:00 and 6:00 P.M. In adults, or with less strenuous activity in children, lowering pump basal rates rather than suspending delivery may be as effective and safer. Insulin reductions may also be necessary during the postexercise recovery period.

An elevation in the pre-exercise blood glucose level can be an indicator of an insulin-deficient state. Supplemental insulin may be necessary to correct a low insulin level and improve metabolic control before exercise is initiated.

If an exercise session is to be initiated within 30 min of an insulin injection, the injection should be administered in an area of the body that will not predominantly be used for the activity. Insulin absorption and peak action time can be accelerated if insulin is injected into an area of working muscle shortly before initiation of exercise. The abdomen is generally the site of choice.

CONCLUSION

Long recognized as a cornerstone of diabetes management, exercise is an all too often underutilized therapeutic modality. Although exercise carries potential risks for people with diabetes, with careful planning it can provide numerous health benefits that far outweigh these risks. Using established, sound guidelines, clinicians and diabetes educators can frame safe and effective exercise programs that will enhance the health and well-being of individuals with type 1 diabetes.

BIBLIOGRAPHY

American Diabetes Association, JDRF. *American Diabetes Association/JDRF Type 1 Diabetes Sourcebook*. Peters A, Laffel L, Eds. Alexandria, VA, American Diabetes Association, 2013

Campbell MD, Walker M, Bracken RM, Turner D, Stevenson EJ, Gonzalez JT, Shaw JA, West DJ. Insulin therapy and dietary adjustments to normalize glycemia and prevent nocturnal hypoglycemia after evening exercise in type 1 diabetes: a randomized controlled trial. *BMJ Open Diabetes Res Care* 2015;3:e000085

Chu L, Hamilton J, Riddell MC. Clinical management of the physically active patient with type 1 diabetes. *Phys Sportsmed* 2011;39:64–77

Colberg SR. *Exercise and Diabetes: A Clinician's Guide to Prescribing Physical Activity*. Alexandria, VA, American Diabetes Association, 2013

Colberg SR, Riddell MC. Physical activity: regulation of glucose metabolism, clinician management strategies, and weight control. In *American Diabetes Association/JDRF Type 1 Diabetes Sourcebook*. Alexandria, VA, American Diabetes Association, 2013, p. 249–292

Gallen IW. Exercise for people with type 1 diabetes. *Med Sport Sci* 2014;60:141–153

Janssen I, Leblanc AG. Systematic review of the health benefits of physical activity and fitness in school-aged children and youth. *Int J Behav Nutr Phys Act* 2010;7:40

Katzmarzyk PT, Church TS, Craig CL, Bouchard C. Sitting time and mortality from all causes, cardiovascular disease, and cancer. *Med Sci Sports Exerc* 2009;41:998–1005

Lumb A. Diabetes and exercise. *Clin Med* 2014;14:673–676

Shugart C, Jackson J, Fields KB. Diabetes in sports. *Sports Health* 2010;2:29–38

Taplin CE, Cobry E, Messer L, McFann K, Chase P, Fiallo-Scharer R. Preventing post-exercise nocturnal hypoglycemia in children with type 1 diabetes. *J Pediatr* 2010;157:784–788

Tsalikian E, Mauras N, Beck RW, Tamborlane WV, Janz KF, Chase HP, Wysocki T, Weinzimer SA, Buckingham BA, Kollman C, Xing D, Ruedy KJ; the Diabetes Research in Children Network DirecNet Study Group. Impact of exercise on overnight glycemic control in children with type 1 diabetes mellitus. *J Pediatr* 2005;147:528–534

U.S. Department of Health and Human Services. 2008 physical activity guidelines for Americans [Internet], 2008. Available from http://www.health.gov/paguidelines/guidelines/default.aspx

Yardley JE, Hay J, Abou-Setta AM, Marks SD, McGavock J. A systematic review and meta-analysis of exercise interventions in adults with type 1 diabetes. *Diabetes Res Clin Pract* 2014;106:393–400

Yardley JE, Sigal RJ. Exercise strategies for hypoglycemia prevention in individuals with type 1 diabetes. *Diabetes Spectr* 2015;28:32–38

Special Situations

Highlights
Special Situations

DIABETIC KETOACIDOSIS

- Diabetic ketoacidosis (DKA) is a life-threatening but reversible complication characterized by severe disturbances in carbohydrate, fat, and protein metabolism.
- DKA is always due to insulin deficiency, either absolute (e.g., in previously undiagnosed diabetes or omission of insulin) or relative (e.g., insufficient insulin and/or excess stress [counterregulatory] hormones).
- Any major stress may precipitate DKA in a patient with diabetes who lacks sufficient circulating insulin.
- The clinical signs and symptoms of DKA are listed in Table 4.1 and usually include polyuria, polydipsia, hyperventilation, dehydration, nausea, abdominal pain, vomiting, the fruity odor of ketones, and disturbances in the conscious state ranging from drowsiness to frank coma.
- The initial goal of therapy should be to correct life-threatening abnormalities, i.e.:
  - volume depletion
  - hyperglycemia
  - metabolic acidosis
  - potassium deficiency
- Upon diagnosis, frequent clinical examination is required every hour initially, with reexamination of laboratory indices every 1–2 h during the first 4 h and at least every 2–4 h thereafter.
- Insulin therapy and hydration will reverse acidosis; routine bicarbonate administration is not recommended. Potassium administration is recommended for all patients, except those who present with hyperkalemia or end-stage renal disease, once urine output, renal function, and initial serum potassium are assessed.
- The cause of DKA must be aggressively pursued. Potential complications of therapy and how to avoid them are outlined.
- DKA can often be prevented with appropriate patient education and prompt physician attention.

HYPOGLYCEMIA

- Hypoglycemia is a common side effect of insulin therapy. Mild hypoglycemic symptoms usually consist of autonomic (sympathetic or neurogenic) symptoms, e.g., tremors, palpitations, sweating, and excessive hunger. Symptoms of moderate and severe hypoglycemia include autonomic as well as neuroglycopenic symptoms, e.g., cognitive impairment, confusion, headache, slurred speech, dizziness,

165

or when quite severe, seizures and coma.

- Mild hypoglycemia may produce only minimal disruption of daily activities. Moderate and severe insulin reactions may severely harm health and morale and should be avoided.
- Certain circumstances favor development of prolonged, incapacitating, and occasionally life-threatening hypoglycemia, including:
  - hypoglycemia unawareness
  - antecedent hypoglycemia
  - failure to notice symptoms because the patient is sleeping or attention is elsewhere
  - intensive glycemic control
  - long duration of diabetes
  - certain medications or drugs, including alcohol and sedatives
- Factors precipitating an episode of hypoglycemia can often be identified, allowing prevention of future episodes in similar circumstances.
- Self-monitoring of blood glucose (SMBG) should be used to full advantage for detection and treatment of hypoglycemia. Those with frequent or severe episodes might consider continuous glucose monitoring. Changes in insulin dosing, eating, or exercise schedules and travel should all be accompanied by increased frequency of monitoring.
- Guidelines for treatment of mild, moderate, and severe reactions should be clearly understood by the patient, family, and school and business associates.
- Hypoglycemia may occasionally lead to rebound hyperglycemia, which should be recognized and appropriately treated if it occurs.

PREGNANCY

- Women with type 1 diabetes who plan their pregnancies, optimize glycemic control, and receive care by an experienced diabetes management team can expect a pregnancy outcome similar to that of women who do not have diabetes.
- Family planning, contraception, retinal exams, and contraindicated medications must be reviewed with the patient during the preconception period.
- Excellent glycemic control during pregnancy has been shown unequivocally to result in improved clinical outcomes to both mother and fetus.
- Poor glycemic control, ketonemia, and vasculopathy are associated with poor perinatal outcomes.
- Patients should be as near to normoglycemia as possible at the time of conception and throughout the first trimester to decrease incidence of congenital malformations, and throughout the remainder of the pregnancy to reduce the risk of macrosomia with resulting shoulder dystocia, birth injury, and/or need for cesarean delivery.
- Frequent SMBG is mandatory during pregnancy. With appropriate patient education, insulin pump therapy and continuous glucose monitoring may aid in achieving optimal glycemic control during pregnancy.
- Most women with type 1 diabetes may be managed as outpatients throughout gestation.
- Tests to assess fetal growth and health should be conducted at appropriate times. Timing of delivery, management during labor and

delivery, and postpartum care are outlined in this section.

SURGERY

- Given appropriate preparation and management, patients with type 1 diabetes are subject to little more than normal risk during surgery.
- Whenever possible, the patient should be in the best possible general health and glycemic control before a surgical procedure.
- The objectives of glycemic management before, during, and after a surgical procedure are to prevent hypoglycemia, excessive hyperglycemia, and ketoacidosis.
- Because hypoglycemia is particularly dangerous in the unconscious patient, plasma glucose should generally be kept between ~100 and 180 mg/dL (~5.3 and 9.6 mmol/L) during and after the surgery.
- Intravenous insulin delivery is preferred during surgery, although subcutaneous insulin may be used if the patient has stable glucose control, the procedure is relatively minor and of short duration, and recovery is expected to be rapid.
- In patients with DKA who need emergency surgery, efforts should be made to delay surgery until DKA is managed.
- Guidelines are given for:
  - major surgery
  - minor surgery

CELL REPLACEMENT STRATEGIES

- Significant progress has been made in islet and pancreatic transplantation, but limitations remain. New research on islet encapsulation and cell replacement strategies including stem cell therapy, xenotransplantation, and regenerative medicine with organ bioengineering is ongoing because of a scarcity of available organs and tissue.
- Islet and pancreatic allotransplantation is recommended for certain patients in whom the benefits of improved metabolic control with avoidance of severe hypoglycemia outweigh the risks of the islet allotransplantation procedure, including hepatic bleeding and the ongoing risks of chronic immunosuppression.
- Most islet transplants to date have been done in patients with recurrent, refractory, severe hypoglycemia or marked glycemic instability.
- It is not known yet whether such transplantation will reverse or stop microvascular complications because glucose intolerance persists.

Special Situations

Diabetic ketoacidosis (DKA) is a life-threatening but reversible complication characterized by severe disturbances in protein, fat, and carbohydrate metabolism that result from insulin deficiency, increased levels of counter-regulatory hormones, and proinflammatory cytokines that impair insulin action. DKA is a medical emergency often requiring treatment in a medical intensive care unit or equivalent setting.

In DKA, the blood pH is <7.3, plasma bicarbonate is <15 mEq/L, blood glucose is generally >200 mg/dL (>13.9 mmol/L), and blood and urine ketones are elevated. DKA is always due to absolute or relative insulin deficiency. The counterregulatory or stress hormones include glucagon, catecholamines, cortisol, and growth hormone, and they are markedly elevated in DKA. Acting in concert with the deficiency of insulin, they augment the metabolic derangements characteristic of DKA:

- hyperglycemia secondary to increased glucose production and decreased utilization
- osmotic diuresis and dehydration secondary to hyperglycemia
- ketone body production secondary to increased lipolysis with excess free fatty acids
- acidosis secondary to increased production and decreased clearance of acetoacetic acid and 3-β-hydroxybutyric acid derived from fatty acids
- an increased anion gap secondary to elevated ketoacids and lactate

There are a few key differences between the presentation and management of DKA in pediatrics and adults. These differences are highlighted in Table 4.1 and further information is included in subsequent portions of this section.

PRESENTATION OF DKA

The clinical diagnosis of DKA is usually apparent in a patient known to have diabetes. However, DKA may not be readily considered in new-onset diabetes, particularly in very young children, in whom a delay in diagnosis may result in life-threatening complications. Those at higher risk are children aged <5 years and/or those who, due to social or economic hardships, do not have access to regular medical care. A blood glucose concentration <200 mg/dL (<11.1 mmol/L) usually excludes DKA unless the patient has been partially treated with insulin and

169

Table 4.1 Presentation and Management of DKA in Children and Adolescents vs. Adults

	Children and Adolescents	Adults
Usual source for blood gas measurement	Venous	Often arterial; may be venous
Risk for cerebral edema	Higher	Lower
Insulin bolus at start of IV infusion	No	OK
Initial insulin infusion rate	0.05–0.1 unit/kg/h	0.14 unit/kg/h
ECG is part of the routine workup for a precipitating cause	No	Yes
The preferred route for insulin delivery is intravenous	Yes	For the critically ill
Subcutaneous insulin is an option for uncomplicated patients with mild-moderate DKA	Not usually	Yes
Cautious replacement of phosphate is sometimes used	Yes	Occasionally

fluids before presentation and/or has severely restricted his or her calorie intake (sometimes seen in severe DKA). So-called euglycemic DKA can also occur in pregnancy (see Pregnancy section on page 203) and in patients treated with sodium-glucose transporter-2 (SGLT2) inhibitors (see Adjunctive Therapy in Type 1 Diabetes on page 104).

For patients who already have diabetes, the chances of developing DKA are 1–10% each year; however, unbalanced familial relationships, poor metabolic control, psychiatric diagnosis, eating disorders, diabetes self-management burnout, and limited medical care can cause patients to be at a higher risk of DKA development. To view current rates of DKA from a U.S. research-based registry please go to www.t1dexchange.org.

Clinical Signs and Symptoms

The clinical signs and symptoms of DKA include polyuria, polydipsia, hyperventilation, and dehydration (Table 4.2). Of note: polyuria may not be present but rather oligouria in end-stage renal disease.

The fruity odor of ketones may be apparent, especially on the breath, and disturbances in consciousness may vary from drowsiness to frank coma. Abdominal pain, without referred rebound and point tenderness, in association with an elevated white blood cell count and serum amylase may occur but resolves with therapy. If severe abdominal pain persists, a surgical consultation should be obtained, because an acute condition such as appendicitis, bowel perforation, pancreatitis, or infarction may coexist and may have been the DKA precipitant.

Table 4.2   Common Presenting Symptoms and Signs in DKA

Symptoms	Signs
Weakness	Hypothermia
Headache	Uncoordinated ocular movements
Anorexia	"Acute abdomen"
Thirst and polyuria*	Dehydration
Polyphagia	Thin (or weight loss)
Nausea and vomiting	Hyperpnea or Kussmaul breathing
Abdominal pain	Acetone (fruity) odor
Somnolence	Impaired consciousness and/or coma

*May not be present with polyuria but rather oligouria in end-stage renal disease.

Precipitating Factors

Any major stress may precipitate DKA in a patient with diabetes. Infections such as pneumonia, meningitis, gastroenteritis, urinary tract infection, and influenza are some of the many heterogeneous causes, as are trauma and myocardial infarction. In most patients, it is possible to identify a specific precipitating cause. Among the most common is omission of insulin, deliberately or inadvertently. The latter is particularly common following interruption of insulin pump delivery because of the short duration of action of rapid-acting insulin when it is being used in the pump. Another common cause of DKA is secondary to mismanagement of sick days—i.e., the withholding of insulin in a patient who is vomiting and unable to eat, because he or she mistakenly believes that giving insulin in this situation may result in hypoglycemia (Table 4.3).

ACUTE PATIENT CARE

The initial goal of therapy should be to correct life-threatening abnormalities, i.e., dehydration, insulin deficiency, and potassium deficiency. Fully correcting all biochemical abnormalities may take several days. During the first 12–24 h of therapy, the condition must be reevaluated frequently. Particular attention

Table 4.3   Points to Consider in Treating DKA

- A precipitating cause can be identified in most patients.
- Isotonic saline is initially preferred to rehydrate patients.
- DKA patients are deplete in total-body potassium (an exception is dialysis patients).
- Administration of dextrose is necessary to clear ketosis.
- Bicarbonate is rarely needed.
- Preventing DKA is a long-term goal of sound diabetes management.

should be paid to the plasma potassium concentration as well as frequent assessment of neurologic changes (headache, mood shifts) or other symptoms of cerebral edema. A flow sheet tabulating successive changes in the patient's condition must be maintained for all patients (Table 4.4). The degree of hyperglycemia, acidosis, dehydration, and conscious state is variable. However, patients in DKA often have significant dehydration; the degree of dehydration can be estimated based on a clinical exam and calculated effective osmolality. If the effective osmolality is >320 mOsm/kg H_2O, the patient has a significant water deficit. If the patient's clinical condition deteriorates after initial therapy has begun, help from an appropriate specialist is needed.

Table 4.4   Ketoacidosis Flow Sheet

	Monitoring Interval*
Clinical	
Mental status	1 h
Vital signs (T, P, R, BP)	1 h
ECG	Initially and as indicated for adults
Weight	Initially and daily
Urine output	2–4 h
Laboratory	
Glucose (bedside)	1 h
pH (venous or arterial)**	1–2 h initially
Potassium, sodium, chloride, bicarbonate	2–4 h
Phosphate, magnesium	2–4 h
BUN and creatinine	2–4 h
Ketones	1–4 h
Anion gap	1–2 h
Effective osmolality	1–2 h
Intake fluid/Metabolites	
Fluid administration (ml/h)	1 h
Insulin (units/h)	1 h
Potassium (mEq/h)	2 h
Dextrose (g/h)***	1–4 h
Bicarbonate (if indicated) (mEq/h)	1–4 h
Phosphate (if indicated) (mEq/h)	1–4 h

T = temperature; P = pulse; R = respiration rate; BP = blood pressure.
*Monitoring interval will be more frequent initially and can become less frequent as clinical status improves.
**Arterial blood gas is often used in adults, although the use of venous blood gas has become more common, while venous blood gas is routinely used in pediatrics.
***Dextrose 5% or 10% is often used in adults, while dextrose in a range of concentrations (5–12.5%) is used in pediatric patients.

Fluid and metabolite administration, laboratory data, and clinical assessment should be monitored at frequent intervals for the first 12–24 h. Patients are generally best followed in an intensive care setting, although in adults with uncomplicated mild or moderate DKA, there is good evidence that treatment with IV or SQ insulin in a step-down unit or medical ward is as effective and less costly than in the ICU. For a treatment schedule, see Table 4.5.

Rehydration Process

Significant dehydration is present in all patients with DKA. There are many routes of water and/or electrolyte loss, including *1*) polyuria, *2*) hyperventilation, and *3*) vomiting and diarrhea. The best index of the degree of dehydration in children is the magnitude of acute weight loss, which may be determined if the patient's baseline weight is known. Other clinical indices include orthostatic hypotension, dry mucous membranes, prolonged capillary refill, decreased tissue turgor, and thirst. A decrease in urine output is less reliable because of persistent osmotic diuresis with hyperglycemia. It is reasonable to assume with DKA an average water loss

Table 4.5   Fluid Replacement*

Hour 1–2
- In children, administer 10–20 mL/kg isotonic saline (0.9% normal saline [NS]) .
- In adults, use 1,000 mL/h; if patient has heart disease, administer fluid cautiously, e.g., according to central venous pressure. In cardiogenic shock, use hemodynamic monitoring and pressors as indicated. If the patient has only mild dehydration, administer 0.9% saline (250–500 mL/h) if the sodium is low, and 0.45% saline (250–500 mL/h) if the sodium is normal or high.

Hour 3–4 (until acidosis resolves)
- In children, subsequently rehydrate over 48 h often at a rate of 1.5 times daily maintenance therapy (typically 5–7% dehydration in moderate DKA). Typically need isotonic saline for first few hours then down to half normal saline with potassium, typically at 40 mmol/L once patient has had urine output. The glucose levels shouldn't fall more than 50–90 mg/dL/h; therefore when blood glucose level reaches ~250 mg/dL, IV dextrose is added ranging from D5 to D12.5%.
- In adults, if urine output is adequate, reduce fluid infusion rate to 250–500 mL/h.
- Adjust fluid rate to meet clinical need. The patient's water deficit can be estimated using the following equation: water deficit = 0.6 × (body weight in kg) x (1-corrected sodium)/140, with the goal of replacing half the water deficit in the first 24 h. Do not consider rate of urine output in fluid replacement calculation, except on rare occasions.
- When blood glucose reaches 200–300 mg/dL (11.1–16.0 mmol/L), change fluid to 5% dextrose in 0.45% NS at 150–250 mL/h. The blood glucose threshold of 200 mg/dL is often used in adults, while a threshold of 250–300 mg/dL is usually used in pediatrics.
- Continue intravenous fluids, including insulin, until acidosis is corrected. In adults, there is some research showing the benefit of starting SQ basal insulin earlier in the treatment of DKA to prevent rebound hyperglycemia. Then change to rapid-acting insulin subcutaneously every 2–4 h, giving the first dose ~30 min before discontinuing intravenous insulin.

*These recommendations do not appy to patients on dialysis or those with end-stage renal disease.

of 5–10% of total body weight. In both children and adults, calculation of effective serum osmolality is another important way to assess degree of dehydration.

Adequate rehydration is extremely important in initial therapy. Isotonic saline (0.9% normal saline [NS]) is usually the initial choice of rehydrating fluid (Table 4.5) at a rate of 10–20 mL/kg/h in children and 500–1,000 mL/h in adults in the absence of shock. A child in shock should be given isotonic saline or Ringer's lactate (crystalloid, not colloid) at a rate of 20 mL/kg/h to restore circulation. If circulation is not re-established, repeat boluses of 10 mL/kg/h can be given over 1–2 h, but likely 30–40 mL/kg total will be the maximum required. Adults with DKA should have hemodynamic monitoring and may need pressors; furthermore, they may need a third or fourth liter of IV fluid after the initial 2-liter fluid replacement. For patients who are hypertensive, hypernatremic, or at risk for congestive heart failure, a solution containing 0.45% isotonic saline may be preferable. In young children (age <10 years), calculate fluid replacement according to body surface area, not weight (e.g., a 30-kg child has ~1 m² body surface area).

In pediatrics, because calculations of dehydration are often over- or underestimated, IV and oral hydration should not exceed a rate of 1.5–2 times the required fluid intake for normal hydration for the age/weight/body surface of the patient.

There is a lack of good data to make definitive therapeutic recommendations around fluid replacement, and poorly understood causes of cerebral edema have contributed to high center variability in fluid management for DKA. Therefore the amount, rate, and type of fluid therapy continues to be debated. The Pediatric Emergency Care Applied Research Network (PECARN)–sponsored FLUID (Fluid Therapies Under Investigation in DKA) study underway in the U.S. may help determine the effect of rehydration regimens on neurological outcomes with DKA.

Insulin Replacement

Because the cause of DKA in all patients includes absolute or relative insulin deficiency, insulin must be provided. Insulin is required for suppression of ketone body production and is thus necessary to correct acidosis. Insulin also inhibits glycogenolysis and gluconeogenesis, suppresses lipolysis, and facilitates the conservation of sodium and other electrolytes by the kidney.

Because insulin drives potassium into the intracellular space, insulin therapy should not be instituted before confirming that serum potassium is ≥3.3 mEq/L to avoid precipitating severe hypokalemia with resultant arrhythmias including ventricular tachycardia.

Short-acting (regular) or rapid-acting insulin should be used initially at a rate of 0.1 units/kg/h (or 0.05 units/kg/h for more sensitive patients). In adults, an infusion rate of 0.14 units/h is recommended. Available evidence does not support the use of an initial insulin bolus, which may increase the risk of cerebral edema. Therefore, an insulin bolus should not be used at the start of therapy. Replacing insulin with a continuous intravenous infusion is the most direct route and is preferred in children if methods are available to regulate the infusion rate. In adults with uncomplicated mild or moderate DKA, rapid-acting insulin given every 1 or 2 h can be used: 0.3 units/kg bolus followed by 0.2 units/kg every 2 h. The optimal rate of reduction in glucose for adults is 50–150 mg/dL per hour. In adults, if the blood glucose does not decrease by 10% in the first hour, a 0.14 units/kg bolus of IV insulin is recommended and therapy should be continued.

Insulin therapy should be initiated 1–2 h after fluid replacement/initial volume expansion. Replacement via the intramuscular route is an alternative, but only if unable to give IV insulin; it should not be used in patients with impaired peripheral circulation. This titration method will adapt to any degree of insulin resistance and prevent severe hypoglycemia as insulin resistance wanes.

Insulin therapy must be continued until both hyperglycemia and acidosis are corrected. Treating acidosis requires higher doses of insulin than reversing hyperglycemia, and it will take longer to regulate than hyperglycemia alone. Therefore, when blood glucose levels approach <250 mg/dL (13.9 mmol/L), 5% glucose should be added to the rehydrating fluid to allow continuation of adequate doses of insulin therapy until acidosis resolves. Not giving glucose will delay clearing acidosis. Some clinicians, particularly those treating patients in the pediatric age range, recommend moderating the glycemic target to ~200 mg/dL (~11.1–mmol/L) range for 12 h, fearing that more rapid reduction in blood glucose will increase the risk of cerebral edema.

Particular attention should be paid to the rate of decrease in serum glucose at initial rehydration, as glucose levels will drop with fluid intake. After this initial drop, and with the administration of insulin, the optimal rate of decrease is approximately 50–90 mg/dL per hour in children, 50–150 mg/dL in adults. The addition of 5% glucose to the saline solution can be added before the serum glucose reaches 250 mg/dL if the rate of fall is more rapid.

Potassium Replacement

Patients with DKA are depleted in total body potassium despite a normal or even elevated serum potassium level at the time of presentation. The reasons for this are complex and include the catabolic state, insulin deficiency (causing potassium shift to the extracellular space), acidemia, potassium wasting in urine secondary to polyuria, the inability of the kidneys to rapidly conserve potassium, and often, the effects of vomiting and/or diarrhea. Therefore, potassium replacement therapy is required (however, an exception is made if the patient has end-stage renal disease or is on dialysis). Correct potassium replacement requires both caution and timely action. The following procedure is recommended:

- establish urine output to be certain patient does not have acute renal failure (as this may have resulted acutely from hypotension)
- send blood samples to the laboratory to measure serum potassium
- do an electrocardiogram (ECG) to help evaluate for acute myocardial ischemia/infarction, hypokalemia, or hyperkalemia (high peaked T-waves in hyperkalemia; low T-waves with U-waves in hypokalemia). It is important to note that we do rely upon ECG to infer the existence of hypokalemia or hyperkalemia. Patients who are hyperkalemic should not receive potassium until after initial expansion and with insulin initiation.
- begin potassium replacement at the suggested rate (Figures 4.1 and 4.2)
- when laboratory reports are available, alter rate of potassium replacement with the goal of maintaining the plasma potassium level between 3.5 and 5.5 mEq/L at all times

In adults, if starting potassium at initial volume expansion, a concentration of 20–30 mEq/L in each liter of fluid should be used (if the patient has adequate

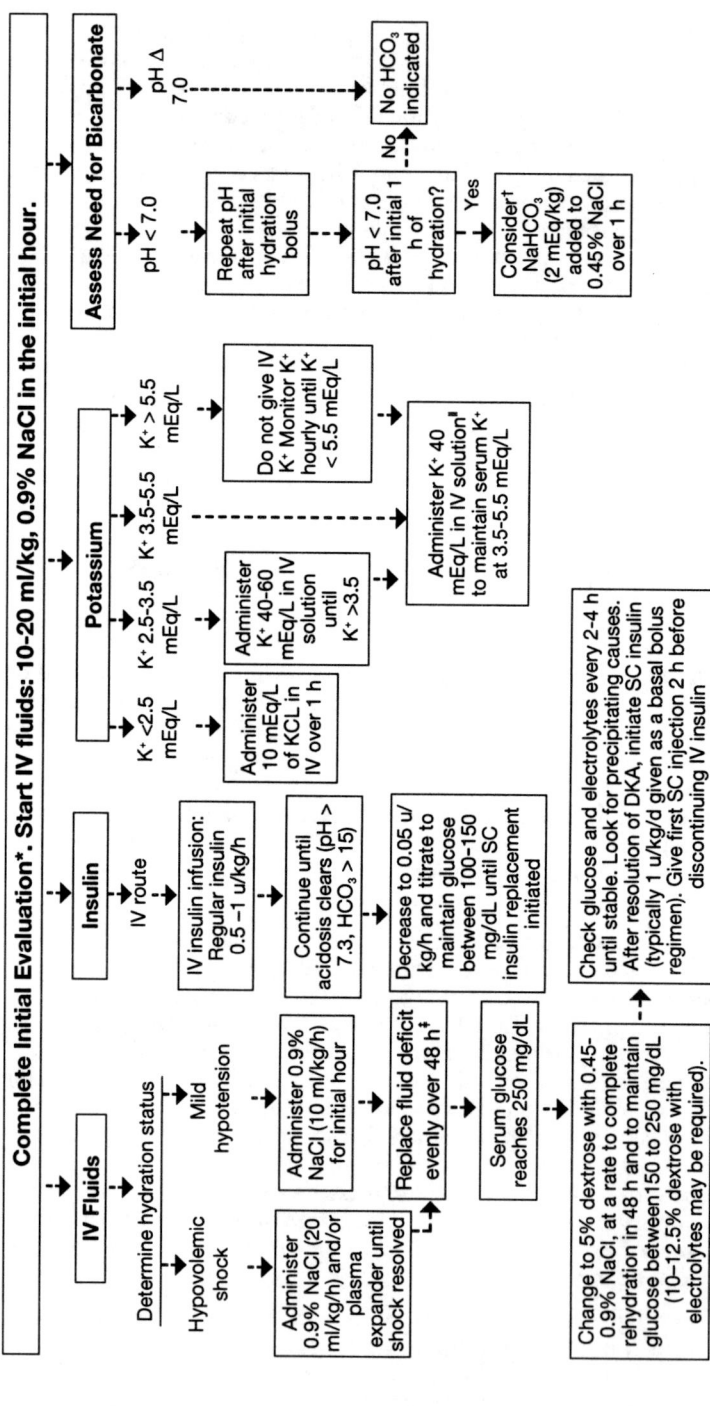

Figure 4.1 Protocol for the management of pediatric patients with DKA. *After the initial history and physical examination, obtain blood glucose, venous blood gases, electrolytes, blood urea nitrogen (BUN), creatinine, calcium, phosphorous, and urine analysis STAT. ‡Usually 1.5 times the 24-h maintenance requirements (~5 ml/kg/h) accomplish a smooth rehydration; do not exceed 2 times the requirement. ‖The potassium in solution can be a combination of KCl and Kacetate or KPO₄. †Bicarbonate therapy may cause paradoxical central nervous system (CNS) acidosis and/or hypokalemia; it is questionable if there is clinical benefit. *Source:* Adapted from Kitabchi AE, Umpierrez GE, Murphy MB, et al. Management of hyperglycemia crisis in patients with diabetes (Technical Review). *Diabetes Care* 2001;24:131–153.

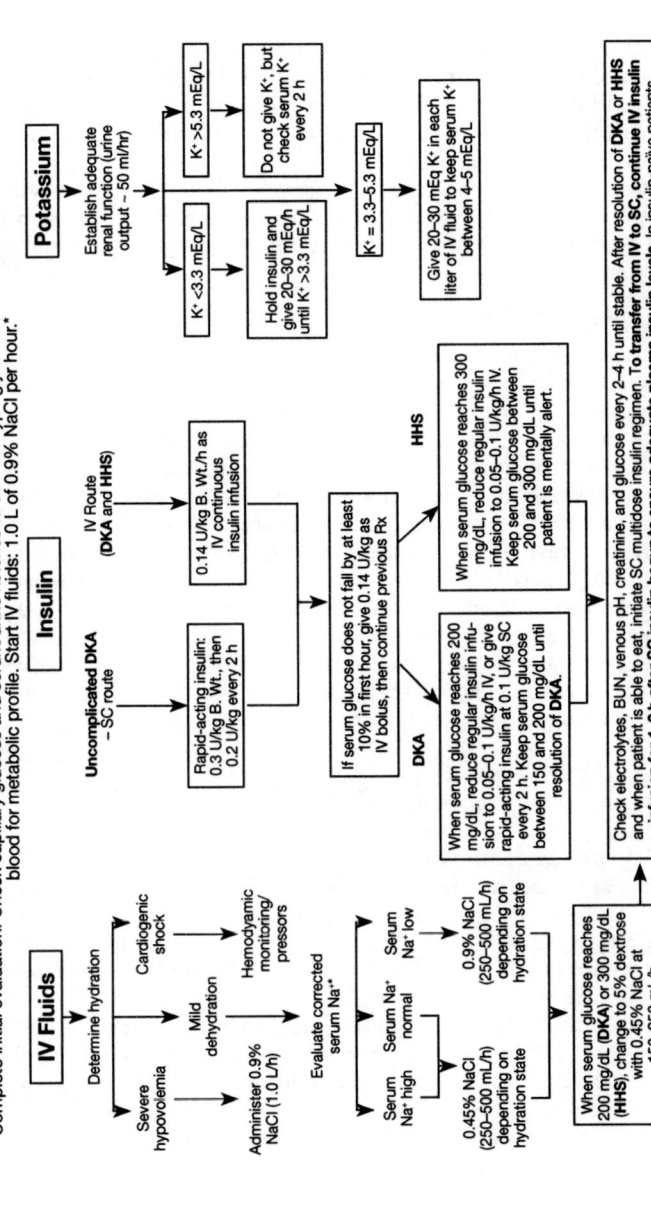

Complete initial evaluation. Check capillary glucose and serum/urine ketones to confirm hyperglycemia and ketonemia/ketonuria. Obtain blood for metabolic profile. Start IV fluids: 1.0 L of 0.9% NaCl per hour.*

IV Fluids

Determine hydration

- Severe hypovolemia → Administer 0.9% NaCl (1.0 L/h)
- Cardiogenic shock → Hemodynamic monitoring/pressors
- Mild dehydration → Evaluate corrected serum Na+*

Evaluate corrected serum Na+*
- Serum Na+ high → 0.45% NaCl (250–500 mL/h) depending on hydration state
- Serum Na+ normal → 0.45% NaCl (250–500 mL/h) depending on hydration state
- Serum Na+ low → 0.9% NaCl (250–500 mL/h) depending on hydration state

When serum glucose reaches 200 mg/dL (**DKA**) or 300 mg/dL (**HHS**), change to 5% dextrose with 0.45% NaCl at 150–250 mL/h

Insulin

Uncomplicated DKA – SC route
Rapid-acting insulin: 0.3 U/kg B. Wt., then 0.2 U/kg every 2 h

IV Route (DKA and HHS)
0.14 U/kg B. Wt./h as IV continuous insulin infusion

If serum glucose does not fall by at least 10% in first hour, give 0.14 U/kg as IV bolus, then continue previous Rx

DKA
When serum glucose reaches 200 mg/dL, reduce regular insulin infusion to 0.05–0.1 U/kg/h IV, or give rapid-acting insulin at 0.1 U/kg SC every 2 h. Keep serum glucose between 150 and 200 mg/dL until resolution of **DKA.**

HHS
When serum glucose reaches 300 mg/dL, reduce regular insulin infusion to 0.05–0.1 U/kg/h IV. Keep serum glucose between 200 and 300 mg/dL until patient is mentally alert.

Potassium

Establish adequate renal function (urine output ~ 50 ml/hr)

- K+ >5.3 mEq/L → Do not give K+, but check serum K+ every 2 h
- K+ <3.3 mEq/L → Hold insulin and give 20–30 mEq/h until K+ >3.3 mEq/L
- K+ = 3.3–5.3 mEq/L → Give 20–30 mEq K+ in each liter of IV fluid to keep serum K+ between 4–5 mEq/L

Check electrolytes, BUN, venous pH, creatinine, and glucose every 2–4 h until stable. After resolution of DKA or HHS and when patient is able to eat, initiate SC multidose insulin regimen. **To transfer from IV to SC, continue IV insulin infusion for 1–2 h after SC insulin begun to ensure adequate plasma insulin levels.** In insulin-naïve patients, start at 0.5 U/kg to 0.8 U/kg body weight per day and adjust insulin as needed. Look for precipitating cause(s).

Figure 4.2 Protocol for the management of adult patients with DKA. DKA diagnostic criteria: serum glucose >250 mg/dL, arterial pH <7.3, serum bicarbonate <18 mEq/L, and moderate ketonuria or ketonemia. Hyperglycemic hyperosmolar syndrome (HHS) diagnostic criteria: serum glucose >600 mg/dL, arterial pH >7.3, serum bicarbonate >15 mEq/L, and minimal ketonuria and ketonemia. Normal laboratory values vary; check local lab normal ranges for all electrolytes. After history and physical exam, obtain capillary glucose and serum or urine ketones (nitroprusside method). Begin 1 liter of 0.9% NaCl over 1 h after blood is drawn for arterial blood gases, complete blood count with differential, urinalysis, serum glucose, blood urea nitrogen (BUN), electrolytes, chemistry profile, and creatinine levels STAT. Obtain electrocardiogram, chest X-ray, and specimens for bacterial cultures, as needed. *Serum Na+ should be corrected for hyperglycemia (for each 100 mg/dL glucose >100 mg/dL, add 1.6 mEq to sodium value for corrected serum sodium value). IV, intravenous; SC, subcutaneous. *Source:* Umpierrez G, (Ed.). *Therapy for Diabetes Mellitus and Related Disorders.* 6th ed. Alexandria, VA, American Diabetes Association, 2014, p. 627.

urine output). The potassium can be a combination of potassium phosphate, potassium chloride, and/or potassium acetate. When combining, use a concentration of 20 mEql/L each of acetate and phosphate. IV administration should not exceed 0.5 mEq/kg/h, and if no response in levels is apparent and hypokalemia persists, reduction in insulin administration should occur until potassium levels begin to rise.

Once insulin infusion is begun, potassium replacement is particularly critical. Insulin lowers serum potassium by enhancing its movement back into cells, and hypokalemia-induced cardiac arrhythmia and/or respiratory paralysis may result from insufficient replacement.

Bicarbonate and Phosphate Replacement

Although it seems reasonable to administer sodium bicarbonate to the patient with DKA to correct the metabolic acidosis with alkali, the potential benefits do not outweigh potential risks. The potential harmful effects are accelerated reduction in plasma potassium concentration from rapid correction of acidosis and exacerbated intracellular acidosis (paradoxical central nervous system acidosis). Randomized trials have shown lack of improved outcomes in patients with DKA given bicarbonate therapy. For these reasons, routine bicarbonate administration is not recommended in most cases of DKA when pH is ≥6.9. In adults with severe acidosis (i.e., arterial pH <6.9), particularly when hypotension, shock, and arrhythmias are also present, or a patient has life-threatening hyperkalemia, 50–100 mmol of bicarbonate can be given as an isotonic solution in 200 mL of water every 2 hr, until the pH rises above 6.9–7.0. The use of bicarbonate is strongly discouraged in children except in cases of severe acidosis with impaired tissue perfusion and life-threatening hyperkalemia (and even then, it should be used with caution).

Patients presenting in DKA are usually phosphate deplete. As with potassium, insulin administration enhances the movement of phosphate into cells, which can further reduce plasma phosphate concentration.

There are pros and cons to administering phosphate, an ion important to many chemical reactions at the cellular level. One potential benefit is that hyperchloremia may be less likely to result when potassium is replaced as potassium phosphate instead of potassium chloride. However, administering too much phosphate can induce hypocalcemia. Therefore, calcium levels should be checked before phosphate is administered.

Randomized controlled trials show that routine phosphate replacement is not of benefit in the treatment of DKA. However, conservative potassium phosphate administration, not to exceed 1.5 mEq/kg/24 h in children or 20–30 mEq/L of potassium phosphate in each liter of fluid in adults, may be recommended, especially in patients with severe hypophosphatemia (<1 mg/dL). The bulk of the potassium should be administered as potassium chloride.

OTHER IMPORTANT CONSIDERATIONS

It is important to pursue other aspects of therapy while correcting the laboratory abnormalities. The cause of DKA must be pursued aggressively. The physician must be certain that there is no coexisting medical condition. In several reported series of adult patients admitted to the hospital with DKA, infection was the most common precipitating factor. Therefore, depending on clinical signs and symptoms, a chest X-ray and cultures of the urine, throat, sputum, and/or blood may be warranted.

An ECG is mandatory in adults to assess potential cardiac effects of hyper- or hypokalemia and also because myocardial infarction may precipitate DKA. The clinician should also carefully investigate all possible causes of abdominal pain, but any surgery should be delayed for several hours, if possible, while attaining metabolic stability; the abdominal pain may improve during DKA treatment.

Malfunction of the continuous subcutaneous insulin infusion system is the most likely and most readily treatable cause of DKA in those on an insulin pump. Recommendations for prevention and treatment of impending DKA in patients on pump therapy are covered more fully on pages 181–182.

In addition to determination of the cause of DKA, other supportive therapy must be considered. Protection of the airway and inserting a nasogastric tube to drain gastric contents in comatose patients are strongly recommended to prevent aspiration pneumonia. Low-dose subcutaneous heparin (5,000 units every 8–12 h) is often recommended to prevent hypercoagulability, especially in elderly patients. However, data that demonstrate the benefit of heparin administration in DKA are lacking.

Be alert to complications of treatment. Potential complications directly attributable to the treatment of DKA must be anticipated. Be aware of the following:

- Generally, glucose will be normalized more quickly than acidosis. Premature discontinuation of insulin may result in persistence and worsening of ketoacidosis.
- Hyperchloremic acidosis can also occur as the result of excessive chloride replacement in the form of both sodium and potassium chloride.
- Failure to give IV glucose or dextrose when blood glucose is <250 mg/dL (<13.9 mmol/L) will cause persistence of ketogenesis due to inability to continue high-dose insulin.
- Hypoglycemia can occur if the insulin infusion rate is not lowered after correction of acidosis, as insulin resistance improves and glucose toxicity clears.
- Nausea and vomiting from gastric atony due to hypokalemia or from feeding the patient before gastric peristalsis has returned can result in aspiration pneumonia.
- Hypokalemia can occur from inadequate or delayed potassium replacement.

Cerebral Edema

Cerebral edema is the leading cause of death from DKA in children and youth; the incidence of cerebral edema is 0.5–0.9% and, once developed, the mortality rate is 21–24%, and 60–90% of DKA deaths are from cerebral edema. Those who have severe DKA appear to be at heightened risk to develop cerebral edema. Common characteristics of patients who develop cerebral edema include young age, new-onset diabetes, and long duration of symptoms. Retrospective studies have shown that risk factors for cerebral edema include severity of acidosis, excess fluid administration over first 3–4 h, insulin administration in the first hour of treatment, a greater degree of hypocapnia, increased serum urea nitrogen, and use of bicarbonate. There is thought that an attenuated rise in measured serum sodium concentrations during treatment is a risk factor for cerebral edema but it has recently been questioned by studies showing that cerebral edema is actually associated with a drop in sodium. The pathophysiology for cerebral edema, previously thought secondary to intracerebral osmotic shifts, may be, in fact, due to cerebral ischemia and reperfusion injury. It remains critical to determine the mechanism of cerebral edema, since this may alter the approach to the initial treatment of DKA and rehydration strategy. Therefore the amount, rate, and type of fluid continues to be debated. In fact, the PECARN-sponsored FLUID (Fluid Therapies Under Investigation in DKA) study underway in the U.S. may help determine the effect of rehydration regimens on neurological outcomes with DKA.

Clinically significant cerebral edema usually develops 4–12 h into therapy, though it can occur before as well, and can be detected by a changing neurologic examination that may include onset of severe headache, pupillary changes, incontinence, vomiting, hypertension and bradycardia, neurogenic respiratory pattern, and decorticate or decerebrate posturing. Once diagnosed, cerebral edema is treated by the administration of mannitol 0.5–1 g/kg IV over 20 min. This is repeated if there is no initial response in 30 min to 2 h. Hypertonic saline (3%), 5–10 mL/kg over 30 min, may be an alternative to mannitol, especially if there is no initial response to mannitol. Intubation may be required. When the patient is stabilized, a cranial CT or MRI scan should be obtained to rule out other possible intracerebral causes of neurologic deterioration (~10% of cases), especially thrombosis or hemorrhage, which may benefit from additional therapy. Since there is no way to completely avert the development of cerebral edema, and approximately 50% of patients who develop cerebral edema suffer permanent neurologic deficit or die, eliminating DKA should be the goal of public and professional awareness campaigns as these campaigns have been found to reduce the frequency of DKA in children, for example, in Parma, Italy, and in two studies in Australia (for more information, see Preventive Care, page 181).

INTERMEDIATE PATIENT CARE

Intravenous fluid and insulin should be continued until vital signs are normal, acidosis has been corrected, nausea and vomiting have stopped, and the DKA precipitating factor has been addressed. When subcutaneous insulin is begun, three points should be considered:

1. Because subcutaneous insulin takes effect more slowly than intravenous insulin loses its effectiveness, the first subcutaneous insulin injection should be given 1–2 h before stopping the intravenous insulin infusion if using regular insulin and 15–30 min before if using rapid-acting insulin. For basal insulin, release from IV insulin should be gradual (e.g., a reduced dose of SC basal insulin begins at night and the patient is completely sus-

pended from IV insulin in the morning). A recent small trial suggested that initiating basal insulin at the home insulin dose or 0.25 units/kg/day at the start of initiating the insulin infusion can significantly reduce rebound hyperglycemia.

2. Higher doses of short- or rapid-acting insulin, every 4–6 h for the first 24–72 h, or increased basal insulin delivery with continuous subcutaneous insulin infusion, should be used to meet the increased insulin demands of continuing stress surrounding DKA, to overcome glucose toxicity, and to facilitate rapid adjustment of the insulin dose to control blood glucose during this transition phase. The patient should be carefully observed to prevent recurrence of acidosis in the transition phase.

3. The patient may remain mildly insulin resistant for several weeks, so doses of subcutaneous insulin may exceed the patient's usual requirements.

PREVENTIVE CARE

Most often, DKA can be prevented given appropriate patient education and prompt attention. All patients with type 1 diabetes should perform self-monitoring of blood glucose (SMBG) regularly or use continuous glucose monitoring in addition to having the resources to perform urine or blood ketone testing when hyperglycemic (>200–250 mg/dL [>111 mmol/L]) and feeling sick. Patients must be taught how to give appropriate corrective doses of insulin when they develop hyperglycemia. A proven method of doing this is to use their normally prescribed correction dose formula and repeat the dose at 2–4-h intervals until hyperglycemia has cleared.

Patients on insulin pumps must know how to change all of their disposable supplies, i.e., infusion set, reservoir, and insulin, at the first evidence of hyperglycemia (>200–250 mg/dL [>11.1–13.3 mmol/L]) that is associated with ketones or does not respond to an initial correction bolus. (In pediatric patients, the higher threshold of 250 mg/dL is usually used.)

Patients must contact their health-care team as soon as they become ill or have nausea and vomiting, fever, or persistent hyperglycemia and ketones in the urine or blood. When contacted early, the clinician is often able to treat impending DKA successfully by prescribing frequent injections of short- or rapid-acting insulin and oral administration of fluids. It may also be possible to rehydrate and adequately replace insulin in the doctor's office or emergency room, thereby preventing hospitalization. However, when there is any doubt that the patient can be successfully treated in the home, doctor's office, or emergency room, hospitalization is indicated.

Attempts are being made to decrease the rates of DKA at the time of diagnosis, particularly in children. The rate of DKA in children at diagnosis varies by age, with children under 2 years of age having the highest rates. Worldwide studies have shown that DKA rates vary by country. But in general, the incidence of DKA at diagnosis has been decreasing. This decrease in DKA is likely due to a number of factors, including increasing public and professional awareness about the signs and symptoms of diabetes and the need for early diagnosis. In Parma, Italy, a public awareness campaign conducted with physicians and schools essentially eliminated DKA at diabetes onset in children. In the U.S., it has been shown that genetic screening combined with monitoring for signs of β-cell autoimmunity has decreased the severity of illness at diagnosis.

CONCLUSION

The pathogenesis of DKA must be understood in the context of insulin deficiency and excessive counterregulatory hormones, which combine to produce a severe state of life-threatening metabolic decompensation. Insulin, fluids, and electrolytes, given judiciously with close monitoring in a hospital setting, form the cornerstone of treatment. A precipitating event, such as infection, infarction, or accidental or deliberate omission of insulin, must be identified and treated. All efforts at prevention should be employed with patients, and awareness should be promoted with the public, so that DKA at diagnosis and in those with known diabetes can eventually be completely avoided.

BIBLIOGRAPHY

Barker JM, Goehrig SH, Barriga K, Hoffman M, Slover R, Eisenbarth GS, Norris JM, Klingensmith GJ, Rewers M. Clinical characteristics of children diagnosed with type 1 diabetes through intensive screening and follow-up. *Diabetes Care* 2004;27:1399–1404

Dunger DE. European Society for Pediatric Endocrinology and the Lawson Wilkins Pediatric Endocrine Society consensus statement on diabetic ketoacidosis. *Pediatrics* 2004;113:33–40

Glaser N. Cerebral injury and cerebral edema in children with diabetic ketoacidosis: could cerebral ischemia and reperfusion injury be involved? *Pediatr Diabetes* 2009;10:534–554

Glaser N, Barnett P, McCaslin I, Nelson D, Trainor J, Louie J, Kaufman FR, Quayle K, Roback M, Malley R, Kuppermann N. Risk factors for cerebral edema in children with diabetic ketoacidosis. *N Engl J Med* 2001;344:264–269

Hsia E, Seggelke S, Gibbs J, Hawkins RM, Cohlmia E, Rasouli N, Wang C, Kam I, Draznin B. Subcutaneous administration of glargine to diabetic patients receiving insulin infusion prevents rebound hyperglycemia. *J Clin Endocrinol Metab* 2012;97:3132–3137

Kaufman FR, Halvorson M. The treatment and prevention of diabetic keto-acidosis in children and adolescents with type 1 diabetes. *Pediatr Ann* 1999;28:576–582

Kitabchi AE, Umpierrez GE, Miles JM, Fisher JN. Hyperglycemic crises in adult patients with diabetes. *Diabetes Care* 2009;32:1335–1343

Kitabchi AE, Umpierrez GE, Murphy MB, Barrett EJ, Kreisberg RA, Malone JI, Wall BM. Management of hyperglycemic crises in patients with diabetes (Technical Review). *Diabetes Care* 2001;24:131–153

Kraut JA, Kurtz I. Use of base in the treatment of severe acidemic states. *Am J Kidney Dis* 2001;38:703–727

Larsson HE, Vehik K, Bell R, Dabelea D, Dolan L, Pihoker C, Knip M, Veijola R, Lindblad B, Samuelsson U, Holl R, Haller MJ; on behalf of the TEDDY Study Group, SEARCH Study Group, DVP Study Group, and Finnish Diabetes Registry Study Group. Reduced prevalence of diabetic ketoacidosis at diagnosis of type 1 diabetes in young children participating in longitudinal follow-up. *Diabetes Care* 2011;34:2347–2352

Marcin JP, Glaser N, Barnett P, McCaslin I, Nelson D, Trainor J, Louie J, Kaufman FR, Quayle K, Roback M, Malley R, Kuppermann N. Factors associated with adverse outcomes in children with diabetic ketoacidosis-related cerebral edema. *J Pediatr* 2002;141:793–797

Savage MW, Dhatariya KK, Kilvert A, Rayman G, Rees JAE, Courtney CH, Hilton L, Dyer PH, Hamersley MS; for the Joint British Diabetes Societies. Joint British Diabetes Societies guideline for the management of diabetic ketoacidosis. *Diabet Med* 2011;28:508–515

Umpierrez GE, Mendez CE. Chapter 37: Diabetic ketoacidosis and hyperglycemic hyperosmolar state in adults. In *Therapy for Diabetes Mellitus and Related Disorders*. 6th ed. Alexandria, VA, American Diabetes Association, 2014

Vanelli M, Chiari G, Ghizzoni L, Costi G, Giacalone T, Chiarelli F. Effectiveness of a prevention program for diabetic ketoacidosis in children: an 8-year study in schools and private practices. *Diabetes Care* 1999;22:7–9

Viallon A, Zeni F, Lafond P, Venet C, Tardy B, Page Y, Bertrand JC. Does bicarbonate therapy improve the management of severe diabetic ketoacidosis? *Crit Care Med* 1999;27:2690–2693

Wolfsdorf J. The International Society of Pediatric and Adolescent Diabetes guidelines for management of diabetic ketoacidosis; do the guidelines need to be modified? *Pediatr Diabetes* 2014;15:277–286

Wolfsdorf J, Craig ME, Daneman D, Dunger D, Edge J, Lee W, Rosenbloom A, Sperling M, Hanas R. Diabetic ketoacidosis in children and adolescents with diabetes. *Pediatr Diabetes* 2009;10(Suppl. 12):118–133

HYPOGLYCEMIA

The precise blood glucose level at which patients develop symptoms of hypoglycemia is difficult to define. Generally, symptoms do not occur until blood glucose is <50–60 mg/dL (<2.7–3.3 mmol/L), though we treat if blood glucose is < 70 mg/dL (3.0 mmol/L). Clinical hypoglycemia is the occurrence of typical autonomic and/or neuroglycopenic symptoms with low blood glucose levels, and its symptoms are relieved by the administration of fast-acting carbohydrate. Because of its sporadic and somewhat unpredictable nature and because of the need for rapid treatment, hypoglycemia is often self-diagnosed on the basis of predominantly autonomic symptoms and may be treated without documentation of the blood glucose level.

PATHOPHYSIOLOGY

Hypoglycemia occurs when there is an imbalance between the rate of glucose removal from the circulation (e.g., uptake into muscle) and the rate of glucose entry into the circulation (e.g., release of glucose from the liver or ingestion of nutrients). Clinically, this most often occurs when there is one of the following:

- a relative excess of insulin (which inhibits hepatic glucose production and stimulates glucose utilization by muscle and adipose tissue)
- a decrease or delay in food intake (which decreases the availability of dietary carbohydrate or gluconeogenic precursors)
- an increase in the level of exercise (which accelerates glucose utilization by muscle)

In individuals without diabetes, as the glucose level declines below normal (typically to 50–60 mg/dL [2.7–3.3 mmol/L]), a complex series of neuroendocrine events occur that raise the plasma glucose concentration back toward normal. Glucagon and epinephrine are thought to be the most important counterregulatory hormones in this process because of their prompt secretion and potent ability to stimulate the release of glucose from the liver. In addition, epinephrine can contribute to glucose recovery by reducing glucose uptake into insulin-sensitive tissues, and it is responsible for many of the autonomic warning symptoms of hypoglycemia (see the symptoms in Mild, Moderate, and Severe Hypoglycemia, page 185). The other major counterregulatory hormones—cortisol and growth hormone—generally are released more slowly than glucagon and epinephrine and appear to have a more permissive role in glucose recovery. Finally, endogenous insulin secretion is typically inhibited by hypoglycemia, also facilitating the rise in plasma glucose levels.

In contrast, the patient with type 1 diabetes has several abnormalities in this feedback system. First, the secretion of glucagon typically becomes deficient within the first 2–5 years of diabetes. Second, with more prolonged duration of the disease, epinephrine secretion may also be impaired as a result of the development of autonomic failure. Epinephrine secretory thresholds can also be lowered by antecedent hypoglycemia or by tight glycemic control, with these effects being reversible. Finally, the rate of absorption of insulin from a subcutaneous depot is not regulated by normal homeostatic mechanisms, such as nutrient availability, and thus, it continues despite the presence of ongoing hypoglycemia. The combination of these and other factors makes the patient with type 1 diabetes particularly susceptible to the frequent development of hypoglycemia.

MILD, MODERATE, AND SEVERE HYPOGLYCEMIA

Signs and Symptoms of Mild Hypoglycemia

Mild low blood glucose reactions usually consist of tremors, palpitations, sweating, blurred vision, mood variations, difficulty with auditory processing, and excessive hunger. These symptoms are mostly mediated through the autonomic (sympathetic) nervous system. Major cognitive deficits usually do not accompany mild reactions, so patients are generally capable of self-treatment. These mild symptoms respond within 10–15 min after oral ingestion of 15–20 g carbohydrate.

Signs and Symptoms of Moderate Hypoglycemia

Moderate low blood glucose reactions include neuroglycopenic as well as autonomic signs and symptoms, e.g., headache, mood changes, irritability, decreased attentiveness, and drowsiness. Because of possible confusion, impaired judgment, and/or weakness, patients may require assistance in treating themselves. Moderate reactions produce longer-lasting and somewhat more severe symptoms and often require a second dose of carbohydrate to treat.

Signs and Symptoms of Severe Hypoglycemia

Severe low blood glucose reactions are characterized by unresponsiveness, combativeness, unconsciousness, or seizures and typically require assistance from another individual for appropriate treatment. Approximately 5–10% of type 1 diabetes patients suffer at least one severe reaction each year that requires emergency measures such as parenteral glucagon or intravenous glucose. Subjects who experience a hypoglycemic seizure with severe hypoglycemia are at risk for recurrence.

Potential Effects of Hypoglycemia

Mild hypoglycemic reactions may produce only minimal disruption of daily activities. Hypoglycemia can cause hunger with consequent overeating, thus contributing to obesity or hyperglycemia. Patients may experience cognitive dysfunction and counterregulatory hormone impairment related to moderate hypoglycemia even if they never reach a critically low blood glucose level if there is a steep rate of fall. Cognitive dysfunction due to rapid rate of fall has been shown to correlate with decreased counterregulatory hormone production.

In contrast, moderate and severe reactions may be seriously disabling in many ways and their prevention is critical. Hypoglycemia that interferes with normal thinking makes taking a school examination an impossible task; riding a bicycle, driving a car, or operating dangerous machinery becomes potentially disastrous. Repeated or prolonged episodes may cause irreparable damage to the central nervous system in very young children. In adults, this is quite rare, and careful cognitive testing of the Diabetes Control and Complications Trial (DCCT) cohort has shown no decrement in cognitive ability in intensively treated subjects or those with severe hypoglycemia. However, despite the DCCT findings, there still remains a potential link between cognitive dysfunction and prolonged or repetitive hypoglycemic events. Severe hypoglycemia is frightening and deleterious for the morale of the patient and family members—a final reason for highlighting the need for prevention.

Some patients develop either an excessive fear of hypoglycemia or an inappropriate lack of concern. Fear of hypoglycemia can lead to chronic overeating, undertreatment with insulin, or both. Maintaining very high blood glucose levels to avoid hypoglycemia increases the risk of metabolic complications, including DKA, and chronic complications of diabetes. Conversely, patients who underestimate the potential for recurrent, prolonged hypoglycemia, may maintain levels of blood glucose that are too low, may take inadequate preventive or treatment steps, and will consequently be at greater risk for recurrent severe hypoglycemia. These patients may sometimes be identified by glycated hemoglobin (A1C) levels that are in the normal or even low range.

Antecedents of Severe Hypoglycemia

Certain circumstances favor the development of prolonged, incapacitating, and occasionally life-threatening hypoglycemia. Patients with hypoglycemia unawareness are always at increased risk for severe reactions. The counterregulatory hormone response to hypoglycemia and the autonomic symptoms tend to decrease after several years of diabetes so that neuroglycopenic symptoms become the first manifestation for many patients. Methylxanthines, β-blockers, selective serotonin reuptake inhibitors (SSRIs), and certain other medications may also diminish early warning signs.

Hypoglycemia occurs more frequently at night, and nocturnal hypoglycemia is more prolonged than realized by most adults and children with type 1 diabetes. Hypoglycemia has been described to occur during 8.5% of nights. The duration of hypoglycemia is >2 h on 23% of nights with hypoglycemia. Risk factors for nocturnal hypoglycemia are lower A1C and the occurrence of prior nocturnal hypoglycemia, but not age or insulin treatment with continuous subcutaneous insulin infusion (CSII) versus multiple daily injections (MDI). The predictors of severe hypoglycemia are a prior severe episode in the preceding 6 months and being female. Studies have also shown that hypoglycemia begets hypoglycemia. In studies done with continuous glucose monitoring (CGM), increased CGM readings <70 mg/dL and greater area under the hypoglycemic threshold increased the risk for severe hypoglycemia.

Intensive insulin therapy also increases the risk of asymptomatic hypoglycemia. Although the increased frequency of low glucose levels can be attributed partly to the more stringent treatment goals associated with intensive regimens, it is now apparent that physiologic alterations occur in the patient's ability to secrete counterregulatory hormones, and thus, the ability to recognize and recover from hypoglycemia is clearly impaired. As few as two moderate episodes of hypoglycemia can blunt counterregulatory hormones. These observations emphasize the importance of SMBG and CGM in such patients to detect and prevent these asymptomatic reactions. Insufficiently intensive insulin therapies (i.e., fixed combination insulins such as twice-daily biphasic insulin, suppertime NPH mixed with short- or rapid-acting insulin, or fixed-dose prandial insulin) carry a greater risk of hypoglycemia since they are less physiologic and provide less flexibility. In such cases, conversion to intensive therapy, with necessary precautions on proper implementation, may ameliorate hypoglycemia.

Delaying treatment of mild hypoglycemia can lead to more severe hypoglycemia as glucose stores are depleted from antecedent episodes. Because early autonomic warning signs such as headache, hunger, mood or behavior changes, or weakness are not specific to hypoglycemia, they are frequently misinterpreted or overlooked. This is especially likely if the patient's attention is directed elsewhere, which may occur during strenuous activity. Hypoglycemia during sleep is particularly difficult to detect as the counterregulatory hormones are suppressed during sleep and therefore do not provide detectable symptoms. The patient should be questioned for the presence of nightmares or nocturnal diaphoresis, and family members should be alert to unusual sounds or activity during the patient's sleep.

COMMON CAUSES OF HYPOGLYCEMIA

The factors precipitating an episode of hypoglycemia can often be identified by looking back over the events of several hours preceding the reactions (see Table 4.6).

Inadvertent or deliberate errors in insulin dose are a frequent cause of hypoglycemia; other causes are changes in timing or schedule of insulin administration

---

Table 4.6 Common Causes of Hypoglycemia

Insulin errors
- Reversal of morning and evening dosage
- Reversal of short- or rapid-acting and intermediate- or long-acting insulin
- Improper timing of insulin in relation to food
- Excessive insulin dosage
- Inadvertent injection into muscle

Intensive blood glucose or A1C targets

Fixed-dose prandial insulin

Fixed combination insulin therapy

Erratic or altered absorption of insulin
- More rapid absorption from exercising limbs
- Unpredictable absorption from hypertrophied injection sites
- Presence of gastroparesis

Changing insulin preparations or regimens

Nutrition
- Omitted or inadequate amounts of food
- Timing errors: late snacks or meals

Exercise
- Unplanned activity
- Prolonged duration or increased intensity of activity

Alcohol and drugs
- Impaired hepatic gluconeogenesis associated with alcohol intake
- Impaired mentation associated with alcohol, marijuana, or other drugs

or meals. For example, sleeping later than usual for patients on fixed regimens is potentially dangerous because it disrupts the balance and timing between insulin and food. Changing insulin type from a short- to rapid-acting preparation or changing the insulin regimen can cause hypoglycemia because of more rapid absorption or other factors.

Vigorous unexpected exercise or activity is commonly associated with hypoglycemia. Aerobic exercise of prolonged duration or increased intensity can cause hypoglycemia up to 24 h after the activity ends or even into the next day.

Alcohol, marijuana, or other drugs often mask a patient's awareness of hypoglycemia in its earliest stages. By inhibiting the liver's gluconeogenic capacity, alcohol also inhibits the body's normal ability to provide glucose and restore low glucose levels toward normal. Some of the most severe hypoglycemic reactions occur during or after parties because the combination of physical activity and the use of alcohol or drugs can mask recognition of the problem and prevent the usual self-correction of hypoglycemia. Drugs used for treatment of depression are linked with increased risk for hypoglycemia. Several other drugs including levothyroxine (liver impairment) and ACE inhibitors are also correlated with more insulin sensitivity and hypoglycemia. Pramlintide used in concert with insulin increases the risk for hypoglycemia.

Anticipating and Preventing Hypoglycemia

Once a situation that leads to hypoglycemia is identified, adjustments can often be made to prevent future episodes.

Sleeping late. Although most patients on regimens of multiple daily injections can safely sleep an extra 30–60 min without particular adjustments, patients who oversleep more than 1 h may need to plan in advance to alter insulin or food intake. For example, if sleeping late is anticipated, a 10–15% reduction of intermediate- or long-acting insulin on the previous evening is an effective means of preventing hypoglycemia. However, it may also lead to excessive morning hyperglycemia. When the patient awakens, the entire day's schedule of insulin and meals is advanced in time. Even the next day's schedule may be affected. All patients should be cautioned against awakening, taking insulin without eating, and then resuming sleep. However, awakening early, performing a blood glucose test, administering insulin, eating breakfast, and then going back to sleep is generally safe. Patients on insulin pumps, and many on long-acting analogs, may be able to sleep late without a problem if their basal insulin doses are appropriate. Before doing so, it would be wise to check the basal rate periodically by skipping or delaying breakfast and observing the glucose changes every 2 h by SMBG.

Exercise. To compensate for the increased caloric needs of exercise, increased absorption of insulin and glucose by exercising muscles, and increased insulin sensitivity induced by extra activity, several strategies to prevent hypoglycemia can be employed. Most important, the exercising patient should always have a source of short-acting carbohydrate immediately available.

If early signs of hypoglycemia develop during exercise, the exercise should be halted and an appropriate amount of carbohydrate eaten (Table 2.9). If similar exercise has previously resulted in hypoglycemia, patients can anticipate and prevent it by snacking before, during, or after exercise, depending on when the episode occurred. Decisions regarding the type and time of extra food can be made based on SMBG.

Alternatively, hypoglycemia can be prevented by anticipatory adjustments of insulin. For example, if a patient usually takes short- or rapid-acting insulin before breakfast but is planning to exercise after breakfast, the insulin dose can be reduced by 10–20%. This strategy may be preferable for patients who do not want to increase the size of a meal before exercise or who are overweight. Patients on insulin pumps can remove their pump or implement a decreased temporary basal rate, with the percentage of the decrease depending on the intensity and duration of the exercise.

Travel. When patients with type 1 diabetes have to travel across time zones, it can be difficult to adjust the timing of basal insulin, whereas bolus insulin can continue to be administered without any changes. Patients on insulin pump therapy should set the time on the insulin pump to the local time. Patients who are traveling shorter distances (across four or fewer time zones) may continue administering basal insulin according to the home time zone. However, patients traveling across five or more time zones and/or traveling for longer than 3 days should adjust the dose of basal insulin by 1/24 or 4% per time zone: reduce by this amount if traveling east, and increase by this amount if traveling west.

Shift work. Patients who switch between day and night shifts may also have difficulty with the timing of basal insulin when not using an insulin pump. Clinicians should have a detailed discussion of the daily and weekly schedule with the patient and find a single time during which he or she can consistently administer a dose of basal insulin. Bolus doses of rapid-acting insulin can be administered without changes.

Role of CSII

It is recommended for patients to switch from MDI to CSII if they are unable to mitigate hypoglycemia. A meta-analysis of 22 randomized controlled trials and before/after studies confirmed that both A1C level and rate of severe hypoglycemia were significantly lower with CSII compared to MDI. The greater improvements from CSII in reducing or preventing severe hypoglycemia were in those with the highest initial rates of hypoglycemia, lower A1C values, younger age, shorter duration of diabetes, and more frequent use of SMBG. Reports of nonrandomized clinic experiences have shown improved glycemic control without increased risk of severe hypoglycemia when patients are switched from MDI to CSII, and with the positive benefit sustained for up to 8 years. In addition, improvement in hypoglycemia unawareness has been reported with CSII.

Role of SMBG and Continuous Glucose Monitoring

The availability of SMBG has made the detection and treatment of hypoglycemia practical, even in the subclinical range. Therefore, the frequency of SMBG should be increased in patients with recurrent hypoglycemia. The addition of continuous glucose monitoring (CGM), with its frequent testing and alarms for low or rapidly decreasing glucose, has demonstrated the ability to further reduce hypoglycemia. Changes in insulin injection, eating or exercise schedules, travel, and other activities recognized as contributors to hypoglycemia call for increased frequency of monitoring. Patients should be instructed to treat asymptomatic hypoglycemia detected by SMBG or continuous monitors.

CGM is able to alert at hypoglycemic thresholds, with rapid rate of change, and with a predictive horizon, allowing the patient to prevent or reduce the time spent in hypoglycemia. A short-term trial using CGM showed that time spent in hypoglycemia decreased by 21% in subjects using real-time CGM compared to controls. Nocturnal hypoglycemia was also significantly reduced, despite that fact that it has been shown that many people sleep through the hypoglycemia alarms. Long-term studies with CGM have shown that it results in a "relative" reduction in hypoglycemia. This occurs because it is expected that as A1C levels decrease, hypoglycemia, including severe hypoglycemia, will increase. But this has not been the case, and lower A1C levels have not been associated with increasing hypoglycemia during CGM usage.

Attempts have been made to develop algorithms to predict risk of severe hypoglycemia. These take into account A1C, hypoglycemia unawareness, ability to mount an autonomic response as glucose levels fall, and the frequency and extent of recent low blood glucose levels on SMBG.

TREATMENT

Mild Hypoglycemic Reactions

For mild reactions, ingesting 15–20 g carbohydrate works quickly to increase the blood glucose and stop classic symptoms. Several sources of short-acting carbohydrate exist. Employing premeasured glucose products instead of juice or food is recommended because patients have a tendency to consume >15 g of juice or food when they have symptomatic hypoglycemia, and also because additional calories from fat or protein may cause weight gain.

Hypoglycemic reactions that occur during the night should be treated initially with 15–20 g carbohydrate, and this can be repeated if needed to treat hypoglycemia. People have often been instructed to combine carbohydrate with protein to prevent further hypoglycemia during the night; however, research does not show that the addition of protein in the treatment of hypoglycemia sustains blood glucose longer than carbohydrate alone; in fact, protein enhances the insulin response which is an undesired effect. However, having a larger snack does make sense, including during the day if the next planned meal is >1–2 h away.

Commercially available glucose tablets have the added benefit of being premeasured to help prevent overtreatment. Glucose gels or small tubes of cake frosting are convenient for children or patients who are uncooperative when hypoglycemic. Chocolate and ice cream should be avoided for treating acute hypoglycemia because the fat content retards absorption of available sugar and could contribute to weight gain from ingestion of unnecessary calories.

Because there is always a risk that mild hypoglycemia will progress to a more severe reaction, all episodes must be treated promptly and patients must test again in 15 min to ensure that they are normoglycemic. Treatment and follow-up testing should be repeated if hypoglycemia persists. Patients should be instructed never to continue driving when they begin to experience hypoglycemia. They should stop, treat the hypoglycemia, and wait 15 min to do SMBG, repeating as needed to ensure full recovery before they resume driving. Patients with type 1 diabetes should always have their meter and glucose products with which to treat hypoglycemia with them. Evaluation of the effect of nonsevere hypoglycemia on work productivity has shown that it is associated with substantial economic consequences. Lost productivity was estimated to be 8.3–15.9 h of lost work time per month, and, therefore, strategies to reduce even mild hypoglycemia could have a major positive impact on lost work productivity for people with diabetes and their employers.

Moderate Hypoglycemia

Individuals with moderate reactions will often respond to the oral carbohydrates listed in Table 2.9 but may require more than one treatment and may take longer to fully recover. These patients may be alert but will frequently be uncooperative or belligerent. Under such circumstances, if it becomes difficult to cajole the patient to take oral carbohydrate, administration of subcutaneous or intramuscular glucagon may be more appropriate.

Severe Hypoglycemia

Patients with impaired consciousness or an inability to swallow may aspirate and should not be treated with oral carbohydrate. These patients require either parenteral glucagon or intravenous glucose. If these are not available, glucose gels, applied between the patient's cheek and gum, may be of some help.

Generally, clinical improvement should occur within 10–15 min after glucagon injection and within 1–5 min of intravenous glucose administration. However, if hypoglycemia was prolonged or extremely severe, complete recovery of normal mental function may not occur for hours to days. Repeated boluses of intravenous glucose do not hasten recovery unless blood glucose measurements show persistent hypoglycemia. If the hypoglycemic event was associated with convulsions, the postictal period may be associated with severe headaches, lethargy, amnesia, or vomiting. Decreased muscle control may also be seen and requires medical evaluation if it persists.

Glucagon. The dose of glucagon needed to treat moderate or severe hypoglycemia for a child <5 years old is 0.25–0.50 mg; for an older child (age 5–10 years), 0.50–1 mg; and for those >10 years old, 1 mg. Glucagon should be given intramuscularly or subcutaneously in the deltoid or anterior thigh region. For children, parents and school or day care providers, and for adults, roommates or spouses should be taught how to mix, draw up, and administer glucagon so that they are properly prepared for emergency situations. Kits that include a syringe prefilled with diluting fluid are available. For mild or moderate hypoglycemia that is associated with nausea or vomiting, administration of a low dose of glucagon should be considered. In general, the dose is 1 unit (0.01 mg or 0.01 mL per unit) per year of age up to about 15–20 units. This can be administered subcutaneously via a normal 30–50-unit syringe rather than the intramuscular syringe provided with the kit. Full doses of glucagon cause nausea or vomiting after recovery from hypoglycemia in some patients.

Intravenous glucose. If medical staff and equipment are available, intravenous glucose should be given as a primary treatment in preference to glucagon. The usual dose is 10–25 g administered as 50% dextrose over 1–3 min. The dose can be titrated according to the patient's response. After the bolus injection, intravenous glucose (5–10 g/h) should be continued until the patient has fully recovered and is able to eat.

HYPOGLYCEMIA UNAWARENESS

In the Diabetes Control and Complications Trial, about one-third of all episodes of severe hypoglycemia seen during waking hours in intensively treated patients were not accompanied by sufficient signs or symptoms so that patients could effectively prevent neuroglycopenia. In the past, hypoglycemia without warning was viewed as a rare condition associated with advanced autonomic neuropathy. This concept is incorrect. Forms of hypoglycemia without warning can occur in recently diagnosed patients, particularly in patients with repeated episodes of recent hypoglycemia and low A1C levels. Repeated episodes of hypoglycemia cause two problems. First, they blunt hormonal defense mechanisms that prevent hypoglycemia. Second, they lower the level at which early hypoglycemic symptoms are perceived.

The key clinical issue is that patients need to be reminded that even with the absence of symptoms of hypoglycemia, a blood glucose level <55 mg/dL (<3.1 mmol/L) should prompt consultation with their diabetes team and increased vigilance. Frequent blood glucose monitoring, particularly before driving and after strenuous exercise, is recommended. Evidence suggests that hypoglycemia unawareness can be reversed by intensive education and self-management training and efforts that successfully avoid hypoglycemia. These efforts may include adopting slightly higher blood glucose targets before meals and during the night and undergoing self-management training to help detect and respond to subtle early signs of hypoglycemia. Continuous glucose monitors with alarms that predict hypoglycemia have also been shown to help reinstate hypoglycemia awareness and the epinephrine response to subsequent hypoglycemia. This suggests that real-time CGM might be a useful tool to reverse the hypoglycemia unawareness associated with type 1 diabetes.

HYPOGLYCEMIA WITH SUBSEQUENT HYPERGLYCEMIA

Hypoglycemia followed by "rebound" hyperglycemia, also called the Somogyi effect, may complicate diabetes management in some patients. The phenomenon originates during hypoglycemia, with the secretion of counterregulatory hormones (glucagon, epinephrine, growth hormone, and cortisol). This hormonal surge, together with decreasing insulin levels, leaves counterregulatory hormones relatively unopposed. Hepatic glucose production is stimulated, thereby raising blood glucose levels. These hormones may cause some insulin resistance for a 12- to 48-h period. Moreover, excessive carbohydrate intake may be a major contributor to rebound hyperglycemia.

The frequency of this phenomenon is debated, and studies suggest that it is much less common than previously reported. It may follow nocturnal hypoglycemia, but it also may occur after hypoglycemia at any time. The hypoglycemic event that precedes the rebound may not produce sufficient symptoms to make it recognizable.

If rebound hyperglycemia goes unrecognized and insulin dosage is increased, a cycle of overinsulinization may result (i.e., more hypoglycemia, more rebound hyperglycemia, more insulin, more hypoglycemia). As a general rule, when hyperglycemia does not respond as expected to treatment adjustments, undetected hypoglycemia and rebound hyperglycemia should be considered as a possible explanation. Rather than increasing insulin dosage day after day, the clinician who suspects rebound hyperglycemia should endeavor to detect (via SMBG) and avoid the initiating hypoglycemic event.

Nocturnal hypoglycemia leading to fasting rebound hyperglycemia should be investigated by measuring blood glucose levels between 2:00 and 4:00 A.M. and again at 7:00 A.M. If blood glucose levels between 2:00 and 4:00 A.M. are <50–60 mg/dL (<2.8–3.3 mmol/L) and those at 7:00 A.M. are >180–200 mg/dL (>10.0–11.1 mmol/L), rebound hyperglycemia may have occurred. The increased blood glucose level may be exacerbated by the waning effect of the previous dose of intermediate-acting insulin or a prominent dawn phenomenon (see Dawn and Predawn Phenomena below). A decrease in presupper intermediate-acting insulin or its deferral to ~9:00 P.M. or a change to a basal analog (glargine) should prevent nocturnal hypoglycemia.

DAWN AND PREDAWN PHENOMENA

The amount of insulin required to normalize blood glucose during the night is less in the predawn period (1:00–3:00 A.M.) than at dawn (5:00–8:00 A.M.). The modest (20–40 mg/dL [1.1–2.2 mmol/L]) increase in plasma glucose commonly seen in patients with type 1 diabetes given enough insulin to avoid hypoglycemia in the predawn period is referred to as the dawn phenomenon. This increment can be greater if insulin levels decline between the predawn and dawn periods or if hypoglycemia occurs during the predawn period. The key clinical implication is that attempts to normalize the prebreakfast glucose level (i.e., 70–115 mg/dL [3.9–6.4 mmol/L]) often result in predawn hypoglycemia.

Several strategies can be used to identify and prevent nocturnal hypoglycemia. These should include monitoring blood glucose at bedtime and at 2:00–3:00 A.M., especially when insulin doses are being adjusted to correct prebreakfast hyperglycemia or when blood glucose level is frequently in the normoglycemic range before breakfast. In the DCCT, >50% of all episodes of severe hypoglycemia occurred during the night or when patients were asleep, even with the use of long-acting insulin preparations given at night or insulin infusion pumps. As a consequence, the median blood glucose before breakfast was 140 mg/dL (7.8 mmol/L), and >75% of all prebreakfast values were over the upper target range of 120 mg/dL (6.7 mmol/L). Adding extra food at bedtime (particularly protein, which helps stimulate glucagon secretion) and giving insulin that does not "peak" between 1:00 and 3:00 A.M. should be considered. Increasing the bedtime snack is particularly important when nocturnal hypoglycemia is most likely (e.g., after sustained exercise during the day or when prebedtime glucose is <100 mg/dL [<5.6 mmol/L]). Among patients taking twice-daily injections, giving the evening intermediate-acting insulin at bedtime or substituting it with long-acting insulin may be effective. Changing the regimen to an insulin pump can also help dramatically; the basal rate can be programmed to prevent nocturnal hypoglycemia as well as cover the dawn rise of glucose.

CONCLUSION

Severe hypoglycemia can be life-threatening if not treated promptly. Even mild and moderate hypoglycemia can cause both short- and long-term problems. All patients should be taught to be aware of the signs of hypoglycemia and should be encouraged to use SMBG frequently to prevent and monitor episodes. Continuous glucose monitoring may be a helpful adjunct in patients, particularly with severe episodes and hypoglycemia unawareness. Patients should know to adjust their regimen with exercise. All families, child care or school personnel, and spouses or roommates of adults, should be taught how to use glucagon and when to call for medical assistance.

BIBLIOGRAPHY

American Diabetes Association. Hypoglycemia and employment/licensure (Position Statement). *Diabetes Care* 2008;31(Suppl. 1):S94

Brod M, Christensen T, Thomsen TL, Bushnell DM. The impact of non-severe hypoglycemic events on work productivity and diabetes management. *Value in Health* 2011;14:665–671

Cox DJ, Gonder-Frederick L, Ritterband L, Clarke W, Kovatchev BP. Prediction of severe hypoglycemia. *Diabetes Care* 2007;30:1370–1373

Cryer PE. Mechanisms of hypoglycemia-associated autonomic failure in diabetes. *N Engl J Med* 2013;369:362–372

Cryer PE. Diverse causes of hypoglycemia-associated autonomic failure in diabetes. *N Engl J Med* 2004;350:2272–2279

Cryer PE, Davis SN, Shamoon H. Hypoglycemia in diabetes (Technical Review). *Diabetes Care* 2003;26:1902–1912

Diabetes Control and Complications Trial Research Group. Hypoglycemia in the Diabetes Control and Complications Trial. *Diabetes* 1997;46:271–286

Fiallo-Scharer R, Cheng J, Beck RW, et al.; Juvenile Diabetes Research Foundation Continuous Glucose Monitoring Study Group. Factors predictive of severe hypoglycemia in type 1 diabetes. *Diabetes Care* 2011;34:586–590

Havlin CE, Cryer PE. Nocturnal hypoglycemia does not commonly result in major morning hyperglycemia in patients with diabetes mellitus. *Diabetes Care* 1987;2:141–147

Jacobson AM, Musen G, Ryan CM, et al.; Diabetes Control and Complications Trial/Epidemiology of Diabetes Interventions and Complications Study Research Group. Long-term effect of diabetes and its treatment on cognitive function. *N Engl J Med* 2007;356:1842–1852

Juvenile Diabetes Research Foundation Continuous Glucose Monitoring Study Group. Prolonged nocturnal hypoglycemia is common during 12 months of continuous glucose monitoring in children and adults with type 1 diabetes. *Diabetes Care* 2010;33:1004–1008

Ly TT, Hewitt J, Davey RJ, Lim EM, Davis E, Jones TW. Improving epinephrine responses in hypoglycemia unawareness with real-time continuous glucose monitoring in adolescents with type 1 diabetes. *Diabetes Care* 2011;34:50–52

McCall AL. Insulin therapy and hypoglycemia. *Endocrinol Metab Clin North Am* 2012;41:57–87

McCoy RG, Van Houten HK, Ziegenfuss JY, Shah ND, Wermers RA, Smith SA. Increased mortality of patients with diabetes reporting severe hypoglycemia. *Diabetes Care* 2012;35:1897–1901

Perlmuter LC, Flanagan BP, Shah PH, Singh SP. Glycemic control and hypoglycemia: is the loser the winner? *Diabetes Care* 2008;31:2072–2076

Pinsker JE, Becker E, Becket Mahnke C, Ching M, Larson NS, Roy D. Extensive clinical experience: a simple guide to basal insulin adjustments for long-distance travel. *J Diabetes Metab Disord* 2013;12:59

Realsen JM, Chase HP. Recent advances in the prevention of hypoglycemia in type 1 diabetes. *Diabetes Technol Ther* 2011;13:1177–1186

Seaquist ER, Anderson J, Childs B, et al. Hypoglycemia and diabetes: a report of a workgroup of the American Diabetes Association and the Endocrine Society. *Diabetes Care* 2013;36:1384–1395

PREGNANCY

Type 1 diabetes complicates ~0.2–0.5% of all pregnancies. During the last 40 years, perinatal outcomes have improved remarkably in this high-risk group. The perinatal mortality rate for women with diabetes who receive optimal care now approaches that of the general obstetric population.

Management of the patient with type 1 diabetes during pregnancy ideally involves an experienced medical management team, including a diabetologist or endocrinologist, obstetrician or maternal-fetal specialist (perinatologist), pediatrician or neonatologist, certified diabetes educator, dietitian, the patient, and her partner. Experience indicates that the outcomes for both mother and baby are generally more favorable when an experienced team is responsible for management during pregnancy, delivery, and the perinatal period. When a team is not conveniently available, phone consultation with individual specialists is of paramount importance. Pregnant women are usually highly motivated; therefore, this time is ideal for teaching self-care skills they can use for the rest of their lives.

RISK FACTORS

What factors help quantify maternal and fetal risk in pregnancies complicated by diabetes? Generally, risk factors fall into two categories: those relating to diabetes and its control and those relating to vascular complications. Thus, pregnancies complicated by type 1 diabetes can be divided into two groups: women with diabetes and women with diabetes and vascular complications.

Diabetes and Its Control

No longer does the onset and duration of diabetes influence the prognosis for good perinatal outcomes. Instead, the degree of glycemic control at conception and the presence or absence of secondary diabetic kidney disease, vasculopathy, albumin levels 30–299 mg/dL/24 h, and hypertension greatly influence the prognosis for a favorable outcome for the mother and the fetus. The quality of maternal glucose control throughout pregnancy is also an important consideration. Poor blood glucose control, including ketoacidosis, is associated with intrauterine death.

Vasculopathy

The greater the degree of vasculopathy, the greater the likelihood of a poor outcome for mother and child. Diabetic kidney disease, particularly if associated with hypertension, appears to bring the greatest hazards, increasing the risk of preeclampsia, fetal growth retardation, and preterm delivery. Pregnancy can contribute to a worsening of retinal disease in women with background or proliferative retinopathy, especially in the presence of hypertension. Women with active proliferative retinopathy are at greatest risk for progression, but visual loss can be minimized with laser therapy. Maternal deaths have been reported in patients with coronary artery disease. Other prognostically bad signs during pregnancy include ketoacidosis, pyelonephritis, preeclampsia, and poor clinic attendance or neglect.

MATERNAL METABOLISM DURING PREGNANCY

During gestation, maternal metabolism adapts to provide the fetus with an uninterrupted supply of fuel. During the first trimester of a normal pregnancy, accelerated utilization of glucose by the developing fetus generally produces a decrease in maternal glucose levels. In addition, pregnancy-associated nausea and vomiting can result in a decrease in food consumption. There is a rapid depletion in glycogen stores while fasting. Women with type 1 diabetes additionally experience relative insulin sensitivity in the first trimester. As a result, women with diabetes are prone to hypoglycemia in the first trimester, especially nocturnal hypoglycemia while fasting, and insulin requirements often decrease. Between 14 and 20 weeks gestation, insulin resistance increases as a result of the changing hormonal milieu, typically resulting in an increase in insulin requirements.

In pregnant women without diabetes, glucose levels are typically lower than in those who are not pregnant. In pregnancy, human placental lactogen, prolactin, and progesterone alter maternal islet cell function, producing β-cell hyperplasia and contributing to maternal hyperinsulinemia. In addition, maternal cortisol is elevated during pregnancy, which potentiates glucose intolerance. Human placental lactogen (hPL), a growth hormone–like protein synthesized by the placental syncytiotrophoblast, produces insulin resistance and augments maternal lipolysis. As placental mass enlarges during pregnancy, hPL levels rise, allowing increased maternal utilization of fats for energy and sparing of glucose for fetal consumption. Additional hormones that have been recently implicated in the decreased responsivity to insulin during pregnancy include leptin, tumor necrosis-factor-α, and resistin. In late pregnancy, the progression of overnight maternal fasting ketosis is so accelerated that delaying breakfast may result in significant ketonuria.

In pregnancy complicated by diabetes, periods of maternal hyperglycemia produce fetal hyperinsulinemia. Larger amounts of maternal amino acids and other fuels also cross to the fetus. Elevated levels of maternal glucose and other nutrients stimulate the fetal pancreas, resulting in β-cell hyperplasia and hyperinsulinemia. This combination of fetal overnutrition and fetal hyperinsulinemia contributes to macrosomia in the infant of the mother with diabetes. In a report describing a 40-year experience in women with type 1 diabetes in Scotland, despite a marked decrease in perinatal mortality (from 225 per 1,000 total births after 28 weeks in the 1960s to 10 per 1,000 births in the 1990s), standardized birth weight (adjusted for gender, gestational age, and parity) did not change, indicating that intrauterine overgrowth of the fetus still occurred due to failure to completely normalize maternal glycemia.

In the postpartum period, the delivery of the placenta withdraws the placental hormones that contributed to insulin resistance and thus immediately drops insulin requirements. Among women with preexisting diabetes who breast-feed, postpartum insulin doses may be lower than prepregnancy doses.

PRECONCEPTION CARE AND COUNSELING

To prevent early pregnancy loss and very costly congenital malformations in infants of mothers with diabetes, optimal medical care and patient education and training must begin before conception. This is best accomplished through a multidisciplinary team comprised of a diabetologist, internist or family practice physician, obstetrician, diabetes educators (including a nurse and registered dietitian), and other specialists as necessary. Ultimately, the woman with diabetes must become the most active member of the team, calling on the other members for specific guidance and expertise to help her toward her goal of a healthy pregnancy and offspring.

Because treatment of the patient with type 1 diabetes must begin before gestation, any regular visit to the physician by a reproductive-age woman, from teenage to middle age, should be considered a preconception visit (Table 4.7). These contacts provide an important opportunity to discuss the patient's contraceptive needs and her thoughts and concerns about a future pregnancy and to establish a database that can be used in assessing perinatal risk. Adolescents in particular should be encouraged to discuss these issues routinely with members of the diabetes management team. Any sexually active woman of childbearing age who is not using reliable contraception should discontinue the use of potentially teratogenic medications including angiotensin-converting enzyme (ACE) inhibitors, angiotensin receptor blockers (ARBs), and statins. Furthermore, any non-insulin adjunctive drugs to lower glucose should be carefully assessed, and

---

Table 4.7   Care before Conception

■ Discuss contraceptive program
■ Establish database for perinatal risk
  • Assess vascular status:
    —Ophthalmologic examination
    —ECG
    —Consider exercise stress test if diabetes >20 years duration
    —Urine albumin excretion
    —Creatinine clearance
    —Peripheral pulses
  • Assess glycemic control via A1C testing
  • Assess thyroid function: TSH, free T4, anti-microsomal (thyroid peroxidase, or TPO) antibodies
■ Optimize glycemic control: A1C as close to normal as possible without significant hypoglycemia
■ Refer for medical nutrition therapy
■ Assess medication regimen and discontinue potentially teratogenic medications including ACE inhibitors, ARBs, and statins, as well as non-insulin adjunctive glucose-lowering therapies
■ Determine immune status against rubella
■ Evaluate psychosocial setting
■ Caution patient against smoking or excessive alcohol
■ Assess exercise program
■ Begin daily folate supplement (600 μg)
■ Consider whether insulin pump therapy may be indicated or advisable and initiate the transition before conception

the regimen transitioned to one without the use of such medications that could be teratogenic.

Important periodic assessments include measurements of blood pressure, dilated eye examinations, and assessments of kidney function and urine albumin excretion. Note that preexisting cardiovascular disease significantly increases morbidity and mortality to the mother and cardiovascular health should be evaluated in women of childbearing age with a long duration of diabetes. A1C testing should be performed routinely and SMBG taught, if needed. Continuous glucose monitoring should be considered. Continuous subcutaneous insulin infusion therapy may also be considered in motivated women with access to sufficient education and support during pump therapy initiation. The optimal time to switch to pump therapy is during preconception planning. The desired outcome of glycemic control in the preconception phase of care is to lower A1C to <6.5%, preferably as close to normal as possible without frequent or severe hypoglycemia, so as to achieve maximum fertility and optimal embryo and fetal development. Poor glycemic control during the period of organogenesis (first 7 weeks after conception) significantly increases the risk of congenital anomalies and early pregnancy loss. Since much of this period may pass before the woman is aware she is pregnant, preconception planning and excellent glycemic control are critical.

Immune status against rubella should also be checked before conception. Consultation with a nutritionist and a review of the patient's exercise program are important. Daily folate supplementation (600 µg) should be advised. The patient must understand that smoking and alcohol are strictly prohibited during pregnancy.

Because pregnancy complicated by type 1 diabetes may cause emotional and financial stress, it is essential to evaluate the psychosocial interactions of the patient and her partner, their support network, and their financial resources.

Women with type 1 diabetes who are contemplating pregnancy often have questions regarding its impact on their health and the possible consequences for the fetus. Some of the most commonly encountered questions, along with suggested answers, are presented below.

Q. How will pregnancy affect my health and life expectancy?
A. Pregnancy is not generally life-threatening, but serious complications can occur if glycemic control is not maintained during pregnancy. There is no evidence that pregnancy shortens the lives of women with type 1 diabetes, except for some with established coronary artery disease. However, women with diabetes do face a higher risk for certain pregnancy complications and for progression of diabetes complications. If ketoacidosis occurs, there is the additional threat of fetal death. Preeclampsia and preterm delivery of the fetus by cesarean section are more common in women with diabetes.

Q. What effect will pregnancy have on diabetic kidney disease?
A. There is no evidence that pregnancy will permanently worsen diabetic kidney disease, although a temporary increase in proteinuria and decrease in creatinine clearance may occur. On the other hand, advanced kidney disease may jeopardize both mother and infant, increasing the risk for early preeclampsia

requiring preterm delivery and/or a smaller-than-normal infant. Factors that point in this direction include:

- proteinuria >2 g/24 h
- creatinine clearance <50 mL/min or serum creatinine >2 mg/dL
- hypertension: blood pressure >130/80 mmHg despite treatment

In some cases, women with severe renal insufficiency may require dialysis during the pregnancy and their kidneys may not recover from the decline in glomerular filtration rate that occurs during the pregnancy.

Q. What effect will pregnancy have on diabetic retinopathy?
A. Women without diabetic retinopathy will not usually develop it during pregnancy. Some women who have background retinopathy at the start of pregnancy experience a worsening of this condition, though rarely to a proliferative stage. Proliferative retinopathy treated by laser photocoagulation that is stable before pregnancy will generally remain so. In contrast, women with active proliferative retinopathy or macular edema that has not been treated with photocoagulation may experience a serious worsening of this complication during pregnancy. Women should have a dilated eye examination prior to conception and during each trimester, though women with no or minimal retinopathy may not need the second trimester retinal eye exam.

Q. Will the baby develop diabetes?
A. The infant is slightly more likely to develop type 1 diabetes later in life because of maternal diabetes, but the risk is not very high (i.e., ~3–4%). If the mother *and* father have type 1 diabetes, the offspring's risk for developing it is higher.

Q. Can I use birth control pills?
A. Young women without vascular complications may use a low-dose estrogen (≤35 µg)/progestin oral contraceptive. Those with hypertension or vasculopathy should use a progestin-only pill (or some other means of birth control). Women who are current smokers should not use hormonal contraceptive methods.

Q. What effect will diabetes have on the baby?
A. The answer to this question appears to hinge largely on the mother's blood glucose control; generally, the better the diabetes control, the fewer the complications. In the first weeks of pregnancy, poor diabetes control appears to increase the occurrence of fetal malformations, fetal macrosomia, intrauterine growth restriction, and miscarriage. Later, high blood glucose levels may bring about other serious consequences. Because glucose crosses from the mother to the fetus but insulin does not, high maternal glucose stimulates the fetus to overproduce insulin, which may:

- cause excessive fetal growth, which increases the risk of shoulder dystocia, birth injury, and need for cesarean delivery
- prevent the baby's lungs (and other organs) from maturing at a normal pace

Table 4.8 Techniques and Purpose of Fetal Assessments Used in Pregnant Women with Preexisting Diabetes According to Gestational Age

Testing modality	Timing	Comments
Ultrasound, transvagina or transabdominal • Crown-rump length • Fetal cardiac activity • Nuchal translucency (NT) thickness at 12–13 weeks; couple with free β-hCG[1], PAPP-A[2]	1st trimester	Important to confirm living fetus, establish gestational age and estimated due date as early as possible; elevated NT measurement is associated with fetal Down Syndrome and specific congenital anomalies (cardiac defects, diaphragmatic hernia, skeletal and neurologic abnormalitites) more common in women with PDM[3]
Maternal serum marker screening	1st trimester (with or without ultrasonic NT measurement) 2nd trimester (triple[4] or quad[5] marker test, or MSAFP alone)	PDM is associated with an increased risk of open neural tube defects (detected by 2nd trimester triple or quad marker test, or MSAFP alone)
Ultrasound, transabdominal • Fetal biometric measurements • Fetal anatomy	2nd trimester	Important to establish gestational age when this has not been done earlier in pregnancy; detailed fetal anatomic examination and fetal echocardiography should be considered in all women with PDM, but particularly in those at highest risk for congenital anomalies[6]
Ultrasound, transabdominal Fetal growth rate (abdominal circumference measurement reflects fetal adiposity) Amniotic fluid volume	3rd trimester	Following fetal growth by ultrasound examinations at regular intervals may be warranted when a pregnancy is at risk for fetal growth restriction (hypertension or vascular complications) or excessive fetal growth (poor glycemic control), or in lower-risk women when a fundal height dates discrepancy is noted
Nonstress test (NST)	3rd trimester	Abnormal NST and BPP tests suggest possible decreased fetal oxygenation status, but are affected by other factors. The optimal testing regimen and the ideal time to initiate testing are not known. However, women with hypertensive disorders, vascular disease, or evidence of fetal growth restriction should begin testing earlier, with a frequency of every 3–7 days
Biophysical profile (BPP)	3rd trimester	
Amniotic fluid markers of fetal lung maturity	Before delivery in indicated cases	Positive tests suggest a low risk of RDS in newborn infant[7]

[1]Free β-hCG, free beta-human chorionic gonadotropin.
[2]PAPP-A, pregnancy-associated plasma protein A.
[3]PDM, preexisting diabetes mellitus.
[4]Maternal serum α-fetoprotein (MSAFP), unconjugated estriol, chorionic gonadotropin.
[5]All components of the triple marker test, plus inhibin.
[6]Elevated 1st trimester hemoglobin A1C value, abnormal multiple marker results, abnormality suspected in basic ultrasound study, or personal history of a prior birth affected by congenital anomalies.
[7]RDS, respiratory distress syndrome.

- give the baby serious hypoglycemia after birth, when it no longer receives glucose from the mother
- cause intrauterine growth restriction resulting in a baby who is small for gestational age

In addition, high glucose levels are associated with sudden unexplained fetal death late in pregnancy. The incidence of preeclampsia is lowest in women with optimal glycemic control and rises as A1C increases. Preeclampsia in women with type 1 diabetes is also correlated with the presence of albumin levels 30–299 mg/dL/24 h.

CONGENITAL MALFORMATIONS AND ABNORMAL FETAL GROWTH: RISK AND DETECTION

The incidence of major congenital malformations in the offspring of women with type 1 diabetes that is well controlled in the first trimester is similar to the 2–3% rate observed in the general population. However, the rate increases with poorer glycemic control to as high as 20–25% among women with markedly elevated A1C in the first trimester. Cardiac and neural tube defects are common classes of malformation in these cases. Elevated A1C in the beginning weeks of pregnancy and second-trimester hypertension have also been linked to early delivery (before 34 weeks).

Much evidence links such malformations with inadequate diabetes control during embryogenesis (gestational weeks 3–7). The magnitude of risk for abnormalities increases proportionally to the degree of elevation of A1C during this period. For this reason, patients should have as close to normal glycemic levels as possible at conception and throughout the first trimester. All women of child-bearing age should be made aware of these risks, and if pregnancy is considered, they should be encouraged to use contraception until excellent glycemic control is achieved (see Philosophy and Goals, page 33). The risk of fetal anomalies should be reviewed at preconception counseling visits and the first prenatal visit.

Fetal anomalies associated with diabetic embryopathy can be detected prenatally in most cases (see Table 4.8 for an overview of fetal assessments). Ultasonography for nuchal translucency (possibly with first trimester biochemical screening with pregnancy-associated plasma protein A and β-human chorionic gonadotropin) should be offered at 11–13 weeks. At 16 weeks, further evaluation for a potential fetal malformation should include a maternal serum β-fetoprotein level, possibly combined with unconjugated estriol and chorionic gonadotropin ("triple screen") or additionally with inhibin ("quadruple screen"). A detailed ultrasound examination of fetal anatomy should be done at 18–20 weeks. In women with a high risk of fetal cardiac anomalies (such as those with poor first-trimester glycemic control), assessment of fetal cardiac structure by echocardiography at 20–22 weeks should be considered. Nonstress testing twice weekly is recommended starting at 32 weeks gestation. Fetal ultrasounds for growth can be considered during the third trimester. All of these studies require interpretation by specialists experienced in prenatal diagnosis.

MATERNAL GLUCOSE CONTROL DURING PREGNANCY

Excellent control of maternal diabetes will reduce the risks of fetal demise, excessive fetal growth, and delayed pulmonary maturation. During a nondiabetic pregnancy, maternal plasma glucose rarely exceeds 100 mg/dL (5.6 mmol/L), ranging from fasting levels of 60 mg/dL (3.3 mmol/L) to postprandial levels <120 mg/dL (<6.7 mmol/L). These values should be therapeutic objectives for pregnancies complicated by type 1 diabetes (Table 4.9).

Maintaining maternal glucose levels in this range throughout gestation is difficult. During the first trimester, when morning sickness may be troublesome, the risk of hypoglycemia is increased; hypoglycemia is most likely to occur during the night, when the mother is fasting but the fetus and placenta continue to consume glucose. Severe hypoglycemia is three times more frequent in early pregnancy (8–16 weeks) compared to the prepregnancy time period. In the third trimester, hypoglycemia decreases when insulin resistance from the counterregulatory hormones of pregnancy is greatest. Insulin needs may rise 50–100% over the final 4–6 weeks, and the total insulin dose at the time of delivery may double or even triple that of prepregnancy.

On the other end of the spectrum, pregnant women with diabetes who have hyperglycemia are more prone to developing diabetic ketoacidosis than when not pregnant, and at a lower blood glucose level (euglycemic DKA). DKA in pregnancy increases the risk of intrauterine fetal demise. Precipitants include infections, lack of insulin, steroids, and tocolytics. Thus, women should be educated about when to test for ketones and how to prevent DKA. Health-care providers and patients should treat DKA promptly and aggressively.

Monitoring Control

SMBG and CGM. During pregnancy, women with type 1 diabetes must use SMBG to assess glycemic control. SMBG has been shown to decrease the need for hospitalization and reduce the cost of care. Patients should monitor in the fasting state, before each meal, 1 h or 2 h after meals, and at bedtime. Testing at 2:00–3:00 A.M. is necessary for most patients, particularly for those who are likely to experience nocturnal hypoglycemia, those who have persistent fasting hyper-

Table 4.9 Optimal Target Blood Glucose Levels in Pregnancy

Time of Measurement	Blood Glucose (mg/dL [mmol/L])
Before breakfast	≤90–95 (5.0–5.3)
1 h after meals	≤130–140 (<7.2–7.8)
2 h after meals	≤120 (<6.7)
A1C*	6.0–6.5% (<6.0% as pregnancy progresses if achievable without hypoglycemia)

*May need to be monitored more frequently than usual.

glycemia, or those who are using continuous subcutaneous insulin infusion. Continuous glucose monitoring (CGM) can be used in pregnancy and may help diagnose high postprandial glucose levels and nocturnal hypoglycemia that are missed with SMBG. Insulin dosing prior to meals should be based on SMBG values, not CGM readings. The patient should be instructed to self-adjust insulin and maintain a careful record of the daily glucose and insulin values with comments about calorie intake and exercise.

Available data are too limited to permit specific recommendations regarding exercise programs in pregnant women with diabetes, but in most women with type 1 diabetes, the general recommendations for all pregnant women apply.

A1C testing. A1C testing should be obtained at the patient's first prenatal visit to assess previous glycemic control. This test should be repeated every 4–6 weeks.

Ketone testing. Patients should be instructed to test for ketones any time glucose levels exceed 200 mg/dL (11.1 mmol/L).

Insulin Regimen During Pregnancy

An insulin regimen tailored to the patient's needs can be developed based on SMBG and CGM data (when available), the meal plan, and the exercise regimen. Almost all women will require preprandial rapid- or short-acting insulin with a basal insulin. In 2015, the U.S. Food and Drug Administration (FDA) mandated that the previous pregnancy categories be eliminated by 2018, and replaced by text that more clearly explains the available information regarding risks of medications to pregnant women and fetuses, and lactating mothers. Currently, the basal insulin detemir is assigned to the FDA pregnancy category B (adverse effects emerged in animal studies, but adequate and well-controlled trials with pregnant women failed to demonstrate a risk to the fetus during the first trimester, and there is no evidence of risk in later trimesters). Although the basal insulin glargine is FDA pregnancy category C (animal reproduction studies have shown an adverse effect on the fetus and there are no adequate and well-controlled studies in humans, but potential benefits may warrant use of the drug in pregnant women despite potential risks), there have been reports of the use of insulin glargine in pregnancy that have shown no increase in morbidity or macrosomia. For women who are well controlled on a long-acting analog prior to pregnancy, the theoretical benefit of switching to NPH insulin (which has a long track record of safety in pregnancy) must be weighed against the risks of a deterioration in glycemic control or increased number of hypoglycemic reactions with a change in regimen. The greatest flexibility and control is provided by insulin pump therapy. Rapid-acting insulin analogs are preferred over regular insulin for premeal boluses.

Some women may be controlled with a morning mixture of intermediate-acting and rapid- or short-acting insulins, rapid- or short-acting insulin before supper, and intermediate-acting insulin near bedtime. This regimen helps avoid glycemic irregularities overnight, decreasing the likelihood of nocturnal hypoglycemia and providing effective prophylactic treatment for the dawn phenomenon and/or the waning of the insulin effect in the early morning hours leading to prebreakfast hyperglycemia. However, postlunch glucose levels may be difficult to control without a prelunch injection of rapid- or short-acting insulin.

During pregnancy, some women prefer the flexibility of a four-injection regimen: a mixture of intermediate-acting and rapid- or short-acting insulins at breakfast, rapid- or short-acting insulin at lunch and supper, with an injection of intermediate- or long-acting insulin at bedtime.

In general, if glucose levels remain elevated pre- or postmeal, the corresponding insulin dose should be increased by 10–20%. Although glycemic goals are lower, strategies for titrating insulin doses are similar in pregnant women to those used in nonpregnant adults (see Optimizing Blood Glucose Control, page 91).

Insulin pump therapy. Pump therapy in pregnancy is best managed by a diabetes team with expertise in this form of therapy. Patients who have used insulin pump therapy before gestation should continue on this program. Patients who are not at goal during preconception should be considered for pump therapy. Transitioning to pump therapy during pregnancy is less preferable; it is best to make the transition prior to conception in order to optimize glycemic control and make sure the woman is comfortable using pump therapy prior to the first trimester.

Pump therapy in pregnancy offers several advantages over multiple daily injections. Rapid-acting insulin is infused continuously for basal requirements with active boluses from the patient for carbohydrate loads and/or correction of high glucose levels. Quick titration of both basal insulin and bolus insulin to achieve the stringent goals of pregnancy without hypoglycemia is relatively easily accomplished. In times of morning sickness in the first trimester, the patient can rely on her basal infusion and take the bolus postmeal once food is consumed. Boluses for snacks are also easily covered without the need of a separate injection. Most pregnant women use at least 2–3 basal infusion rates per 24 h, with an increased rate in the early morning hours to counteract the increased release of the counterregulatory hormones, growth hormone, and cortisol later in pregnancy. The pump also allows the nocturnal basal infusion to be decreased early in pregnancy if needed to reduce the risk of hypoglycemia. Insulin infusion rates can be temporarily increased or decreased for short periods of time to prevent hypo- or hyperglycemia.

Pump therapy is not without risks during pregnancy. Most important, since pregnancy is already a ketogenic state, should there be an interruption of insulin delivery, rapid development of ketoacidosis may occur. All pregnant patients on pumps must be instructed at each visit how to troubleshoot hyperglycemia and change the infusion set and insulin reservoir if hyperglycemia (>200 mg/dL [>11.1 mmol/L]) does not respond to a correction bolus. All women should be educated regarding ketone monitoring at home should hyperglycemia persist. This is particularly important because pregnant women with diabetes are at increased risk for euglycemic diabetic ketoacidosis. Changing of the infusion site every 2 days is often needed in addition to rotation of the sites away from the abdominal area in the third trimester—to the the upper buttocks or thighs, for example. Skin irritation can be more common in pregnancy, and appropriate troubleshooting must be instituted.

NUTRITION NEEDS

The daily nutrition needs of pregnant women with type 1 diabetes should be based on a nutrition assessment by a dietitian. SMBG results, ketone tests, appetite, and weight gain can be a guide to developing and evaluating an individualized meal plan.

For most patients, 10% of their daily calories should be consumed at breakfast, 30% at lunch, and 30% at supper. The remaining 30% of calories can be distributed among several snacks, particularly at bedtime to decrease the risk of nocturnal hypoglycemia. Nutrient-dense, high-fiber foods should be predominant in the maternal diet. Additional snacks may be added if the patient anticipates an increase in physical activity. Patients with persistently elevated midmorning glucose levels should reduce the calorie and/or fat content of breakfast and redistribute the calories to lunch and supper. Fat can slow digestion, resulting in elevated blood glucose levels later than when carbohydrate alone is eaten. The presence of morning ketonuria with normal glucose levels indicates the need to increase the calorie content of the bedtime snack or to consider adding a snack around 3:00 A.M. However, there is no evidence that starvation ketosis has an effect on outcome. The calorie content of the meal plan may be reduced in women who are obese, who demonstrate early excessive weight gain, or who have a sedentary lifestyle. Guidelines for calorie needs for women who begin pregnancy at a desirable weight can be obtained from appropriate references (also see Nutrition, beginning on page 125 in the Tools of Therapy chapter). Attention should be paid to providing sufficient intake of folate (in the form of supplementation of 800 µg daily), calcium, other vitamins, and iron, although these vitamins and minerals are important for all pregnant women and not specific to women with diabetes.

OUTPATIENT CARE

Most women with type 1 diabetes may be managed as outpatients throughout gestation. Some may benefit from early hospitalization to evaluate cardiovascular and renal status and glucose control. Failure to maintain acceptable glucose levels, worsening hypertension, or infectious complications, such as a viral illness or pyelonephritis, may necessitate hospitalization. A urine culture may be ordered in the first trimester because up to 25% of women with type 1 diabetes can have asymptomatic urinary tract infections in the first trimester.

Clinic visits can be scheduled at monthly intervals early in pregnancy if glycemic control is good, but should be scheduled at 1- to 2-week intervals if glycemic control is poor during the first trimester. At each visit, the patient's SMBG meter, log, or uploaded data should be reviewed, problems with hyperglycemia and/or hypoglycemia discussed, and the patient's weight gain and blood pressure checked. The patient should also be instructed to contact the team promptly if there are any recurrent episodes of hypoglycemia (<50 mg/dL [<2.8 mmol/L]) or hyperglycemia (>200 mg/dL [>11.1 mmol/L]) so that appropriate immediate remedial action may be taken.

Throughout gestation, the physician coordinating the patient's management must communicate regularly with other members of the medical management team. If background retinopathy has been detected, repeat ophthalmologic examinations should be obtained in the second or third trimester; proliferative retinopathy requires more intensive follow-up. If rapid normalization of blood glucose is needed, then monthly visits to the ophthalmologist are necessary to treat any development of neovascularization. Renal function studies, including creatinine clearance and protein excretion, should be repeated in each trimester if baseline values are abnormal.

Assessment of Fetal Condition

Significant advances have been made in the ability to assess fetal growth and well-being. The detection of fetal malformations between 16 and 20 weeks is discussed above (see Congenital Malformations and Abnormal Fetal Growth: Risk and Detection, page 202). In the third trimester, attention should be directed toward the assessment of fetal well-being, growth, and pulmonary maturation. Several approaches should be used to assess fetal condition to prevent sudden intrauterine death, a catastrophe most likely to occur during the final 4–6 weeks of gestation.

Patient self-assessment. Maternal monitoring of fetal activity has proved to be a simple yet valuable screening approach in high-risk pregnancies. Daily assessment of fetal movement may be started at 28 weeks' gestation. The patient counts fetal activity for several 30- to 60-min periods throughout the day or records the time of day at which she has felt a total of 10 fetal movements. A significant decrease in fetal activity demands further evaluation.

Nonstress test. The nonstress test (NST) is an ideal screening technique that is easily performed in an outpatient setting and usually requires no more than 20 min. Fetal heart rate is recorded with an external heart rate monitor. A normal response is the presence of two or more accelerations of at least 15 beats and lasting at least 15 sec during 20 min of observation. This "reactive" test is considered a reassuring finding. In a metabolically stable patient, a reactive NST will predict fetal survival for up to 1 week.

The NST may be performed weekly after 28 weeks of gestation and then twice weekly after 32 weeks. Because normal fetal activity and a reactive NST are rarely associated with an intrauterine fetal death, the primary value of surveillance is to allow the clinician to delay delivery safely while the fetus gains further maturity. However, because the screening tests have significant false-positive rates, an abnormal test, e.g., a decrease in fetal activity, must be further evaluated.

Biophysical profile. Some clinicians have turned to the biophysical profile to assess fetal condition. The biophysical profile utilizes real-time ultrasound to observe fetal activity, fetal breathing movements, amniotic fluid volume, and fetal tone. Like the NST, the biophysical profile can usually be completed quickly (in 15 min) and, if normal, indicates fetal well-being.

Assessment of Fetal Growth

Fetal growth assessment with serial ultrasound examinations may be warranted during the third trimester in women at risk for fetal growth restriction (due to maternal hypertension or vasculopathy) or excessive fetal growth (due to poor glycemic control), or in lower-risk women if there is a discrepancy between fundal height and pregnancy dates. Delivery by cesarean section should be considered if the ultrasound suggests excessive fetal size. In pregnancies complicated by diabetes, an infant >4,000 g increases the risk of shoulder dystocia. At 18–20 weeks, an anatomic ultrasound may help detect congenital malformations and a maternal Doppler may be a good early assessment for preeclampsia.

The techniques utilized today for antepartum fetal surveillance permit most patients to remain out of the hospital even during the final 4–6 weeks of gestation, as long as maternal control is acceptable and fetal evaluation is reassuring. Nevertheless, hospitalization may be necessary if the patient has kidney disease and/or hypertension, if she has not adhered to the regimen, or when fetal jeopardy is suspected.

TIMING OF DELIVERY

In the past, preterm delivery was often elected to avoid the risk of intrauterine fetal death. In many instances, such infants, although born alive, succumbed to respiratory distress syndrome (RDS). An increased incidence of RDS due to the combined effects of prematurity and diabetes, which may retard normal maturation of pulmonary surfactant production, was observed in infants of mothers with diabetes.

Today, delivery can be safely delayed until 38 weeks in most pregnancies complicated by type 1 diabetes. Labor may then be induced after 38 weeks without amniocentesis to confirm lung maturity, or the onset of spontaneous labor may be awaited. Patients must continue excellent glycemic control, and all parameters of antepartum fetal surveillance should remain normal.

In women who have vasculopathy, who have had poor glycemic control, who have had a prior stillbirth, or who have not adhered to the program of care, early elective delivery to prevent a late fetal death may be planned provided that fetal pulmonary maturation has been confirmed by the analysis of amniotic fluid obtained by amniocentesis. RDS is highly unlikely when the amniotic fluid lecithin-to-sphingomyelin ratio is >2.0 and phosphatidylglycerol is present.

If the fetal lungs are immature, delivery may be postponed as long as the results of fetal assessment remain reassuring. It is essential that the obstetrician know the reliability of the analytical technique used for phospholipid analysis in the reporting laboratory, particularly in pregnancies complicated by diabetes.

Delivery despite fetal lung immaturity may be necessary when testing suggests fetal compromise or if the pregnant patient develops preeclampsia, rapidly worsening retinopathy, or renal failure. As is the case in nondiabetic pregnancies, antenatal glucocorticoids are indicated to enhance lung maturity for preterm delivery at 24–33 weeks' gestation; however, there are no clinical trials specifically in diabetic pregnancies or in deliveries at 33–38 weeks if indices of fetal lung maturity are abnormal. Administration of high-dose corticosteroids will cause hyperglycemia in the mother with diabetes, and this should be treated aggressively.

LABOR AND DELIVERY

The timing and site of delivery must be discussed and coordinated with the neonatologists who are to be present. If delivery is anticipated and adequate maternal or neonatal care cannot be provided, the patient should be transferred to a hospital with an appropriately equipped nursery. Expert care is required to deal with the various complications that may arise in the infant of the mother with diabetes.

Intrapartum electronic monitoring of the fetal heart rate is mandatory. Labor should be allowed to progress as long as cervical dilation and descent follow the established curves for normal labor. Any evidence of an arrest pattern should alert the physician to the possibility of cephalopelvic disproportion and fetal macrosomia.

Maternal Glucose Levels During Delivery

Maintenance of normal maternal glucose levels (60–100 mg/dL [3.3–5.6 mmol/L]) during labor and delivery is important in eliminating hypoglycemia for the mother and keeping both mother and child safe. Though a more recent study shows a stronger correlation of maternal A1C during the second trimester to neonatal hypoglycemia than maternal glucose levels during labor and delivery, other studies show normal maternal glucose levels will reduce the risk of subsequent neonatal hypoglycemia. A glucose and insulin infusion can be used to maintain glucose levels in this range. Below are insulin infusion rates deemed safe and effective in maintaining maternal glucose levels during labor.

Infuse a 10% dextrose solution at an 80 mL/h rate and with hourly capillary blood glucose monitoring:

- constant 1 unit/h with a blood glucose level of 61–140 mg/dL (3.4–7.8 mmol/L)
- increase to 1.5 units/h for blood glucose of 140–180 mg/dL (7.8–10.0 mmol/L)
- increase to 2 units/h for blood glucose of 180–220 mg/dL (10.0–12.2 mmol/L)
- increase to 2 units/h for blood glucose of 220 mg/dL (10.0–12.2mmol/L)

OR

Infuse a 5% dextrose solution at a 100–150 mL/h rate (2.5 mg/kg/min) and with hourly capillary blood glucose monitoring:

- constant 1.25 units/h if glucose level >110 mg/dL (5.6 mmol/L)
- adjust insulin or dextrose infusion rate hourly to achieve a ~100 mg/dL (5.6 mmol/L) glucose level

During active labor in most patients, insulin requirements typically decrease substantially, with most patients requiring a reduction in their basal insulin. Glucose levels should be determined hourly with SMBG or CGM techniques at the bedside, because even small doses of insulin may produce hypoglycemia during active labor. Adjustments in the delivery of insulin and/or glucose should be made based on the glucose determinations. See *Medical Management of Pregnancy Complicated by Diabetes* for more information (also see Bibliography, page 211).

If labor is electively induced or a cesarean section is planned, the procedure should be scheduled for the early morning and the patient's usual morning rapid- or short-acting insulin dose withheld. Further glycemic control can be achieved if the patient is fasting. If using an insulin pump, the basal insulin may be continued at lower rates with further decreases in the basal rates at the time of delivery to avoid maternal hypoglycemia. Epidural anesthesia is preferred in patients scheduled for cesarean section. After the operation has been completed, glucose levels should be monitored every 1–2 h, and an intravenous solution containing 5% dextrose should be continued. Because human placental lactogen and its counterregulatory actions fall rapidly after removal of the placenta, no or very little insulin may be required for the remainder of the day if the previous injection of long-acting insulin is still in effect.

POSTPARTUM CARE

In the immediate postpartum period, the patient's insulin requirements are usually lower than her prepregnancy needs for the first 24–48 h. The antepartum objective of physiologic glycemic control is usually relaxed at this time and returned to prepregnancy levels (90–130 mg/dL [5.0–7.2 mmol/L]). If the patient uses an insulin pump, the basal rate should be reset at or below the prepregnancy rate. Breast-feeding is encouraged. The meal plan for the breast-feeding mother should be 30–37 kcal/kg desirable body weight. Breast-feeding may induce hypoglycemia and, thus, basal insulin requirements may be lower in women who breast-feed than they were prepregnancy and women may require a small carbohydrate snack with each feeding or breast-pumping session.

If the patient delivered vaginally, and if glucose levels are ≥200 mg/dL, short-acting insulin should be administered as necessary as a correction bolus based on prepregnancy requirements, or an insulin infusion can be continued or started. Once eating, the insulin regimen can be resumed but lowered to or below the prepregnancy insulin requirements. The doses should be adjusted based on SMBG.

In patients who have undergone a cesarean section, minimal insulin may be required for the first 2 postoperative days because calorie intake is limited. By day two or three, the prepregnancy insulin schedule may be resumed and the dose adjusted using SMBG. Further adjustment of insulin needs in the postpartum period should always be individualized based on SMBG results.

FAMILY PLANNING AND CONTRACEPTION

Family planning and contraception must be reviewed with the patient during the postpartum period. The most effective methods for contraception that are reversible include intrauterine devices (IUD), contraceptive implants, and progestin-only injections, in decreasing order of effectiveness. Oral contraceptives are commonly used, but the increased risk of thromboembolic disease and vasculopathy require that combined estrogen/progestin oral contraceptive preparations be used with caution; they are contraindicated in women who have macrovascular disease, vasculopathy, or hypertension, and the risks may outweigh the benefits in women who have had diabetes for longer than 20 years. For these women, low-dose (≤35 μg) estrogen agents, progestin-only agents (pills or injections), etonogestrel implants, or IUDs should be prescribed. For women planning to breastfeed, progestin-only agents are recommended. After >20 years of diabetes, women, regardless of the presence of macrovascular disease, retinopathy, kidney disease, or neuropathy, should be removed from a combination hormone treatment and placed on a single hormone treatment or an IUD. Risk for weight gain and user error should be considered in the case of progestin-only pills or injections. Condoms should be encouraged in all patients as a secondary/dual form of contraception as they also help protect against sexually transmitted diseases.

Motivated patients may do well with one of the barrier methods of contraception, such as the diaphragm, although their efficacy is significantly lower than that of oral contraceptives. Sterilization of the patient or her partner should be discussed with the patient when she has completed her family or if she has serious vasculopathy. All contraception discussions should be in accordance with the patient's religious and cultural beliefs.

CONCLUSION

Advances in prenatal care and diagnosis, fetal surveillance, and perinatal care have markedly improved maternal and fetal well-being in pregnancy complicated by diabetes. Meticulous metabolic control before and during pregnancy holds the key to a successful outcome and to minimizing fetal malformations or perinatal complications. A team approach is more likely to achieve a desirable result.

BIBLIOGRAPHY

ACOG Practice Bulletin: Clinical Management Guidelines for Obstetrician-Gynecologists. Number 60. March 2005. Pregestational diabetes mellitus. *Obstet Gynecol* 2005;105:675–685

American Diabetes Association. *Medical Management of Pregnancy Complicated by Diabetes.* 4th ed. Jovanovic L, Ed. Alexandria, VA, American Diabetes Association, 2009

American Diabetes Association. Preconception care of women with diabetes (Position Statement). *Diabetes Care* 2004;27(Suppl. 1):S76–S78

Blumer I, Hadar E, Hadden DR, Jovanovič L, Mestman JH, Murad MH, Yogev Y. Diabetes and pregnancy: an Endocrine Society clinical practice guideline. *J Clin Endocrinol Metab* 2013;98:4227–4249

Codner E, Soto N, Merino PM. Contraception, and pregnancy in adolescents with type 1 diabetes: a review. *Pediatr Diabetes* 2012;13:108–123

Jensen DM, Beck-Nielsen H, Damm P, Westergaard JG, Ovesen P, Moeller M, Mølsted-Pedersen L, Mathiesen ER. Microalbumenuria, preeclampsia and preterm delivery in pregnant women with type 1 diabetes: results from a nationwide Danish study. *Diabetes Care* 2010;33:90–94

Johnstone FD, Lindsay RS, Steel J. Type 1 diabetes and pregnancy: trends in birth weight over 40 years at a single clinic. *Obstet Gynecol* 2006;107:1297–1302

Jovanovic L, Peterson CM, Reed GF, Metzger BE, Mills JL, Knopp RH, Aarons JH. Maternal postprandial glucose levels and infant birth weight: the Diabetes in Early Pregnancy Study. The National Institute of Child Health and Human Development—Diabetes in Early Pregnancy Study. *Am J Obstet Gynecol* 1991;164:103–111

Kitzmiller JL, Block JM, Brown FM, et al. Managing preexisting diabetes for pregnancy: summary of evidence and consensus recommendations for care. *Diabetes Care* 2008;31:1060–79

Lepercq J, Abbou H, Agostini C, Toubas F, Francoual C, Velho G, Dubois-Laforgue D, Timsit J. A standardized protocol to achieve normoglycaemia during labour and delivery in women with type 1 diabetes. *Diabetes Metab* 2008;34:33–37

Mukherjee MS, Coppenrath VA, Dallinga BA. Pharmacologic management of types 1 and 2 diabetes mellitus and their complications in women of child-bearing age. *Pharmacotherapy* 2015;35:158–174

Price N, Bartlett C, Gillmer MD. Use of insulin glargine during pregnancy: a case-control pilot study. *BJOG: An International Journal of Obstetrics and Gynaecology* 2007;114:453–457

Trujillo AL. Insulin analogs and pregnancy. *Diabetes Spectrum* 2007;20:94–101

Vargas R, Repke JT, Ural SH. Type 1 diabetes mellitus and pregnancy. *Rev Obstet Gynecol* 2010;3:92–100

Yogev Y, Chen R, Ben-Haroush A, Phillip M, Jovanovic L, Hod M. Continuous glucose monitoring for the evaluation of gravid women with type 1 diabetes mellitus. *Obstet Gynecol* 2003;101:633–638

The physician caring for patients with type 1 diabetes must become familiar with perioperative management; factors that affect decisions about glycemic management include duration of surgery and anticipated duration of nothing-by-mouth (NPO) status. In the critical care setting, continuous intravenous insulin infusion has been shown to be the best method for achieving glycemic targets and should be administered based on validated written or computerized protocols that allow for predefined adjustments in the infusion rate, accounting for glycemic fluctuations and insulin dose. The target glucose range for the perioperative period should be 80–180 mg/dL (4.4–10.0 mmol/L).

On the morning of the surgery or procedure, any non-insulin hypoglycemic agents should be held. Patients should administer only half of the usual NPH dose, or a full dose of a long-acting analog or pump basal insulin. Blood glucose needs to be monitored every 4–6 h while NPO and patients should be dosed with short-acting insulin as needed.

GENERAL PRINCIPLES

The objectives of glycemic management during surgery are to maintain good glycemic control to avoid metabolic derangements while also avoiding hypoglycemia. Insulin resistance and gluconeogenesis increase during stress. For this reason, the customary basal insulin dosage is the *minimum* requirement during the perioperative period. Additional insulin will be needed to prevent excessive hepatic glucose production and decreased peripheral glucose uptake while maintaining good glycemic control and normal fluid and electrolyte balance. Perioperative hyperglycemia leads to delayed healing and increased risks of infection and ischemia. Although one large study suggested that critically ill, postoperative patients receiving ventilator support in the intensive care unit have lower morbidity and mortality with tight glycemic control on an insulin infusion as compared with less intensive glycemic control, it is unclear whether this applies to patients with type 1 diabetes or those who do not require ventilator support. An operative/postoperative team guided by frequent glucose monitoring, using a simple and safe algorithm for intravenous insulin administration, can maintain good glycemic control and metabolism.

Omission of basal insulin will precipitate DKA in patients with type 1 diabetes and should be avoided. Furthermore, when transitioning from a continuous intravenous infusion of insulin to subcutaneous insulin, the first basal dose of insulin should be administered at least 2 h prior to discontinuation of the insulin infusion. A particular concern in the hospital setting is the inadvertent discontinuation of all or part of the insulin order set including basal insulin during transfer to a different unit. Clinicians should be alert to this possibility and take measures to make sure the appropriate orders are in place during and after each transition.

MAJOR SURGERY

Elective Surgery

The patient scheduled for elective surgery should be placed on intravenous insulin and dextrose infusion several hours preoperatively and maintained at a blood glucose level between 100–180 mg/dL (5.3–9.6 mmol/L). Appropriate preoperative evaluation should be performed before surgery, including assessment of the patient's metabolic state, renal function, and myocardial function. Once this evaluation is complete, surgery can be performed at any time of the day based on the urgency of the surgical condition.

Intravenous infusion of insulin rather than subcutaneous insulin administration is indicated during the perioperative period. Intravenous infusion allows careful control of the amount and speed of insulin delivery and circumvents problems with subcutaneous absorption in the event of shock.

Emergency Surgery

In the event of emergency surgery requiring general anesthesia, there is usually sufficient time to optimally evaluate and stabilize the patient before surgery. In the event of DKA in a patient who needs emergency surgery, e.g., trauma and ketoacidosis, the condition can be treated concurrently with surgery.

MINOR SURGERY

Patients undergoing elective surgery with local anesthesia (e.g., dental work) should fast prior to surgery. The ideal management during these circumstances is to withhold food, withhold short-acting insulin, and continue long-acting basal insulin via subcutaneous injection or insulin pump. If the person with type 1 diabetes is being managed in some other manner, they should be switched to a basal-bolus regimen before the elective procedure. Alternatively, the morning dose of NPH can be decreased by one-third and supplemental rapid-acting insulin analog can be used as needed.

CONCLUSION

Medical management of the patient with diabetes requiring major surgery must focus on provision of dextrose and insulin in amounts to maintain good glycemic control and avoid metabolic derangements during and after surgery, while avoiding hypoglycemia. Intravenous insulin and dextrose infusions at a rate adjusted for the individual's insulin requirement titrated from frequent blood glucose values can safely keep blood glucose levels between 100–180 mg/dL (5.3–9.6 mmol/L).

BIBLIOGRAPHY

ACE/ADA Task Force on Inpatient Diabetes. American College of Endocrinology and American Diabetes Association Consensus Statement on inpatient glycemic control: a call to action. *Diabetes Care* 2006;29:1955–1962

Jacobi J, Bircher N, Krinsley J, Agus M, Braithwaite SS, Deutschman C, et al. Guidelines for the use of an insulin infusion for the management of hyperglycemia in critically ill patients. *Crit Care Med* 2012;40:3251–3276

Pittas AG, Siegal RD, Lau J. Insulin therapy for critically ill hospitalized patients: a meta-analysis of randomized controlled trials. *Arch Intern Med* 2004;164:2005–2011

Umpierrez GE, Hellman R, Korytkowski MT, Kosiborod M, Maynard GA, Montori VM, Seley JJ, Van den Berghe G; Endocrine Society. Management of hyperglycemia in hospitalized patients in non-critical care setting: an Endocrine Society clinical practice guideline. *J Clin Endocrinol Metab* 2012;97:16–38

Van den Berghe G, Wouters P, Weekers F, Verwaest C, Bruyninckx F, Schetz M, Vlasselaers D, Ferdinande P, Lauwers P, Bouillon R. Intensive insulin therapy in critically ill patients. *N Engl J Med* 2001;345:1359–1367

Zerr KJ, Furnary AP, Grunkemeier GL, Bookin S, Kanhere V, Starr A. Glucose control lowers the risk of wound infection in diabetics after open heart operations. *Ann Thorac Surg* 1997;63:356–361

CELL REPLACEMENT STRATEGIES

Significant progress in the field of islet and pancreatic transplantation has occurred, including research on islet encapsulation and cell replacement strategies including stem cell therapy, xenotransplantation, and regenerative medicine with organ bioengineering (because of a scarcity of available organs and tissue). In July 2000, a team from University of Alberta in Edmonton reported success in achieving up to 14 months of insulin independence with normalization of A1C and resolution of recurrent severe hypoglycemia in seven patients with type 1 diabetes, using human islet allotransplantation from cadaver pancreases. Their success was attributed to improved human islet isolation and purification procedures, along with different immunosuppression regimens that avoided the use of glucocorticoids and cyclosporine, which had been shown to be toxic to islets. After their initial report, hundreds of other islet allotransplantations into the portal vein of the liver have been performed in designated research centers around the world using variations of the Edmonton Protocol. Individual centers reported good success; however, the 2006 results of a carefully conducted multicenter trial of the Edmonton Protocol were somewhat mixed: 44% of patients achieved insulin independence and normalization of A1C at 1 year post–islet transplantation, but the majority of patients required resumption of insulin therapy 3–5 years after transplantation. More than one cadaver pancreas was used in staged procedures in most patients, with some requiring islets from three or more cadaver pancreases. However, patients with residual islet function are protected from severe hypoglycemia. With ongoing research, newer immunomodulatory regimens and other improvements, including identification of optimal donor tissue, have resulted in 5-year graft survival and higher rates of insulin independence.

However, islet and pancreas allotransplantations are associated with significant surgical risks and complications to patients. The most significant complication has been hepatic bleeding, with two reported cases of portal vein thrombosis. Other complications include mouth ulcerations from sirolimus, transient rise in liver enzymes, the need for statin therapy, renal dysfunction, severe neutropenia, and rare cases of pneumonitis, with one death from pneumonitis reported in a European center. No cancers or infection with cytomegalovirus have been reported, but these remain theoretical risks with longer-term immunosuppression.

As a result of these risks, islet and pancreatic allotransplantation is only recommended for certain patients in whom the benefits of avoiding severe hypoglycemia outweigh the risks of the islet allotransplantation procedure and the ongoing risks of chronic immunosuppression. Most transplants have been done in patients with recurrent, refractory, severe hypoglycemia or marked glycemic instability. It is not known yet whether such transplantation will reverse or stop microvascular complications, because glucose intolerance persists.

Additional research is ongoing in multiple areas to improve the current clinical results. These areas involve:

- improving islet yield from cadaver pancreases
- refining the protocol to improve islet survival and engraftment
- encapsulation to protect transplanted islets

- improving immunomodulation strategies
- achieving donor-specific immune tolerance

If success is achieved in these areas, the critical challenge will be to identify sufficient and suitable sources of insulin-producing tissue to treat the large number of patients who could benefit from this therapy. For these reasons, research on xenogeneic islets, embryonic and adult stem cells, islet regeneration and proliferation, and engineering of insulin-producing cells continues. It is important to identify the ideal source of insulin-producing tissue that can be utilized on a large scale once the current limitations of immunosuppression are resolved.

BIBLIOGRAPHY

Cogger K, Nostro MC. Recent advances in cell replacement therapies for the treatment of type 1 diabetes. *Endocrinology* 2015;156:8–15

McCall M, Shapiro AM. Islet cell transplantation. *Semin Ped Surg* 2014;23:83–90

Orlando G, Gianello P, Salvatori M, Stratta RJ, Soker S, Ricordi C, Dominguez-Bendala J. Cell replacement strategies aimed at reconstitution of the β-cell compartment in type 1 diabetes. *Diabetes* 2014;63:1433–1444

Shapiro AM, Ricordi C, Hering BJ, Auchincloss H, Lindblad R, Robertson RP, Secchi A, Brendel MD, Berney T, Brennan DC, Cagliero E, Alejandro R, Ryan EA, DiMercurio B, Morel P, Polonsky KS, Reems JA, Bretzel RG, Bertucci F, Froud T, Kandaswamy R, Sutherland DE, Eisenbarth G, Segal M, Preiksaitis J, Korbutt GS, Barton FB, Viviano L, Seyfert-Margolis V, Bluestone J, Lakey JR. International trial of the Edmonton Protocol for islet transplantation. *N Engl J Med* 2006;355:1318–1330

Shapiro AMJ, Lakey JRT, Ryan EA, Korbutt GS, Toth E, Warnock GL, Kneteman NM, Rajotte RV. Islet transplantation in seven patients with type 1 diabetes using a glucocorticoid-free immunosuppressive regimen. *N Engl J Med* 2000;343:230–238

Psychosocial Factors Affecting Adherence, Quality of Life, and Well-Being: Helping Patients Cope

Highlights
Psychosocial Factors Affecting Adherence, Quality of Life, and Well-Being: Helping Patients Cope

PERIODS OF INCREASED EMOTIONAL DISTRESS

- Emotional distress can be high at the time of diagnosis, when the honeymoon period is over, when planning pregnancy, and at the onset of complications. Psychological equilibrium can generally be reestablished with early identification of distress; initiation of medical, psychological, and social supports; and monitoring of intervention effects. Initiation of multidisciplinary intervention can improve adaptation and adherence and prevent deterioration in metabolic control.

- Monitoring of emotional status, quality of life, and well-being is an ongoing component of comprehensive diabetes care.

MAINTAINING ADHERENCE

- Over time or periodically, motivation to maintain optimal diabetes control may wane. Maintenance strategies include planning a lifestyle-based diabetes regimen, improving patient/care provider communication, addressing barriers, screening for depression, and employing research-tested educational and behavioral strategies.

DIABETES COMPLICATIONS

- Psychosocial factors should be suspected in the case of extreme poor control and/or recurrent diabetic ketoacidosis.

- Repeat episodes of severe hypoglycemia can have serious psychosocial consequences, which call for medical, educational, behavioral, and family intervention.

- When chronic complications begin, feelings of anger and guilt are common. Interventions that include psychological counseling and adaptive coping strategies can help resolve these emotional reactions. Family members should be included in the intervention whenever possible.

DEVELOPMENTAL CONSIDERATIONS IN CHILDREN

- Although a diagnosis of diabetes during childhood can be a devastating experience for parents and children, families are usually resilient and adapt to the demands of the regimen within the first year.

- Because children and adolescents are growing, developing, and acquiring new motor skills, cognitive abilities, and emotional maturity, the management priorities and self-management issues change over time. However, continued parental involvement is necessary throughout childhood and adolescence. Caution should be exercised in forcing too much self-care too soon or abandoning parental oversight during adolescence. Sharing diabetes care responsibilities produces the best glycemic outcomes and reduces individual burden.

DEVELOPMENTAL CONSIDERATIONS IN ADOLESCENTS

- For adolescents, peer influences, together with family support and supervision, play an important role in adherence and glycemic control.
- Many aspects of the treatment regimen are at odds with adolescents' normal drive for independence and peer acceptance. New technologies have enabled adolescents to maintain a flexible lifestyle but at the cost of increased monitoring and diabetes care tasks.

ADULTS

- Misunderstandings about diabetes on the part of the patient or parent can interfere with young adult patients' carrying out usual developmental tasks such as developing an independent life from parents.
- Adults with diabetes must deal with a disease and care regimen that complicates their interpersonal relationships and their attempts to establish a family and career, and presents a financial burden as well. Thorough and anticipatory education of patients, family members,

and significant others can facilitate normalization of expectations.

THE ELDERLY

- Older adults with long-standing diabetes can often benefit from reeducation regarding newer technologies and care regimens.
- The demands of the diabetes regimen may be especially burdensome for the elderly, who face other difficult life events such as retirement, loss of physical function, living on a fixed income, the death of a spouse and/or friends, and their own mortality.
- The goal of diabetes care is to maximize physical and psychosocial functioning while respecting the patient's autonomy and independence as much as possible. Availability and maintenance of social support can be particularly difficult for the elderly, who often find themselves dependent on family and friends when physical capacities and financial resources diminish.

EMOTIONAL AND BEHAVIORAL DISORDERS AND DIABETES

- Ongoing monitoring of the psychological status of patients will help with detection of diabetes-related distress and nondiabetes-related psychopathology. It is important to determine whether psychopathology is diabetes related or due to other causes.
- Whenever possible, it is recommended that the health-care team include a mental health professional familiar with diabetes and its care regimen.

- Depression and anxiety disorders have been found to occur frequently in patients with diabetes. Some disorders, such as fear of hypoglycemia, needle phobia, and fear of complications and premature death, are specifically related to having diabetes.
- Eating disorders should be suspected in individuals, especially young women with a history of unstable or poor metabolic control, recurrent ketoacidosis, or recurrent severe hypoglycemia, and in girls with growth retardation, pubertal delay, and/or amenorrhea.

STRESS AND DIABETES

- Results of studies investigating the relationship between stress and blood glucose control have been inconclusive. The impact of stress on glycemia seems to be highly individualized.
- It is important to establish a patient's stress reactivity to develop coping strategies to maintain good glycemic control up to, during, and after stressful events.
- Stress can indirectly affect blood glucose control by undermining adherence to the diabetes treatment regimen.

Psychosocial Factors Affecting Adherence, Quality of Life, and Well-Being: Helping Patients Cope

Diabetes is a demanding chronic disease. Although it is true that type 1 diabetes affects the patient's psychosocial well-being, the converse is also true: psychosocial factors can affect diabetes management. The unrelenting demands, inconveniences, frustrations of treatment, and possibilities of disability or death put tremendous emotional and financial strain on patients with diabetes and their significant others. Patients must struggle continuously to achieve a balance between the demands of their everyday lives and those of their diabetes regimen. To help patients cope successfully with diabetes in their everyday lives, the diabetes management team must consider the patient's daily schedule, lifestyle, and developmental stage, social and financial supports, motivations, and values and preferences when working collaboratively to make diabetes management decisions and set treatment goals. Maintaining quality of life is as important an outcome as good glycemic control.

PERIODS OF INCREASED EMOTIONAL DISTRESS

Psychological and emotional distress is high at the time of diagnosis, after the honeymoon period ends, and at the onset of complications (Table 5.1). At diagnosis, initial shock, denial, and anger often give way to mild depression and anxiety. Studies of newly diagnosed children and their families have found, however, that the initial reactions of both parents and children resolve rather quickly, and psychological equilibrium is reestablished within the first year. More extreme or long-lasting psychological reactions may indicate a need for referral to a mental health professional for evaluation and treatment.

Ongoing monitoring of the emotional status of the patient is part of comprehensive diabetes care. Initiation of an intervention as soon as emotional distress is identified may improve adaptation, prevent psychosocial maladjustment, improve adherence, and prevent deterioration in metabolic control. All members of the diabetes management team can be a great help during these periods by being accessible and sensitive to the patient's and family's need for information, support, and resources. When indicated, a referral to a mental health professional who specializes in working with patients with diabetes is suggested.

The following are intervention suggestions aimed at facilitating adjustment and enhancing metabolic control.

Table 5.1   Factors Causing Emotional Distress

- Uncertainty about the outcome of the immediate situation
- Feelings of intense guilt and/or anger about the occurrence of diabetes, poor glycemic control, and/or complications
- Feelings of incompetence and helplessness about the responsibility of managing the illness
- Fears about future complications and early death
- Loss of valued life goals and aspirations because of illness
- Anxiety about planning for an uncertain future
- Recognition of the necessity for a permanent change in living pattern as a result of diabetes
- Fear of loss of insurance coverage

Source: Adapted from Hamburg SA, Inoff GE: Coping with predictable crises of diabetes. *Diabetes Care* 1983;6:409–416.

- It is essential that the patient and his or her significant others are involved in the initial and ongoing discussions and education regarding diabetes care behaviors and regimens, lifestyle accommodations, sharing of diabetes care tasks, and the need to balance family needs with diabetes care tasks. Both parents in the case of a child, the patient's spouse, the adult children in the case of an elderly patient, or any significant others should be included. This is important given the wealth of research showing significant associations between family and peer support and adherence, problem-solving, and glycemic control. Research with families of children who have diabetes has shown that sharing diabetes care tasks and responsibilities reduces burdens and can improve glycemic control.
- A comprehensive approach to diabetes education and management can be achieved if the roles of the diabetes management team are coordinated and regular communication takes place between care providers. Led by a physician or health professional who specializes in diabetes care, involvement of a diabetes educator, a dietitian, a social worker, and/or a psychologist will ensure that the patient and family receive the educational, dietary, and psychosocial support they need.
- Self-management education and support with newly diagnosed children and their families in the months after diagnosis prevents deterioration in metabolic control during the first 2 years after diagnosis of type 1 diabetes. Close follow-up by the diabetes management team in the weeks after the initial education will increase, reinforce, and clarify diabetes knowledge. Furthermore, emphasis on developing self-management strategies during these weeks appears to enhance adaptation and metabolic control. Self-management education and support includes reinforcement of accurate glucose monitoring and recording and the use of these data to understand

blood glucose fluctuations and make appropriate insulin and behavioral treatment changes. The goal is to help patients adopt a problem-solving approach to diabetes self-management. (See also Patient Self-Management Education and Support, page 45.)

■ Self-management education and support must be ongoing and accommodate the developmental lifestyle and agreed-on treatment goals of the patient and/or family members if the patient is a child, adolescent, or elderly person who requires assistance with care.

■ Goals of treatment, diabetes care regimen tasks, and expectations for glycemic control should be negotiated with the patient and/or supervising adult so that unrealistic goals do not cause diabetes-related distress and feelings of failure.

MAINTAINING ADHERENCE

Expectations that an individual and/or family will make multiple and significant behavior changes at one time may be unrealistic and unfeasible. Focusing on "survival skills" at the time of diagnosis (self-monitoring of blood glucose [SMBG], insulin dosing, and monitoring and treatment of hypo- and hyperglycemia and ketosis) and clearly communicating about the expectation of working toward intensive management of glucose control provide the foundation for success in diabetes self-management. Explaining the significance of each of these survival skills and how they will affect short- and long-term health is important. A step-by-step approach to behavior change is often most successful, although highly motivated patients and parents will attempt to implement health provider recommendations when they are presented.

Failure to maintain self-care behaviors in diabetes management and resultant poor metabolic control are frequently due to a lack of attention to maintenance issues. Caution is needed to monitor diabetes burnout—a state in which patients grow tired of managing their disease and then ignore it for a period of time—and feelings of being "controlled" by the disease.

INDIVIDUALIZED TREATMENT REGIMENS

Regardless of age, a patient's treatment regimen should be individually tailored. Patients have been shown to follow complex treatment regimens when the regimens meet the needs and requests of the patient and quality of life is maintained. Flexibility of lifestyle has become an important consideration in diabetes care, and advances in monitoring technology, insulins, and delivery systems have facilitated this aim. Holding a patient with diabetes to an inflexible diabetes care routine might seem to providers to be an easier way to achieve good glycemic control, but the negative impact on family and individual functioning should not be underestimated and may actually undermine success.

The priorities and personality of the patient and his or her inherent organizational proclivities should help shape the diabetes care regimen that is adopted. For example, forcing a child or adult with attention-deficit/hyperactivity disorder

(ADHD) to keep detailed glucose records may be an exercise in frustration for all involved. Conversely, if such a patient prioritizes good glucose control, the diabetes care regimen may provide structure by which the individual organizes his or her daily routines. The adolescent, in particular, may be motivated to perform more frequent monitoring, take additional insulin injections, and adhere to a specific meal plan if it is perceived that he or she can participate in desired activities or be granted special requests. Many adolescents and young adults are attracted to and comfortable with technology, so tools such as software for organizing SMBG readings may facilitate adherence and self-care. Conversely, some adolescents and adults will attain better metabolic control with more adherence to a simplified regimen than little or no adherence to a more complex or demanding regimen, such as being placed on the insulin pump or continuous glucose monitoring.

Negotiations regarding treatment regimens should be viewed by the care provider as an accommodation of the patient's treatment to lifestyle realities and the patient's value system and preferences. Patients are people who happen to have diabetes, and these people are the ones who must carry out the vast majority of management tasks. This is a departure from the philosophy of diabetes care in the past and may present difficulties for the care provider who wishes to enforce a one-size-fits-all formula for good glycemic control. Adoption of a patient-centered point of view is not only more likely to facilitate long-term successful patient self-management, but also may help providers avoid burnout and frustration as well.

DIABETES COMPLICATIONS

SHORT-TERM COMPLICATIONS

Recurrent diabetic ketoacidosis can be the consequence of underdosing or omission of insulin that occurs because of psychosocial problems, e.g., burnout, depression, psychiatric illness, financial stress, parental neglect, lack of family involvement, chronic family conflict, weight concerns, or eating disorders. Psychosocial factors should always be suspected in the case of recurrent ketoacidosis, especially after it has been established that good glycemic control can be achieved under monitored conditions. A mental health evaluation should be considered for these patients.

SEVERE HYPOGLYCEMIA

Most patients with well-controlled type 1 diabetes experience frequent hypoglycemia that is asymptomatic in addition to several mildly symptomatic low blood glucose reactions each month. In general, these symptomatic mild reactions, although distracting and uncomfortable, do not pose a serious problem for the patient. Severe hypoglycemia, however, defined as an episode in which patients are unable to treat themselves, lose consciousness, and/or have seizures, can be frightening and may have serious cognitive, neurological, and psychosocial consequences. The patient may develop fear of hypoglycemia and decide to maintain blood glucose values at unacceptably high levels, which feel emotionally acceptable to the patient. The family may also become overly fearful, watchful, or angry, blaming the patient for the disturbing glycemic episodes. Because nights are a difficult time to monitor blood glucose levels, patients and parents may also become anxious about nighttime lows, affecting sleep, which has other psychosocial impacts. Patients who experience severe hypoglycemia at work may jeopardize their job or chances for advancement.

Many patients with long-standing, well-controlled type 1 diabetes fail to recognize the early warning symptoms of hypoglycemia (hypoglycemia unawareness). These patients are at risk for repeated episodes of severe hypoglycemia and attendant medical and psychosocial consequences. Efforts should be made to prevent these episodes through reeducation and adjustments in the diabetes regimen.

The health-care provider should discuss the patient's attitudes regarding hypoglycemia and help to establish safe blood glucose goals. Target blood glucose levels may need to be raised to restore hypoglycemic awareness and the patient's confidence in recognition of symptoms. A program called Blood Glucose Awareness Training (BGAT) successfully reduces the incidence of severe hypoglycemia. The patient's family or significant others should be trained to recognize early or subtle hypoglycemic signs and provide adequate prevention and treatment measures, including the administration of glucagon. If the family is angry and blames the patient, the diabetes management team will need to help the family understand the difficulty many patients have in recognizing and avoiding hypoglycemia. The family should also understand that the patient frequently cannot control his or her behavior during a severe low blood glucose reaction.

LONG-TERM COMPLICATIONS

Although most patients are aware of the possibility of long-term complications of diabetes, the detection of the first evidence of retinopathy, kidney disease, or neuropathy can be a devastating event. When the onset of a severe complication occurs, the patient and family must cope with the grief associated with the potential or actual loss of body function. Once again, the patient and family may experience feelings of shock, denial, and anger. Feelings of anger at the health-care provider for "letting this happen" or guilt ("I should have taken better care of myself") are common. These feelings can be eased by emphasizing the positive steps that can still be taken to forestall or prevent serious problems. When complications cause disability and restrictions in lifestyle, the treating physician or health-care provider may need to refer the patient to a rehabilitation program that includes expert care or suggest counseling by an experienced mental health professional who is familiar with the disease and its treatment. Support groups or contact with people who have successfully adapted to complications can provide useful information and role models for patients and help them maintain a hopeful outlook. It is important to note that the risk of complications and the discussion of possible complications are not usually motivating factors that increase adherence; in fact, they often create feelings of anxiety and hopelessness that have the reverse of their desired effect. Broaching complications is a necessary component of diabetes education, but should be discussed carefully and at the right time for the family.

Care providers and patients may be hesitant to broach the issue of sexual dysfunction—a common complication of diabetes in all adults, both men and women. Though it is widely accepted that men with diabetes experience sexual dysfunction, women (especially older women) with type 1 diabetes can experience a wide range of symptoms as well. It is critical to ask patients routinely about sexual function in a straightforward manner. Patients may be more likely to confide in the physician or another member of the diabetes management team if they know that sexual problems are common in diabetes and that a variety of treatment options are available. Along with issues of sexual functioning, issues of reproductive health should be addressed with teens, young adults, and adults of childbearing age. As modern diabetes care has enabled women with diabetes to have healthy babies, misinformation about the inevitability of poor pregnancy outcomes needs to be counteracted. However, tight glycemic control is necessary for a healthy pregnancy and baby. Patients with diabetes must plan pregnancies and achieve excellent glycemic control *before* conception and maintain it throughout pregnancy. This information should be incorporated into routine diabetes care so that patients can make informed decisions regarding childbearing.

DEVELOPMENTAL CONSIDERATIONS IN CHILDREN

Although a diagnosis of diabetes during childhood is a devastating experience for parents and children, families are usually resilient and adapt to the demands of the regimen within the first year. Some of those demands, viewed from a developmental and family perspective, are outlined in Table 5.2.

Generally, children's responsibilities for care should increase in tandem with cognitive, motor, emotional, and psychological development. Children who share responsibility for their diabetes care are generally more knowledgeable about their diabetes and are in better metabolic control. When treating a school-age child, the diabetes management team should be attuned to his or her cognitive maturity and abilities with regard to accurately interpreting results of SMBG or continuous glucose monitoring, calculating carbohydrate intake, and preparing the correct amount of insulin with a pen, syringe, or pump. If cognitive abilities are questioned, referral for testing by a psychologist familiar with the treatment of diabetes should be considered.

Self-esteem is built through mastery of the developmental tasks of childhood and the positive regard of significant others. Children feel good about themselves when they succeed in tasks children their age are expected to master—school work, sports, social relationships, etc. Having diabetes presents children with opportunities to build self-esteem when they learn to perform diabetes-related tasks. These tasks may be as simple as setting up supplies for blood glucose tests or as advanced as calculating the correct dose and giving their own injections or wearing and/or operating an insulin pump. This is especially true if parents, the diabetes management team, and others provide positive reinforcement for their achievements. Conversely, expectations of independent functioning in diabetes care tasks without the foundation of skill mastery, parental support and monitoring, and adequate time-management skills or structure can predispose the child to feelings of failure, low self-esteem, and feeling controlled by their illness.

Table 5.2 Major Developmental Issues, Management Priorities, and Family Issues in Type 1 Diabetes in Children and Adolescents

Developmental stages (approximate ages)	Normal developmental tasks	Type 1 diabetes management priorities	Family issues in type 1 diabetes management
Infancy (0–12 months)	• Developing a trusting relationship or bond with primary caregiver(s)	• Preventing and treating hypoglycemia • Avoiding extreme fluctuations in blood glucose levels	• Coping with stress • Sharing the burden of care to avoid parent burnout
Toddler (13–36 months)	• Developing a sense of mastery and autonomy	• Preventing hypoglycemia • Avoiding extreme fluctuations in blood glucose levels due to irregular food intake	• Establishing a schedule • Managing the picky eater • Limit-setting and coping with toddler's lack of cooperation with regimen • Sharing the burden of care
Preschoolers and early elementary school (3–7 years)	• Developing initiative in activities and confidence in self	• Preventing hypoglycemia • Coping with unpredictable appetite and activity • Positively reinforcing cooperation with regimen • Trusting other caregivers with diabetes management	• Reassuring child that diabetes is no one's fault • Educating other caregivers about diabetes management
Older elementary school (8–11 years)	• Developing skills in athletic, cognitive, artistic, and social areas • Consolidating self-esteem with respect to the peer group	• Making diabetes regimen flexible to allow for participation in school or peer activities • Child learning short- and long-term benefits of optimal control	• Maintaining parental involvement in insulin and blood glucose management tasks while allowing for independent self-care for special occasions • Continuing to educate school and other caregivers
Early adolescence (12–15 years)	• Managing body changes • Developing a strong sense of self-identity	• Increasing insulin requirements during puberty • Diabetes management and blood glucose control becoming more difficult • Weight and body image concerns	• Renegotiating parent and teenager's roles in management to be acceptable to both • Learning coping skills to enhance ability to self-manage • Preventing and intervening in diabetes-related family conflict • Monitoring for signs of depression, eating disorders, risk-taking behaviors
Later adolescence (16–19 years)	• Establishing a sense of identity after high school (decisions about location, social issues, work, and education)	• Starting an ongoing discussion of transition to a new diabetes team (discussion may begin in early adolescent years) • Integrating diabetes into new lifestyle	• Supporting the transition to independence • Learning coping skills to enhance ability to self-manage • Preventing and intervening with diabetes-related family conflict • Monitoring for signs of depression, eating disorders, risk-taking behaviors

Source: Chiang JL, Kirkman MS, Laffel LM, Peters AL; on behalf of the Type 1 Diabetes Sourcebook Authors. Type 1 diabetes through the lifespan: a position statement of the American Diabetes Association. *Diabetes Care* 2014;37:2034–2054.

A child's comfort with self-care tasks should be monitored, because although a skill may be mastered, the child's desire to perform the task can change over time (e.g., during adolescence).

THE FAMILY

Diabetes affects every aspect of family life and affects all family members. Research has shown that shared responsibility within the family is associated with improved adherence and metabolic control. These results underscore the importance of educating family members regarding the treatment of diabetes and defining diabetes care tasks for each family member. Facilitating open discussion of the problems encountered in day-to-day diabetes management will help prevent blaming the child for poor diabetes control and enlist family support. Siblings, who commonly feel neglected or left out because of the extra attention given to the child with diabetes, may feel more involved if they are a part of the family's diabetes management effort, especially because they may be on the front lines with regard to recognition of hypoglycemia and its treatment. Fathers may be more likely to be involved if they, too, have clearly defined tasks. Full family involvement may help prevent over-involvement of one parent and unhealthy dependence between either parent and the child with diabetes.

DIABETES, SCHOOL, AND PEERS

Although school-aged children begin doing more diabetes management tasks, it is important that parents and children continue to share diabetes care responsibilities. A child's early independence in diabetes management can lead to poor diabetes control. School entry can be a difficult experience for parents and children. It is often more traumatic for the parent and child with diabetes, as they must now depend on school nurses, teachers, and other school staff members (who often are not knowledgeable about diabetes) to monitor the child's well-being and potentially handle situations that could be life-threatening. The student's diabetes management team can help by providing diabetes literature and training for school nurses, teachers, and school staff and by being advocates for the child and family. Many school districts incorporate diabetes training for school nurses into their overall training curriculum. Every effort should be made for the school nurse and the diabetes management team to be familiar with each other and to work collaboratively to manage the student/patient. There are programs that can help bring nurses, teachers, administrators, other parents, and diabetes educators together for training, such as the American Diabetes Association's Safe at School program. Often there can be resistance from school personnel when accommodating a child with diabetes due to fear of responsibility or misunderstanding of the disease itself. Proper training can make everyone, families and faculty alike, feel more at ease that a child with diabetes will be attending school and ensure a safe and optimal learning environment for the child.

An important goal of diabetes management during childhood is to prevent the diabetes regimen from disrupting the child's school experience. Every effort should be made to ensure the child's safety at school and ability to participate in all school activities. An individualized Diabetes Medical Management Plan, developed by the student's health-care team (with input from the parent/guardian), outlines what is required for diabetes management at school. Specific issues outlined in the Diabetes Medical Management Plan are insulin administration; signs, symptoms, and treatment of hypoglycemia and hyperglycemia; the timing of meals; management of exercise; where and when SMBG occurs; and which tasks need to be done by school personnel, which can be done independently, and which require supervision. The school, mainly the school nurse, should determine how to execute the plan. Federal laws such as Section 504 of the Rehabilitation Act of 1973, the Americans with Disabilities Act, and the Individuals with Disabilities Education Act prohibit schools from discriminating against children with disabilities—including diabetes. Parents should work with their child's school to document required accommodations in a written plan developed under applicable federal law such as a Section 504 Plan or an Individualized Education Program (IEP). In addition, some states have laws that provide additional legal protections to students with diabetes.

The student's health-care team should work with parents, teachers, and school nurses to minimize absences and missed class time and school activities. Some children may quickly learn to use their diabetes to avoid difficult school situations. Allowing children to check blood glucose levels and treat hypoglycemia at their desks or in the classroom will help prevent missed classroom time. Children who are frequently allowed to stay home for minor diabetes problems may fall behind in school and lose motivation to return to school. Social stigmatization can also occur because of being "sick" or "different." Children and adolescents with diabetes should be able to participate in all school-sponsored activities, including field trips and sports.

During the elementary school years, peer relationships become increasingly important. This means that the student's health-care team must work with parents to ensure that children attend birthday parties and slumber parties, actively participate in school and recreation league sports, and participate in other normal childhood activities. This does not mean relaxing treatment goals. Use of basal-bolus insulin injection regimens or an insulin pump make adjusting to calorie, activity, and timing changes in the child's diabetes care routine feasible and straightforward. Adequate preparation and planning—including dosing of insulin for excessive calorie consumption or consuming extra calories to balance high levels of exercise—can allow the child to incorporate almost any usual childhood activity into their routine.

DEVELOPMENTAL CONSIDERATIONS IN ADOLESCENTS

The adolescent years are known for difficulty with glycemic control—in part because of innate insulin resistance associated with puberty, and in part because of limited adherence to self-care regimens—and increased distress on the part of clinicians, parents, and the children themselves. Research has shown, however, that these difficulties can be lessened and that strategies can be developed to maintain glycemic control during this period of transition to early adulthood.

For the young child with diabetes, successful adherence to the treatment regimen depends largely on parental interest, management skills, and other resources.

For adolescents, peer influences, together with family support and supervision, play an increasingly important role in adherence and glycemic control. Many aspects of the treatment regimen are at odds with adolescents' normal drive for independence and peer acceptance. Adolescents may neglect monitoring, dietary considerations, insulin administration, and even visits to the clinic to avoid drawing attention to their illness or disturbing their daily activities. These actions can have negative short-term consequences, such as feeling sluggish and unfocused or developing ketoacidosis or severe hypoglycemia, as well as potentially negative long-term consequences in terms of future onset of chronic complications. The diabetes management team can use various strategies to help the adolescent patient and his or her family keep diabetes control within acceptable limits.

UNDERSTANDING THE SCOPE OF THE CHALLENGE

Almost all adolescents display characteristic behaviors and attitudes that reflect their drive for independence. Adolescents with diabetes are no exception. They undergo the same developmental process but with the added burden of diabetes. Do not assume that major difficulties are inevitable. There is no evidence that adolescents with diabetes suffer from serious psychological problems any more frequently than their peers without diabetes, though adults with diabetes show a higher incidence of psychological distress than adults without diabetes. There is evidence that interventions can be suggested that are acceptable to the adolescent, parents, and health-care providers and preserve glucose control and the adolescent's sense of autonomy. Use of the peer group and the diabetes management team to support and monitor the health status and behaviors of adolescents holds promise for affecting the decay in glycemic control often seen during these years. Inclusion of the adolescent in devising a solution for their limited adherence and/or poor control is highly recommended.

Many hormonal changes occur at puberty, some of which can adversely affect blood glucose levels. Puberty is associated with decreased sensitivity to insulin, which may result in increased insulin requirements. Poor control may be due to underinsulinization, lack of adherence, depression or other psychopathologies, or poor understanding of required health-care behavior on the part of the adolescent. Do not assume limited adherence to care behaviors over a physiological reason until good glycemic control has been achieved under supervised conditions utilizing the current insulin and diabetes care regimen. Blaming the adolescent for poor control can set the stage for further struggles with the adolescent and negatively affect communication, which is essential to problem-solving. Empower the adolescent as an agent of his or her own good health outcomes. It is important to work with the adolescent to establish motivating goals specifically for them and then to pair adherence steps with these goals. For example, adolescents may not be motivated by reducing blood glucose levels, but instead may be motivated by earning time with peers, time on phones, videogames, or other technology, learning to drive, or performing well at an activity. Leveraging these goals can help create reinforcement for diabetes management tasks and, ultimately, increase adherence. Discovering an individual adolescent's motivating goals is an important step to establishing their treatment protocol.

FAMILY AND PATIENT FACTORS

Because family routines overlap with various aspects of the diabetes treatment regimen (e.g., timing and content of meals, need for monitoring and exercise), family factors and adherence to treatment are strongly interrelated. Adherence to treatment is better among adolescents if their families are characterized by lower levels of general and diabetes-related conflict and greater cohesiveness (i.e., family members interact more and are supportive of one another), and if clear assignments are made among family members for diabetes care tasks.

Effective clinical interventions with adolescents with diabetes and their families should target (for change) negative family interactions, especially those that focus on adherence with the care regimen. Whenever blood glucose values are outside of a target range, rather than blaming the adolescent, it is important for the family to problem-solve regarding actions to take to lower glycemic values. Viewing blood glucose values as numbers to help guide next steps is a useful strategy for parents who often feel there are "good" and "bad" numbers, which can create blame and shame in the adolescent. Parents may need guidance in setting realistic expectations for their teen's self-management behaviors and blood glucose levels. Parents face a difficult balancing act wherein they must respect their teen's growing independence but remain responsible for their child's health and well-being. Negative family interactions may have the inadvertent effect of undermining the teen's attempts at independence in diabetes care. Education and problem-solving intervention efforts with adolescents should include parents, peers, and other acceptable support people, including the diabetes care team (at least as external monitors of glycemic status). Focus on the identification and development of coping strategies that decrease diabetes-related conflicts and tensions in the family and facilitate mastery of diabetes care skills is recommended.

DIABETES MANAGEMENT TEAM FACTORS

In addition to acquiring an understanding of normal adolescent development, members of the diabetes management team should enjoy working with adolescents and show a genuine interest in them as individuals. Patient valuation of their health-care providers has been shown to be associated with better control. It is important for diabetes care providers to directly interact with and involve the adolescent in his or her care, not just direct communication to parents.

Try to develop rapport. The diabetes management team should work toward rapport with the teen. Clinicians should avoid being placed in a parental role and make every effort to remain nonjudgmental and supportive in encouraging mastery and success in diabetes care behavior. Recommendations that are viewed by the adolescent as "parental" demands may be rejected. Clinicians are advised to adopt a child advocacy stance when interacting with adolescents, only assuming an authoritarian position when the child's health is at risk or risk-taking behavior is being demonstrated.

To avoid being viewed as parental figures, members of the diabetes management team should make it clear to both the parents and the adolescent that they have responsibilities to each other. The clinician may agree or disagree with either the parents or the adolescent about different aspects of diabetes care. An attempt should be made to convince the adolescent and family that the clinician-patient relationship is not just one between clinician and child, but an evolving one.

Be willing to compromise. Each member of the diabetes management team must be willing to compromise on almost all aspects of diabetes care and must clearly demonstrate respect for the adolescent's views. If a clinician becomes frustrated and angry when the adolescent does not adhere to the regimen, it will be difficult to retain the ability to influence the patient's self-care. It is not necessary to agree with the adolescent's views, but the clinician should at least listen to the patient and make an effort to accommodate the patient's wishes whenever possible.

Be consistent. An important factor known to affect adherence across all age-groups is consistency in caregiving. The adolescent whose outpatient care is provided by any one of several different diabetes management team members with different management styles is not as likely to adhere to the regimen as the patient seeing a diabetes management team with a consistent and predictable management style. Often, an adolescent will form a bond with one team member while professing to dislike another care provider. This may be face-saving when the adolescent is nonadherent with care and gives health-care providers the opportunity to play "good cop–bad cop." This situation is often found in adults struggling with adherence as well.

MONITORING

The adolescent should receive SMBG training (see Monitoring in the Tools of Therapy chapter, page 114) independent of his or her parents and demonstrate independent mastery. Adolescents will be more likely to monitor if these results are used to make management decisions and are perceived as increasing flexibility and safety while maintaining metabolic control. It is important that when an adolescent becomes independent in SMBG, a mechanism is set in place to communicate blood glucose results to parents and health-care providers independent of parental oversight. Parents and adolescents should review glucose results from SMBG using memory in the meter or by downloading at set times during the week. Using multiple meters can make this assessment more difficult. If the adolescent agrees to keep a logbook, this can be reviewed, but SMBG results should be verified from the meter. The goal is to assess the frequency of monitoring, the degree of hyperglycemia and hypoglycemia, and to review patterns and trends. This review can take place daily, weekly, or at some frequency in-between. A similar review should take place at each clinic visit with the diabetes management team. When discussing the importance of monitoring with an adolescent, the diabetes management team should emphasize that it is done primarily for the patient's benefit and not to placate or please the parents or clinicians. In addition, parents should be warned that negatively shaming the adolescent for numbers seen from downloads will likely result in the adolescent monitoring less frequently.

The same training procedures should occur if the adolescent is using continuous glucose monitoring (CGM) so that they may gain independent mastery. Parents and health-care providers should assess the amount of time the teen is wearing the sensor, how they are responding to glucose alarms, and if they are following calibration instructions. It is important to emphasize that treatment decisions must still be made from SMBG results, and that CGM is an adjunct

(CGM may become nonadjunctive or rather replace SMBG in the near future) and meant to show trends and patterns. Studies have confirmed that use of CGM in adolescents can be beneficial, and the more that sensors are worn, the better the glycemic outcome.

Periodically, the adolescent patient may refuse to monitor at all. The healthcare team should not give up, but instead renegotiate. If the adolescent is willing to perform one test, another can be added at a future office visit. This step-by-step approach often yields good results among adults as well as adolescents. Stress to patients that they need to resume more frequent monitoring if they become ill or are concerned about hypoglycemia.

Adolescents with diabetes can misrepresent glucose monitoring results. In the past, it was possible to manipulate the glucose meter results by reusing an old strip that had a "good" result, by diluting the blood specimen, or by using control solution. However, it has become increasingly difficult to falsify SMBG. Adolescents may choose to tell their parents a false number as they are doing a blood test when they are rushed, it is meal time, or as they are going out. If the parents suspect that they were told a false number, they should ask to see the meter and check its memory on the spot. Repeated misrepresentations should be suspected when the mean glucose values recorded or reported are much lower than would be expected from a very high glycated hemoglobin (A1C) level or when safe round numbers appear to have been neatly recorded at the same time with the same pen.

When approaching the adolescent with an A1C out of target, insufficient numbers of blood tests, or high values on SMBG, the diabetes management team should not be judgmental. Accusations should not be made, but rather a problem-solving approach will work best to engage the adolescent. Avoid accusatory discussions about nonideal glycemic control as this may cause the patient to avoid the desired actions or change out of spite or rebellion.

This nonjudgmental approach may provide a good model for the parents, who should be encouraged not to punish the adolescent for having high glucose monitoring results and A1C. The diabetes management team should also remind parents that other adolescents with diabetes (and even adults) have problems adhering to the treatment regimen and that blood glucose values are difficult to keep steady, with a number of factors influencing fluctuations. Remind parents and the treatment team that diabetes is not the adolescent's "fault," nor are high or low blood glucose values.

Parents often have great difficulty "letting go" of their role as primary manager(s) of their child's diabetes. Parental worry for the child's well-being is to be expected, especially if parental responsibility for complications consequent to poor control have been warned against since diagnosis. Parents and teens may also be so used to interdependence in diabetes care that the child may view the parents as "not caring anymore" if they appear to withdraw from active participation in diabetes management. Unless the parents are assured that diabetes care tasks and reasonable glucose control are being maintained, they may be unable to let their adolescent proceed to independence in care. The need for communication, the method and frequency to be negotiated between parent and child, should not be underestimated. This developmental task is probably the most difficult of the adolescent years, and diabetes exacerbates the dilemma. Keeping the issue in a developmental framework can help patients, family members, and caregivers be more tolerant of the uncertainties produced by transition in care responsibilities.

Comprehensive and coordinated planning is needed for the transition of diabetes care from parents or other adults to the youth with diabetes, as well as shifting from pediatric to adult health-care providers. This planning should begin in early to mid-adolescence, at least 1 year before the date of transition to avoid lapses in health care, deterioration of glycemic control, increased incidence of acute complications, and development of chronic complications.

ADULTS

Marriage, family, employment, and finances are aspects of adulthood that the individual with type 1 diabetes must handle while living with a disease that often complicates interpersonal relationships and attempts to establish a family and career, and often presents a financial burden. Adults may not be prepared to include the diabetes care team in the most intimate aspects of their lives, even though every aspect of their lives is affected by having diabetes.

Development of intimate relationships can be burdened by the self-care regimen of the individual with diabetes and/or by short- and long-term complications such as hypoglycemia and erectile dysfunction. Men in particular may be reluctant to be seen in the role of a patient with their significant others. With the patient's agreement, the significant other can and should be incorporated into the diabetes care routine with proper education and knowledge of the treatment regimen. It is strongly advised that as a relationship becomes more important and central in a patient's life, the patient be encouraged to include the significant other in the diabetes care visits. It is especially important that the new person learn about the management of diabetes crises and methods of supporting adherence to the treatment regimen without demeaning the patient or treating him or her as disabled. Family planning counseling for couples planning a long-term commitment and the possibility of children will provide crucial information as the couple decides whether and/or when to have a child. Both partners should understand the risks of pregnancy for the woman with diabetes and the need for optimal metabolic control at the time of conception (see Pregnancy, page 196). Genetic counseling should be included with education to dispel misunderstandings about the genetic propensity to develop type 1 diabetes.

The diabetes management team should provide psychosocial help in other ways during the adult years. They can offer education and counsel when misunderstandings and conflicts arise in a marriage or other relationship because of diabetes; refer patients to community, state, and federal programs to help with financial difficulties; and educate and reassure children who worry about their parents' diabetes. Physicians can work with patients to match the treatment regimen to the realities of their job, act as a resource if problems arise with diabetes management or employer misunderstanding of the disease, or direct patients if issues related to diabetes threaten a patient's job security. The American Diabetes Association provides resources for health-care providers and patients dealing with discrimination issues in the workplace.

THE ELDERLY

Because of increased survival rates, there is a growing number of older adults with type 1 diabetes, in addition to an increasing number of older patients with type 2 diabetes who require insulin. The elderly are often overlooked when new technologies and medicines are offered. The assumption is that more complex care is not feasible or desirable for this group of patients. However, many older people are active and functional and may wish to increase rather than decrease the intensity of their diabetes care. Retired individuals may have more time and resources to devote to diabetes self-care skills. Because of the availability of Medicare coverage, older people may have greater access to health services and be able to afford to participate more actively in their care.

On the other hand, the demands of the diabetes regimen may be especially burdensome for some elderly individuals, especially those who face a reduction in financial resources due to retirement, the loss of physical function and mobility, the death of a spouse and/or friends, and comorbid conditions that may shorten life expectancy. Aging leads to declines in physical capacity due to decreases in visual and auditory acuity. Although aging has been thought to lead inexorably to diminished muscle mass, bone strength, joint flexibility, and aerobic capacity, accumulating evidence from clinical studies is beginning to show that much of what was regarded as age-related decreases in strength, muscle mass, and physical status can be ameliorated with appropriate resistance training and physical activity. In addition to physical deterioration, as many as 20% of the elderly may also have a diagnosable mental disorder, such as anxiety, severe cognitive impairment, or depression. The elderly are more prone to hypoglycemia due to blunting of counterregulatory hormonal responses, concomitant medications and polypharmacy, decreased renal function with associated decreases in renal contribution to gluconeogenesis and clearance of insulin, alterations of taste and appetite, and decreased physical capacity to eat because of fine or gross motor dysfunction and/or dental conditions. It may be more difficult to keep physician appointments, fill prescriptions, and purchase diabetes supplies because of driving restrictions leading to difficulties with transportation and financial limitations. Before assumptions are made about the needs or wishes of an elderly patient, a periodic evaluation should be conducted that includes factors such as functional status, interpersonal support, financial resources, and assessment for cognitive impairment. The diabetes management team should be aware that errors in insulin administration and blood glucose testing may be due to failing eyesight or poor coordination, cognitive impairment or early dementia, and/or a lack of understanding of new treatment modalities.

It is essential for the diabetes management team to carefully assess each older patient to identify and address these potential barriers to sound diabetes care and, whenever possible, to identify a support person who is willing to monitor the elderly person's health status and provide concrete assistance. Inevitably, there are changes in social support as one ages. Those who have helped in the past may no longer be able or available to do so. Social support is important to the health and well-being of older adults, but the needs will vary according to the individual. It is important to determine the type of help needed to maintain respect for and the autonomy of the older person. The goal is to provide support while safeguarding the patient's autonomy and independence as much as possible. Home-care agencies and special programs, such as Meals on Wheels, are often helpful.

As emphasized for other age-groups, the relationship between the diabetes management team and patient has a major influence on patient adherence. Patients who are satisfied with their care team are more likely to adhere to their diabetes care plan. However, older adults are less likely than individuals in other age-groups to express dissatisfaction directly to the provider. Therefore, it is even more essential to encourage open communication by asking and responding to questions and by taking time to show concern, troubleshoot problems, and develop effective strategies for diabetes care.

EMOTIONAL AND BEHAVIORAL DISORDERS AND DIABETES

It is important that care providers recognize emotional and behavioral disorders in patients with diabetes and refer these patients for evaluation and counseling. Some caregivers mistakenly view psychiatric symptoms, especially those of depression and anxiety, as expected or even normal in people coping with an illness as serious and difficult to treat as diabetes. Unfortunately, when psychiatric symptoms are seen as the norm, therapeutic intervention may not be recommended, and the patient will continue to suffer psychological distress. This situation is especially disturbing in light of the high prevalence of depression and anxiety disorders in individuals with diabetes and the availability of effective treatment options.

DEPRESSION

Individuals with diabetes have higher rates of diagnoses of depression than the general population of the U.S. and of other developed countries. It is not known whether depression predisposes to diabetes, glucose toxicity predisposes to depression, or some other central mechanism is operating that affects both conditions. Depression in a patient with diabetes leads to an average increase of 0.5–1.0% in the A1C level. Regardless, depression is still underdiagnosed, especially in teens and the elderly, and limited adherence due to depression is often underrecognized. Untreated or inadequately treated depression markedly increases the risk of suicide. Ongoing monitoring of patients' mental status by a multidisciplinary team will help with prompt diagnosis and treatment of depression. When depression is suspected, referral to a mental health provider is recommended. Pharmacologic and behavioral treatments have both been shown to be effective in treating depression. Incorporating the family and/or significant others into psychological care is also recommended.

ANXIETY DISORDERS

Anxiety disorders such as needle phobia and fear of hypoglycemia may be a consequence of treatment with insulin. Other disorders, such as obsessive-compulsive disorder, may be exacerbated by having diabetes. When symptoms are identified that suggest these disorders, referral to specialists who can initiate behavioral interventions while working with health-care providers to maintain diabetes care behaviors is imperative. The goal is to prevent deterioration in metabolic control while reducing symptoms that limit the patient's ability to carry out diabetes care tasks and that negatively affect quality of life. An anxiolytic medication in concert with behavioral intervention can also be utilized to diminish symptoms. Once again, it is important not to mistake anxiety for willful noncompliance, especially when the patient expresses distress in association with specific diabetes care tasks (such as injections).

Fear of hypoglycemia may result in patients wishing to raise their glucose levels to avoid the unpleasant feelings and loss of control associated with hypoglycemia. As mentioned earlier, Blood Glucose Awareness Training has been shown to improve patients' recognition of their glycemic status and reduce the incidence of severe hypoglycemia. Other forms of behavior therapy, used while temporarily raising glycemic targets, can improve glycemic awareness in those who have lost feelings of hypoglycemia. Increased blood glucose monitoring, use of continuous glucose monitoring, and compensatory external cues can be enlisted to maintain glycemic status in those with hypoglycemia unawareness.

It is important to treat the disorders in addition to looking for compensatory management strategies (such as pump use, increased SMBG, or addition of continuous glucose monitoring). Parents in particular may respond to their own anxiety by discussing "hurting" their child with insulin injections or SMBG. This inadvertently fosters anxiety and solidifies a child's fear. It is particularly important to include parents in treatment when children express anxiety over diabetes care behaviors, as the child/patient's fears may mirror the parent's fears.

EATING DISORDERS

Eating disorders are common in (but not exclusive to) adolescent or young adult women with type 1 diabetes and are associated with poor metabolic control, poor adherence to the diabetes regimen, and more severe complications. Eating disorders are often related to the regain of and/or increasing weight associated with successful treatment of diabetes with insulin, and they may be exacerbated by the more intense focus on food that occurs in families of children with diabetes. Diagnostic criteria for anorexia nervosa include weight loss and maintenance of body weight 15% below normal, impaired body image, intense fear of weight gain, and absence of menses. Diagnostic criteria for bulimia nervosa include recurrent episodes of binge eating, feelings of loss of control over eating during binges, frequent self-induced vomiting and/or laxative use, and over concern with body image and weight.

Many young people with type 1 diabetes may have eating disturbances that compromise their diabetes control yet do not meet stringent diagnostic criteria. They may lose calories by intentional glycosuria rather than vomiting or laxative use. This is accomplished by decreasing insulin doses or missing meal insulin boluses. The seriousness of these subclinical cases should not be underestimated because they can result in short- and long-term metabolic complications. Eating disorders, clinical and subclinical, should be suspected in young women with persistently unstable or poor metabolic control, recurrent ketoacidosis resulting from insulin omission to induce glycosuria and weight loss, recurrent severe hypoglycemia resulting from food restriction while continuing insulin, anxiety or avoidance about being weighed, or binging with food or alcohol, and in girls with growth retardation and pubertal delay. It is important that members of the diabetes team routinely ask about eating behavior and insulin omission in a nonthreatening and nonjudgmental manner. These patients may require referral to an experienced mental health professional for psychological evaluation and treatment if an explanation for their problems is not found.

STRESS AND DIABETES

Although caregivers and patients have long observed a relationship between stress and blood glucose levels, the results of numerous studies attempting to define this relationship have yielded contradictory results. Some studies have shown an association between stress and hyperglycemia, whereas others have not. In some studies, this relationship has been idiosyncratic, with patients varying dramatically in their glucose response to the same or different stressors. The only way to establish an individual's stress reactivity is to monitor blood glucose before, during, and after a stressful life event. Compensatory strategies should be developed according to the patient's individual response. Parents and teachers need to be made aware of a child's stress reactivity as it applies to schoolwork and sports activities in order to plan a strategy to achieve glycemic targets during stressful times in the child's everyday life.

Stress can also have indirect effects on diabetes. Patients under stress may be less able to follow their diabetes regimen, may give a low priority to their diabetes care, or may respond to the stress by overeating or increasing their use of alcohol or illicit drugs. Care providers should explore possible explanations for poor metabolic control. While some patients may find support through family, friends, religious community, or support groups, others can learn to cope through stress management counseling or relaxation training.

BIBLIOGRAPHY

Anderson RJ, Grigsby AB, Freeland KE, De Groot M, McGill JB, Clouse RE, Lustman PJ. Anxiety and poor glycemic control: a meta-analytic review of the literature. *Int J Psychiatry Med* 2002;32:235–247

Brod M, Kongsø JH, Lessard S, Christensen TL. Psychological insulin resistance: patient beliefs and implications for diabetes management. *Qual Life Res* 2009;18:23–32

Chiang JL, Kirkman MS, Laffel LM, Peters AL; on behalf of the Type 1 Diabetes Sourcebook Authors. Type 1 diabetes through the lifespan: a position statement of the American Diabetes Association. *Diabetes Care* 2014;37:2034–2054

Corathers SD, Kichler J, Jones NH, et al. Improving depression screening for adolescents with type 1 diabetes. *Pediatrics* 2013;132:e1395–e1402

Enzlin P, Rosen R, Wiegel M, et al.; DCCT/EDIC Research Group. Sexual dysfunction in women with type 1 diabetes: long term findings from the DCCT/EDIC study cohort. *Diabetes Care* 2009;32:780–785

Ducat L, Philipson LH, Anderson BJ. The mental health comorbidities of diabetes. *JAMA* 2014;312:691–692

Hamburg SA, Inoff GE. Coping with predictable crises of diabetes. *Diabetes Care* 1983;6:409–416

Kovacs J, Brent D, Steinberg TF, Paulauskas S, Reid J. Children's self-report of psychologic adjustment and coping strategies during first year of insulin-dependent diabetes mellitus. *Diabetes Care* 1986;9:472–479

Lustman PJ, Anderson RJ, Freedland KE, de Groot M, Carney RM, Clouse R. Depression and poor glycemic control: a meta-analytic review of the literature. *Diabetes Care* 2000;23:934–942

Lustman PJ, Penckofer SM, Clouse RE. Recent advances in understanding depression in adults with diabetes. *Curr Diab Rep* 2007;7:114–122

Peters A, Laffel L; American Diabetes Association Transitions Working Group. Diabetes care for emerging adults: recommendations for transition from pediatric to adult diabetes care systems: a position statement of the American Diabetes Association, with representation by the American College of Osteopathic Family Physicians, the American Academy of Pediatrics, the American Association of Clinical Endocrinologists, the American Osteopathic Association, the Centers for Disease Control and Prevention, Children with Diabetes, The Endocrine Society, the International Society for Pediatric and Adolescent Diabetes, Juvenile Diabetes Research Foundation International, the National Diabetes Education Program, and the Pediatric Endocrine Society (formerly Lawson Wilkins Pediatric Endocrine Society). *Diabetes Care* 2011;34:2477–2485

Peyrot M, Rubin RR. Behavioral and psychosocial interventions in diabetes: a conceptual review. *Diabetes Care* 2007;30:2433–2440

Rodin G, Olmsted M, Rydall A, Maharaj S, Colton P, Jones J, Biancucci L, Daneman D. Eating disorders in young women with type 1 diabetes mellitus. *J Psychosom Res* 2002;53:943–949

Schmitz N, Wang J, Lesage A, Malla A, Strychar I. Psychological distress and short-term disability in people with diabetes: results from the Canadian Community Healthy Survey. *J Psychosom Res* 2008;65:165–172

Silverstein J, Klingensmith G, Copeland K, Plotnick L, Kaufman FR, Laffel L, Deeb L, Grey M, Anderson B, Holzmeister LA, Clark N; American Diabetes Association. Care of children and adolescents with type 1 diabetes mellitus: a statement of the American Diabetes Association. *Diabetes Care* 2005;28:186–212

Weissberg-Benchell J, Wolpert H, Anderson BJ. Transitioning from pediatric to adult care: a new approach to the post-adolescent young person with type 1 diabetes. *Diabetes Care* 2007;30:2441–2446

Complications

Neuropathy
    Overview of Neuropathies
    Distal Symmetric Sensorimotor Polyneuropathy
    Late Complications of Polyneuropathy
    Management of Distal Symmetric Polyneuropathy and Complications
    Autonomic Neuropathy
    Focal Neuropathies
    Conclusion

Macrovascular Disease
    Prevalence and Risk Factors
    Assessment and Treatment
    Symptoms and Signs of Atherosclerosis
    Conclusion

Musculoskeletal Complications
    Osteoporosis
    Limited Joint Mobility (Cheiroarthropathy)

Abnormal Linear Growth
    Subtle Growth Abnormalities
    Determining Growth Rate
    Conclusion

Highlights
Complications

SCREENING

■ Ongoing assessment for acute and chronic complications of diabetes is an important part of comprehensive care and management of type 1 diabetes.

■ The assessment must be focused, age-appropriate, and based on the likelihood of abnormality.

■ A brief overview of general screening recommendations is provided in this section.

RETINOPATHY

■ Significant retinopathy in patients with type 1 diabetes is a major cause of visual disability.

■ Long-term data from the Diabetes Control and Complications Trial/Epidemiology of Diabetes Interventions and Complications (DCCT/EDIC) and the Pittsburgh Epidemiology of Diabetes Complications Experience demonstrates the importance of good glycemic control early on in the course of type 1 diabetes, with a 50% cumulative incidence of proliferative retinopathy in the DCCT conventional treatment group and 21% in the intensive therapy group.

■ The clinician should assure that patients receive their initial ophthalmologic examination within

5 years of onset of type 1 diabetes; sooner if there are visual symptoms or in adults when the true date of diabetes onset is unclear. Indications for more urgent ophthalmologic referral are described in Table 6.1.

■ High-risk characteristics of proliferative retinopathy greatly increase the risk of blindness and include:
  • new vessels on the optic disk (NVD) involving greater than ~25% of the optic disk area
  • any NVD with preretinal or vitreous hemorrhage
  • new vessels elsewhere covering an area ≥50% of the optic disk area (totaled for the entire retina) with preretinal or vitreous hemorrhage

■ When high-risk characteristics are present, photocoagulation therapy should generally be performed promptly. An eye with severe nonproliferative diabetic retinopathy, or worse, should be considered for photocoagulation.

■ Lesions typical of nonproliferative retinopathy, proliferative retinopathy, and macular edema are described in Clinical Findings in Diabetic Retinopathy (page 252).

■ Treatment for diabetic retinopathy can be highly effective in preserv-

ing vision. Treatment modalities include:
- scatter (panretinal) photocoagulation
- focal/grid laser photocoagulation
- vitrectomy
- anti-vascular endothelial growth factor (VEGF) therapies
■ Medical therapies are discussed under Treatment (page 257).

DIABETIC KIDNEY DISEASE

■ Epidemiologic studies suggest that up to 20–40% of patients with type 1 diabetes will eventually develop kidney failure and require dialysis, although more recent data suggest that this rate may be decreasing with implementation of intensive glycemic control and more effective screening and treatment.

■ Possible mechanisms by which diabetes damages the kidney are discussed in Pathogenesis (page 264). Elevated blood glucose, genetic susceptibility, elevated blood pressure, and abnormal glomerular hemodynamics are key factors.

■ Renal function and albuminuria should be monitored annually in all patients with type 1 diabetes after a diabetes duration of 5 years or more.

■ Patients with persistent albuminuria are at a higher risk for developing renal insufficiency and may benefit from more intensive glycemic control and ACE inhibitor or ARB therapy.

■ The management of more advanced diabetic kidney disease includes strict blood pressure control, minimizing factors that are known to accelerate the natural progression of renal disease or that may oth-erwise jeopardize the kidney, and assisting patients in responding to changing insulin needs (Table 6.3).

■ If kidney failure ensues, dialysis and kidney transplantation are available options.

NEUROPATHY

■ Diabetic neuropathy is classified into a set of discrete clinical syndromes, each with a characteristic presentation and clinical course (Table 6.5). The syndromes overlap clinically and may occur simultaneously.

■ Distal symmetrical polyneuropathy is the most common form of diabetic neuropathy.

■ Patients with chronic unrecognized neuropathy may present with late complications, e.g., foot ulceration, foreign objects embedded in the foot, unrecognized trauma to the extremities, or neuroarthropathy (Charcot's joints). All of these conditions are avoidable with proper early diagnosis of neuropathy and institution of appropriate foot care.

■ Treatment for diabetic distal symmetrical polyneuropathy is symptomatic, palliative, and supportive, with primary emphasis on preventing the late complications.

■ Persistent and severely painful neuropathy has been treated with various drugs, including standard analgesics and drugs normally used to treat other conditions (antidepressants, anticonvulsants). Narcotics should be avoided.

■ Although autonomic neuropathy produces diffuse subclinical dysfunction, autonomic symptoms are usually confined to one or two organ systems, producing the discrete autonomic syndromes listed in Table 6.8.

- Erectile dysfunction in men with diabetes is usually neuropathic but can also be psychogenic, endocrine, vascular, or drug- or stress-related.
- Other dysfunctions related to autonomic neuropathy include diabetic cystopathy and hypoglycemia unawareness.
- Mononeuropathies comprise neural deficits corresponding to the distribution of single or multiple peripheral nerves and are usually acute in onset and resolve spontaneously within weeks to months.
- Screen for diabetic peripheral neuropathy (DPN) starting 5 years after the diagnosis of type 1 diabetes and at least annually thereafter.

MACROVASCULAR DISEASE

- Coronary heart disease, peripheral arterial disease, and cerebrovascular disease are more common, tend to occur at an earlier age, and are more extensive and severe in people with diabetes.
- Physicians should systematically assess patients for risk factors for atherosclerotic cardiovascular disease, question them about symptoms, and be alert for signs of atherosclerosis.
- A program for modifying risk factors should be started at the appropriate point in the patient's diabetes course.
- Recommendations for treatment of cerebrovascular disease, coronary heart disease, and peripheral arterial disease appear in Symptoms and Signs of Atherosclerosis (page 292).

MUSCULOSKELETAL COMPLICATIONS

- Type 1 diabetes is associated with low bone density, particularly in the radius in children and adolescents.
- Patients with diabetes are at higher risk for fractures at all sites despite similar bone mineral density (BMD), so dual-energy X-ray absorptiometry (DEXA) scores may not accurately represent bone strength and risk for fractures in this population.
- Risk factors for fragility fractures appear to include degree of glycemic control and presence and severity of vascular complications (particularly neurologic and renal), although in some studies, age and BMI appear to play a role while A1C, duration of diabetes, and vascular complications do not. There may be a higher risk for falls, and fractures are slower to heal with higher risk for infection.
- It is important to identify patients at risk prior to development of fractures.
- Treatment should include good glycemic control with prevention of and screening for vascular complications, assessing risk for and prevention of falls, adequate calcium and vitamin D supplementation if needed, and if indicated, osteoporosis-specific therapy. The latter is usually not indicated in children and adolescents. In women of childbearing age, you must take into consideration the prolonged half-life of bisphosphonates in the bone, which may have unintended long-term consequences. Furthermore, anabolic therapies should

be reserved for patients with clear evidence of osteoporosis and/or osteoporotic fractures.

■ Limited joint mobility (LJM), which is not restricted to children, now occurs less often than in the past and is a potentially important clinical marker for diabetes complications such as retinopathy, diabetic kidney disease, neuropathy, and other disorders. Glycation of tissue proteins may be responsible for LJM, which is painless, can cause some disability, and is marked by a scleroderma-like stiffness of the skin and joints.

ABNORMAL LINEAR GROWTH

■ Subtle abnormalities of growth and development affect 5–10% of young patients with type 1 diabetes and usually result from inadequate metabolic control.

■ Signs of growth abnormalities include a lag in height or weight or a falling away from the patient's previously established growth curves.

■ Children most likely to be affected are those with the earliest onset of diabetes and the worst glycemic control. Boys are two to three times more likely to be affected than girls.

■ To detect growth abnormalities, the physician should regularly plot height and weight on standard growth charts. Other growth-impairing conditions should be considered in assessing growth abnormalities including hypothyroidism and celiac disease.

Complications

Ongoing assessment of the patient for both acute and chronic complications is an important part of care and management in type 1 diabetes. This assessment needs to be focused, age-appropriate, and based on the likelihood of an abnormality. An example described in Type 1 Diabetes Through the Lifespan: A Position Statement of the American Diabetes Association is that of screening for macrovascular disease, which might be more focused on lifestyle assessment and changes in a young adult at low risk versus risk evaluation in an older adult, with or without longer duration of disease, who would need more intensive laboratory and vascular screening and management.

Screening can help prevent and/or delay both micro- and macrovascular complications in type 1 diabetes. When patients are first diagnosed with type 1 diabetes, the elements of the initial evaluation that also serve as a baseline for future assessment of complications include height, weight, BMI (percentile in children and adolescents), blood pressure, general physical exam, comprehensive foot exam, A1C, creatinine clearance/estimated glomerular filtration rate (eGFR), and fasting lipid panel soon after diagnosis for patients ≥10 years of age (or beginning at 2 years of age if there is significant family history of cardiovascular disease).

The initial assessment of a random urine sample for albumin-to-creatinine ratio should be performed annually, beginning 5 years after diagnosis of diabetes.

Screening for microvascular complications includes annual evaluation and quarterly follow-up of blood pressure and A1C. A retinal exam by an eye care specialist should be performed within 5 years after diagnosis, unless there are visual symptoms, in which case it should be performed earlier. In adults, the true date of diabetes diagnosis is sometimes unknown, and the initial retinal exam should be performed earlier. Follow-up retinal exams should be performed annually, but if there are two consecutive negative yearly exams, one might consider lengthening the time between retinal exams to 2 years. For prevention and detection of diabetic kidney disease, an annual creatinine clearance/estimated glomerular filtration rate and urinary albumin-to-creatinine ratio should be performed. In children, subsequent urine albumin-to-creatinine ratios may be performed more often than once a year as needed based on treatment.

To prevent foot complications, foot inspections by visual foot exam should be performed at each visit. Annual foot exams should be considered for the child who is ≥10 years of age or at the time of puberty, whichever is earlier, after he or she has had diabetes for at least 5 years. Adults should undergo a comprehensive foot exam annually. A comprehensive foot exam includes inspection, palpation of dorsalis pedis and posterior tibialis pulses, presence or absence of patellar and Achilles tendon reflexes, an examination for proprioception vibration, and pinprick or monofilament sensation. In children and adults, more frequent follow-up visual foot exams should be performed based on high-risk characteristics, and patients should be advised to perform self-exams if any high-risk characteristics are present.

People with type 1 diabetes are at increased risk for atherosclerotic cardiovascular disease (ASCVD) but often have a different risk profile as compared to patients with type 2 diabetes. The vast majority of available data on risk of cardiovascular disease in diabetes is based on individuals with type 2 diabetes, who often have additional risk factors for ASCVD such as hypertension, diabetic dyslipidemia, obesity, and metabolic syndrome. Risk factors for ASCVD including age, smoking, weight, family history, hypertension, hyperlipidemia, and albuminuria are known to increase the risk of ASCVD in individuals with type 1 diabetes. Screening should include assessment and management of lifestyle factors. However, even in the absence of classic risk factors, adults with childhood-onset of type 1 diabetes, with duration of 20 years or more have a markedly increased coronary artery disease risk and should undergo annual evaluation of fasting lipid profile, as should those with type 2 diabetes.

More details regarding evaluation and management of each complication are presented in subsequent sections of this chapter.

BIBLIOGRAPHY

Chiang JL, Kirkman MS, Laffel LM, and Peters AL; on behalf of the Type 1 Diabetes Sourcebook Authors. Type 1 diabetes through the lifespan: a position statement of the American Diabetes Association. *Diabetes Care* 2014;37:2034–2054

RETINOPATHY

Diabetic retinopathy is one of the most common causes of blindness in the U.S., particularly in those 20–74 years old, and is a major cause of visual disability. A person with diabetes has a 5–10% chance of becoming legally blind, and this risk is greater in people with type 1 than type 2 diabetes. Thirty-year data from the Diabetes Control and Complications Trial/Epidemiology of Diabetes Interventions and Complications (DCCT/EDIC) and the Pittsburgh Epidemiology of Diabetes Complications Experience (EDC) studies, encompassing the years 1983–2005, showed the differential risk by conventional and intensive treatment groups for the DCCT/EDIC compared to the EDC cohort. After 30 years of diabetes, the cumulative incidences of proliferative retinopathy were 50% in the DCCT conventional treatment group, 47% in the EDC cohort, and 21% in the DCCT intensive therapy group, with fewer than 1% legally blind. The EDIC follow-up data show that the intensive therapy group also had a reduction in risk of any diabetes-related ocular surgery of 48% (95% confidence interval [CI], 29 to 63; P<0.001) and a reduction in risk of all ocular procedures, such as cataract extraction, vitrectomy, and retinal detachment surgery, by 37% (95% CI, 12 to 55; P = 0.01).

Vision-threatening retinopathy virtually never appears in patients with type 1 diabetes in the first 3–5 years of diabetes or before puberty. Retinopathy detected by fundus photography reaches a prevalence of 50% by the 10th year of diabetes. By the 15th year, up to 28% of patients have proliferative retinopathy, with new blood vessels developing from the retinal circulation, carrying with it a substantial risk of hemorrhage and retinal detachment. After 20 years' duration of diabetes, nearly all patients have some form of retinopathy. Earlier age at diagnosis, puberty, pregnancy, rapid intensification of blood glucose control, hypertension, hypercholesterolemia, anemia, use of tobacco, and presence of cataracts or cataract surgery may exert an accelerating influence on the progression of retinopathy. Limited data has suggested that vitamin D deficiency might be associated with an increased prevalence of retinopathy in young people with type 1 diabetes. To reduce the risk or slow the progression of retinopathy, optimization of glycemic control is important, and it is critical to optimize blood pressure control.

EYE EXAMINATION

Diabetic retinopathy appears primarily in the posterior retina and mid-periphery. Many but not all lesions may occur within an area viewable by the non-ophthalmologist with the monocular direct ophthalmoscope. However, this examination is not an adequate substitute for an annual retinal examination by an ophthalmologist or optometrist who is knowledgeable and experienced in the detection of diabetic retinopathy. It has been demonstrated that non–eye care professionals will miss a substantial amount of retinopathy, especially if pupils are not dilated. Although the finding of retinopathy by indirect ophthalmoscopy is well correlated with presence of disease and is important for prompt referral of the patient, lack of observed retinopathy does not obviate the need for comprehensive ophthalmologic evaluation in patients with diabetes. In many centers, retinal photographs are performed and the images transmitted for review by an eye specialist—this may be a good option for individuals, especially those in areas not supported by enough eye specialists for in-person visits to undergo retinal exam, but is not a substitute for comprehensive ophthalmologic evaluation.

CLINICAL FINDINGS IN DIABETIC RETINOPATHY

Mild to Moderate Nonproliferative Retinopathy

The earliest lesion visible through the ophthalmoscope is the microaneurysm, a pouch-like dilation of a terminal capillary. Ophthalmoscopically, microaneurysms look like tiny red dots. Dot hemorrhages may be indistinguishable from microaneurysms unless specialized techniques, such as fluorescein angiography, are used, but blot hemorrhages may be recognized because they are larger (Figure 6.1). Hard exudates are another common feature of nonproliferative retinopathy. Early nonproliferative retinopathy does not cause visual symptoms unless it is associated with macular edema.

Severe to Very Severe Nonproliferative Retinopathy

Multiple, extensive, clustered blot hemorrhages throughout the retina suggest progression to the severe nonproliferative stage. At this stage, substantial portions of the capillary circulation may have become nonfunctional, and retinal tissue is nonperfused. This nonperfusion may result in retinal hypoxia, which is thought to stimulate new retinal blood vessel development.

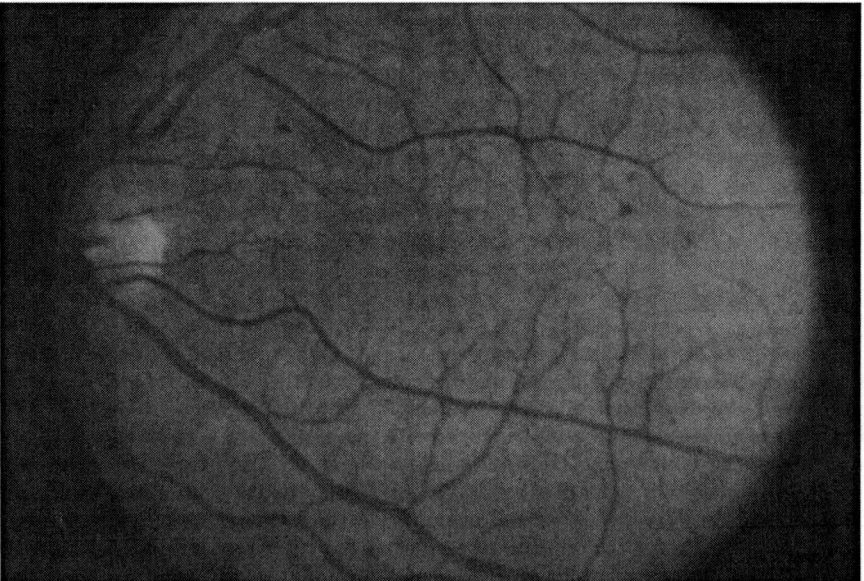

Figure 6.1 Nonproliferative retinopathy, with microaneurysms, dot, and blot hemorrhages. For color image, please visit the National Eye Institute (NEI) Photos and Images Catalog available from http://nei.nih.gov/photo.

Veins may appear dilated, tortuous, and irregular in caliber. Intraretinal microvascular abnormalities are other signs of significant nonproliferative retinopathy. These small loops of fine vessels usually extend from a major artery or vein and probably represent early new-vessel formation within the retina. Fluffy white lesions, commonly referred to as cotton-wool spots, were formerly associated with this stage of retinopathy. Evidence suggests that these lesions, when they appear alone, may be poor prognostic indicators.

Proliferative Retinopathy

Proliferative diabetic retinopathy involves the formation of new blood vessels, extending from within the retinal substance onto the inner surface of the retina or into the vitreous cavity. These vessels commonly occur on the optic nerve head, where they are called new vessels on the disk (NVD) (Figure 6.2). They may also occur elsewhere in the retina, usually extending from major vessels, where they are called new vessels elsewhere (NVE). New vessels are fragile and carry a substantial risk of rupture with hemorrhage. The vessels also eventually undergo fibrosis and contraction, which are capable of producing retinal detachment from the tractional forces exerted.

Certain findings were defined as high-risk characteristics (HRC) by the national Diabetic Retinopathy Study (DRS), a large-scale randomized controlled clinical trial

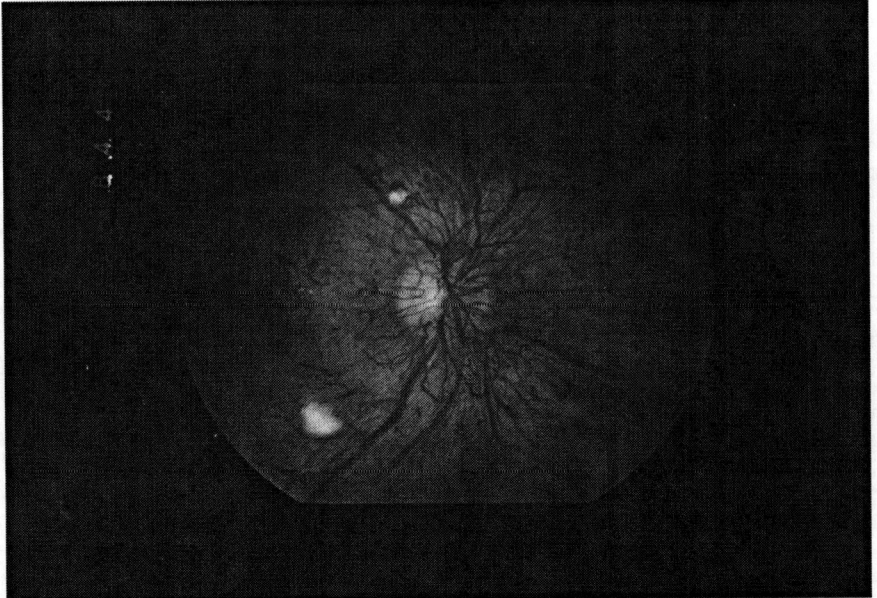

Figure 6.2 Proliferative retinopathy, with abnormal new blood vessels and scar tissue on the surface of the retina. For color image, please visit the National Eye Institute (NEI) Photos and Images Catalog available from http://nei.nih.gov/photo.

completed in 1981. The presence of HRC increases an eye's risk of severe vision loss (<25/200 on two consecutive visits at least 3 months apart) to 30–50% within 3–5 years of detection if appropriate treatment is not provided. HRC include:

- NVD greater than ~25% of the optic disk area
- any NVD with preretinal or vitreous hemorrhage
- NVE greater than or equal to 50% of the optic disk area (totaled for the entire retina) with preretinal or vitreous hemorrhage

When HRC are present, photocoagulation therapy (Figure 6.3) is indicated to preserve vision.

Diabetic Macular Edema

Macular edema involves thickening of the central portion of the retina. The macula occupies an area of ~5 disk diameters just temporal to the optic nerve head (Figure 6.4). Visual acuity can be decreased in this condition, particularly when the center of the macula (the fovea centralis) is involved. Macular edema is difficult to diagnose with the direct ophthalmoscope because this instrument does not allow the stereoscopic vision necessary to determine retinal thickening. However, the presence of hard lipid exudates—yellowish-white, often glistening, deposits of round or irregular shape lying within the retina, usually in the macular region—strongly suggests macular edema. This is particularly true if the exudates assume

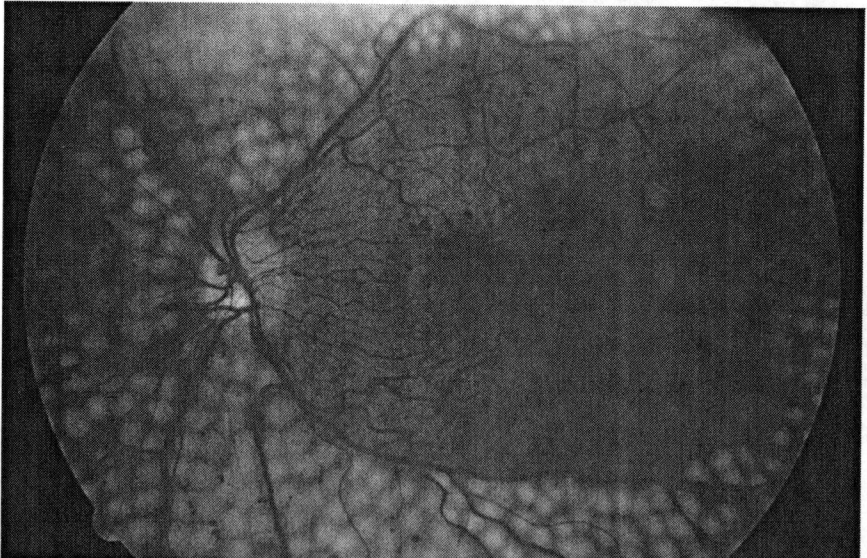

Figure 6.3 Scatter laser photocoagulation therapy for proliferative diabetic retinopathy. For color image, please visit the National Eye Institute (NEI) Photos and Images Catalog available from http://nei.nih.gov/photo.

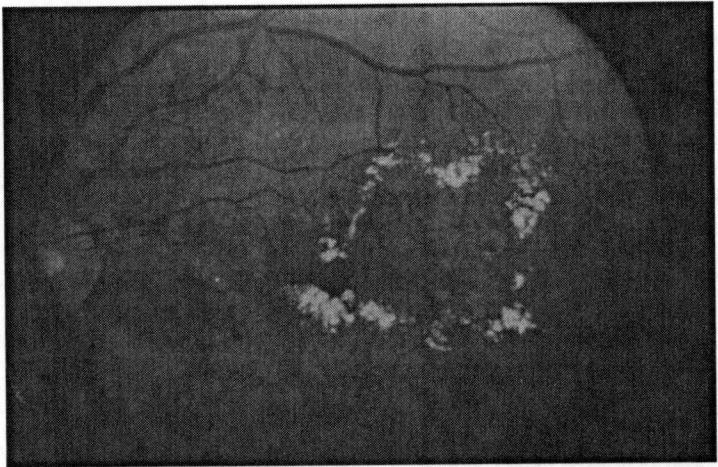

Figure 6.4 Diabetic macular edema. For color image, please visit the National Eye Institute (NEI) Photos and Images Catalog available from http://nei.nih.gov/photo.

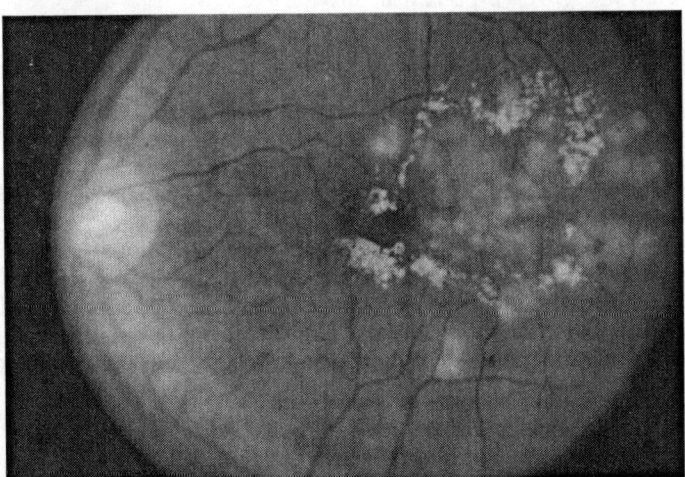

Figure 6.5 Focal laser photocoagulation therapy for clinically significant macular edema. For color image, please visit the National Eye Institute (NEI) Photos and Images Catalog available from http://nei.nih.gov/photo.

Figures 6.1–6.5 provided by National Eye Institute, Institute of Health website: http://www.nei.nih.gov/photo/diabetic-eye-disease. Accessed March 2012.

a ring-shape, or circinate, configuration. The features of clinically significant macular edema are:

- retinal thickening at or within 500 μm of the macular center
- hard exudates at or within 500 μm of the macular center with adjacent retinal thickening
- retinal thickening involving retinal area >1 disk diameter, with any part within 1 disk diameter of the macular center

When clinically significant macular edema is present, focal laser therapy (Figure 6.5) is indicated to preserve vision. In addition, intravitreal injections of anti-vascular endothelial growth factor (anti-VEGF) agents are indicated for diabetic macular edema that involves the retinal center, since this may threaten reading vision. This is defined as macular edema that affects the area just beneath the foveal center.

Glaucoma

Sometimes, in advanced (usually proliferative) diabetic retinopathy, new vessels may also form on the surface of the iris and extend into the "angle" of the anterior chamber of the eye, where the cornea and iris come together. Here, fibrous scar tissue extending from the new vessels may block the outflow of aqueous humor from the eye, causing a rise in intraocular pressure (neovascular glaucoma), severe pain, and loss of vision. Angle-closure glaucoma, a major complication, is a rare disorder in any age-group, especially before the age of 40 years.

EVALUATION

Patients with type 1 diabetes should have an initial dilated and comprehensive eye examination within 3–5 years after the onset of diabetes, at age ≥10 years or at the onset of puberty, whichever is earlier. For adults diagnosed with type 1 diabetes, the initial exam should be performed earlier if the patient has visual symptoms and/or the true date of diagnosis is unknown. In general, this examination is not necessary before 10 years of age. However, some evidence suggests that the prepubertal duration of diabetes may be important in the development of microvascular complications, so clinical judgment should be used when applying this recommendation to individual patients. The screening examination should be done by an experienced ophthalmologist or optometrist and should include:

- determination of visual acuity of each eye
- refraction, especially if visual acuity is impaired
- gross external examination of the eyes
- evaluation of ocular motility
- examination of the eyes by slit-lamp microscopy
- examination of the retina with monocular direct and binocular indirect ophthalmoscopy after dilation of the pupils
- slit-lamp ophthalmoscopy to exclude macular edema
- in adult patients, measurement of intraocular pressures

Patients with any level of macular edema, severe nonproliferative retinopathy, or any proliferative retinopathy require the prompt care of an ophthalmologist who is knowledgeable and experienced in the management of diabetic retinopathy.

Further examinations may be carried out for specific indications. These include retinal photography, which is used to document lesions, and intravenous fluorescein angiography. During angiography, a fluorescent dye is injected into a vein and rapid-sequence photography of the retinal circulation is carried out. Both eyes are typically evaluated at a single injection sequence.

Fluorescein angiography is useful clinically to plan photocoagulation treatment for macular edema. Although it is more sensitive than ophthalmoscopy or color photography for detecting very early lesions of retinopathy, the minute lesions detected with angiography are rarely critical for making decisions regarding treatment. Therefore, intravenous fluorescein angiography should not be used as a screening test in the annual ocular examination of patients with diabetes. Guidelines for care and referral are described in Table 6.1.

TREATMENT

Clinicians should always refer patients to an ophthalmologist for treatment of retinopathy, preferably one who is an expert in retinal disease (a retinal specialist).

Table 6.1 Guidelines for Care

Routine Care by Physician

- Examine retina with direct ophthalmoscope annually and when indicated by symptoms or previous findings

Referral to Optometrist or Ophthalmologist

- Examine retinas through dilated pupils once a year (this need not be done before puberty unless the patient has eye symptoms or other complications of diabetes)

Referral to a Retinal Specialist*

- At the beginning of pregnancy or if planning pregnancy within 12 months
- Moderate nonproliferative diabetic retinopathy, or worse
- Any level of macular edema (suggested by hard exudates within the macula)
- Immediate referral is mandatory (preferably to an ophthalmologist specializing in retinal disease) if any of the following are present:
  - NVD greater than ~25% of the optic disk area
  - any NVD with preretinal or vitreous hemorrhage
  - NVE greater than or equal to 50% of the disk area with preretinal or vitreous hemorrhage
- Reduced vision from any cause
- Immediate referral is strongly urged when the following are present:
  - proliferative retinopathy without HRC
  - severe nonproliferative retinopathy, which includes
    - —dilated irregular veins
    - —multiple dot and blot hemorrhages
    - —intraretinal microvascular abnormalities

*An ophthalmologist knowledgeable and experienced in the management and treatment of diabetic retinopathy.

If laser treatment has been recommended, the clinician should ensure that the treatment has been implemented and that the patient maintains the recommended follow-up.

Photocoagulation

Scatter (panretinal) photocoagulation. The principal method used to treat diabetic retinopathy is laser or light photocoagulation. For patients with proliferative retinopathy and HRC, scatter photocoagulation with the laser is standard therapy based on the Diabetic Retinopathy Study results and subsequent results from the Early Treatment Diabetic Retinopathy Study (ETDRS), another large-scale randomized controlled clinical trial.

In this procedure, a series of 1,200–1,600 (or sometimes more) laser burns, 500 μm in diameter and spaced one-half burn diameter apart, are placed throughout the midperipheral retina, avoiding the macular region (see Figure 6.3). The DRS demonstrated that this procedure reduced the rate of progression to blindness by 50% in eyes with HRC over a 5-year follow-up. The ETDRS study suggested that >95% of severe visual loss could be prevented if all patients received scatter photocoagulation just as they exhibit HRC.

Many eyes with proliferative retinopathy but without HRC, or with severe nonproliferative retinopathy also will require scatter photocoagulation. The factors determining whether such patients should receive treatment include type of diabetes, progression rate, contralateral eye status, systemic status, etc., and should be discussed with the patient by the retinal specialist.

Patients undergoing scatter photocoagulation should have a clear understanding of what to expect from the procedure in terms of their vision. Often prevention of severe visual loss is the goal, rather than improvement in vision. The procedure itself may result in some loss of peripheral and/or night vision.

Focal/grid laser photocoagulation. Diabetic macular edema is treated by focal/grid laser photocoagulation. With this technique, leaking microaneurysms and other vascular abnormalities in the macular region, determined by fluorescein angiography, are treated by direct application of small (50- to 100-μm) laser burns or laser burns placed in a grid-like pattern (Figure 6.5). The ETDRS showed that this treatment reduced the rate of visual loss from diabetic macular edema by 50% over a 3-year follow-up.

Vitrectomy

Vitrectomy is a surgical procedure used primarily to *1*) remove vitreous humor filled with blood, *2*) cut fibrous traction bands, *3*) peel contractile fibrous membranes from the inner retinal surface, and *4*) repair some types of complex retinal detachments. Vitrectomy is particularly effective in certain cases of advanced proliferative diabetic retinopathy. Although it can restore useful vision to eyes that would otherwise have severe visual impairment, vitrectomy is usually used only in more diseased eyes, as there are significant potential surgical complications.

Anti-VEGF Injections

Vascular endothelial growth factor (VEGF) is implicated in the pathology of neovascularization, permeability, and inflammation, which are key mechanisms of pathogenesis in diabetic macular edema and proliferative diabetic retinopahy. Biologic therapies directed against VEGF have been demonstrated to improve visual acuity significantly in patients with diabetic macular edema. In addition, these therapies may also be effective for proliferative diabetic retinopathy, and a trial comparing the three currently available therapies is due to be completed in 2016. However, risks of therapy with VEGF inhibitors, such as geographic atrophy and endophthalmitis, must be weighed against potential benefits. A recent meta-analysis shows that this issue has not been well studied, with most studies lasting for only 1 year. However, ocular events (such as infectious endophthalmitis; 3.9 patients per 1000) appear to be rare, and nonocular events were not different between the anti-VEGF treated subjects and the comparative risk group.

Medical Therapy

It is important to maintain normal blood pressure levels and near-normal blood glucose levels in patients with retinopathy because diabetic retinopathy progresses more rapidly in patients with uncontrolled hypertension and hyperglycemia than in those whose blood pressure and blood glucose are controlled. Control of systemic lipid levels is also important, as dyslipidemia is associated with increased risk of hard exudates in the macula. The addition of fenofibrate therapy has been shown to slow progression of retinopathy in patients with dyslipidemia and mild nonproliferative diabetic retinopathy.

Therapies under Evaluation

Other medical treatments for diabetic retinopathy have been evaluated.

- Aspirin (650 mg/day) was tested in the ETDRS because it inhibits platelet aggregation. Platelet microthrombi have been proposed as a factor in the cause of diabetic retinopathy. Aspirin was shown to be of no benefit or risk for retinopathy in this study.
- Two experimental classes of drugs, both targeting pathways involved in the pathogenesis of microvascular complications, may be useful in preventing or reducing the progression of diabetic retinopathy: aldose reductase inhibitors and protein kinase C inhibitors. Aldose reductase inhibitors have shown promise in animal studies but have not yet shown good efficacy or safety in human retinopathy trials. Similar findings have resulted from studies of protein kinase C inhibitors. Anti-VEGF therapies are being studied for potential use in proliferative diabetic retinopathy.

CONCLUSION

Diabetic retinopathy is a common complication of long-term diabetes that ranks as a leading cause of blindness and visual disability. Appropriate care includes optimization of blood glucose, blood pressure, and serum lipid levels and routine, lifelong ophthalmic examinations. Although treatment strategies cannot totally prevent or cure this complication, there is clear evidence that they can substantially retard its progression if used appropriately and provided promptly when indicated. Accordingly, careful, early, persistent optimization of glycemic control and other risk factors by the primary care physician, together with annual screening by an eye care professional and referral of patients with significant retinopathy to an ophthalmologist who is knowledgeable and experienced in the management of diabetic retinopathy, is a standard of care for all patients with diabetes.

BIBLIOGRAPHY

Aiello LP, Cahill MT, Wong JS. Systemic considerations in the management of diabetic retinopathy. *Am J Ophthalmol* 2001;132:760–776

Antonetti DA, Klein R, Gardner TW. Diabetic retinopathy. *N Engl J Med* 2012;366:1227–1239

Cheung N, Wong IY, Wong TY. Ocular anti-VEGF therapy for diabetes retinopathy: overview of clinical efficacy and evolving applications. *Diabetes Care* 2014;37:900–905

Chew EY, Davis MD, Danis RP, et al.; Action to Control Cardiovascular Risk in Diabetes Eye Study Research Group. The effects of medical management on the progression of diabetic retinopathy in persons with type 2 diabetes: the Action to Control Cardiovascular Risk in Diabetes (ACCORD) Eye Study. *Ophthalmology* 2014;121:2443–2451

DCCT/EDIC Research Group, Aiello LP, Sun W, Das A, et al. Intensive diabetes therapy and ocular surgery in type 1 diabetes. *N Engl J Med* 2015;372:1722–1733

DCCT Research Group. The effect of intensive treatment of diabetes on the development and progression of long-term complications in insulin-dependent diabetes mellitus. *N Engl J Med* 1993;329:977–986

DCCT Research Group. The relationship of glycemic exposure (HbA1c) to the risk of development and progression of retinopathy in the Diabetes Control and Complications Trial. *Diabetes* 1995;44:968–983

Diabetes Control and Complications Trial/Epidemiology of Diabetes Interventions and Complications Research Group. Retinopathy and nephropathy in patients with type 1 diabetes four years after a trial of intensive therapy. *N Engl J Med* 2000;342:381–389

Diabetes Control and Complications Trial/Epidemiology of Diabetes Interventions and Complications Research Group, Nathan DM, Zinman B, Cleary PA, et al. The modern-day clinical course of type 1 diabetes mellitus after 30 years' duration: the Diabetes Control and Complications Trial/Epidemiology of Diabetes Interventions and Complications and Pittsburgh Epidemiology of Diabetes Complications Experience (1983–2005). *Arch Intern Med* 2009;169:1307–1316

Early Treatment Diabetic Retinopathy Study Research Group. Early photocoagulation for diabetic retinopathy: ETDRS report number 9. *Ophthalmology* 1991;98(Suppl. 5):766–785

Early Treatment Diabetic Retinopathy Study Research Group. Photocoagulation for diabetic macular edema: Early Treatment Diabetic Retinopathy Study report number 1. *Arch Ophthalmol* 1985;103:1796–1806

Fong DS, Aiello LP, Ferris FL, Klein R. Diabetic retinopathy (Technical Review). *Diabetes Care* 2004;27:2540–2553

Hietala K, Harjutsalo V, Forsblom C, Summanen P, Groop PH; on behalf of the FinnDiane Study Group. Age at onset and the risk of proliferative retinopathy in type 1 diabetes. *Diabetes Care* 2010;33:1315–1319

Kaur H, Donaghue KC, Chan AK, Benitez-Aguirre P, Hing S, Lloyd M, Cusumano J, Pryke A, Craig ME. Vitamin D deficiency is associated with retinopathy in children and adolescents with type 1 diabetes. *Diabetes Care* 2011;34:1400–1402

Klein R, Lee KE, Gangnon RE, Klein BE. The 25-year incidence of visual impairment in type 1 diabetes mellitus: the Wisconsin Epidemiologic Study of Diabetic Retinopathy. *Ophthalmology* 2010;117:63–70

Nordwall M, Abrahamsson M, Dhir M, Fredrikson M, Ludvigsson J, Arnqvist HJ. Impact of HbA1c, followed from onset of type 1 diabetes, on the development of severe retinopathy and nephropathy: the VISS Study (Vascular Diabetic Complications in Southeast Sweden). *Diabetes Care* 2015;38:308–315

Sheetz MJ, Aiello LP, Shahri N, Davis MD, Kles KA, Danis RP; Mbdv Study Group. Effect of ruboxistaurin (RBX) on visual acuity decline over a 6-year period with cessation and reinstitution of therapy: results of an open-label extension of the protein kinase C diabetic retinopathy study 2 (PKC-DRS2). *Retina* 2011;31:1053–1059

Virgili G, Parravano M, Menchini F, Evans JR. Anti-vascular endothelial growth factor for diabetic macular oedema. *Cochrane Database Syst Rev* 2014;10:CD007419

White NH, Sun W, Cleary PA, Tamborlane WV, Danis RP, Hainsworth DP, Davis MD; for the DCCT-EDIC Research Group. Effect of the prior intensive therapy in type 1 diabetes on 10-year progression of retinopathy in the DCCT/EDIC: comparison of adults and adolescents. *Diabetes* 2010;59:1244–1253

DIABETIC KIDNEY DISEASE

About 40% of individuals starting dialysis in the U.S. have diabetes, and almost half of these have type 1 diabetes. In the past, epidemiological studies suggested that 20–40% of patients affected by type 1 diabetes would eventually develop kidney failure and require dialysis. More recent evidence suggests that the frequency of diabetic kidney disease may be decreasing in the type 1 diabetes population with increased implementation of intensive glycemic control and wide application of early screening and effective preventive measures. Thirty-year data from the DCCT/EDIC and the Pittsburgh Epidemiology of Diabetes Complications Experience (EDC) studies, encompassing the years 1983–2005, showed the differential risk by conventional and intensive treatment groups for the DCCT/EDIC compared to the EDC cohort. After 30 years of diabetes, the cumulative incidences of diabetic kidney disease were 25% in the DCCT conventional treatment group, 17% in the EDC cohort, and 9% in the DCCT intensive therapy group with fewer than 1% requiring kidney replacement therapy.

CLINICAL SYNDROME

In its fully established form, diabetic kidney disease is a distinct clinical entity characterized by proteinuria, hypertension, edema, and renal insufficiency; in its most severe form, nephrotic syndrome can be present. Diabetic kidney disease occurs in type 1 diabetic patients with long-standing diabetes (usually over 10 years).

Histopathological Changes

Three classes of renal histopathological changes characterize diabetic kidney disease: *1)* glomerulosclerosis; *2)* structural vascular changes, particularly in the small arterioles; and *3)* tubulointerstitial disease. Glomerular damage, e.g., mesangial expansion and basement membrane thickening, is the most characteristic feature of diabetic kidney disease and most often takes the form of diffuse scarring of entire glomeruli. The tubulointerstitial changes are the hallmark for progression of diabetic kidney disease with worsening glomerular filtration rate (GFR). These changes also interfere with potassium ion and hydrogen ion secretion and may be at least partly responsible for the hyperkalemia and metabolic acidosis, i.e., type IV renal tubular acidosis, that can accompany diabetic kidney disease.

NATURAL HISTORY

Shortly after diabetes is diagnosed, the GFR and renal blood flow are characteristically elevated, typically with a corresponding increase in kidney weight and size related to the degree of hyperglycemia. The serum creatinine and urea nitrogen concentrations are slightly reduced when renal hyperfiltration is present. Improvement in glycemic control can normalize GFR and reduce renal hypertrophy. Although a slight increase in urine protein is common when a patient initially presents in diabetic ketoacidosis, once glycemia is well regulated by insulin therapy proteinuria disappears and remains absent for many years.

Early in the course of diabetes, the renal histology is normal despite renal hypertrophy. However, within 2–3 years, many kidneys demonstrate some histological evidence of mesangial expansion and basement membrane thickening. Despite these histological changes, GFR and renal blood flow may remain elevated, and proteinuria is not detectable. The earliest clinical evidence of diabetic kidney disease is the appearance of low but abnormal levels (>30 mg/day or 30 µg/mg creatinine) of albumin in the urine. This subclinical range of increased albumin excretion goes undetected with routine urine dipstick testing, but is detectable with more sensitive techniques. Poor glycemic control is the main precipitant in the development of albuminuria via activation of the renin-angiotensin system (RAS). RAS activation via volume loss and sodium depletion leads to increased glomerular filtration and podocyte apoptosis permitting increased protein loss.

Hyperglycemia, infection, vigorous exercise, and smoking can each lead to elevated urine albumin in the absence of kidney disease. The presence of even microscopic hematuria (or contamination by menstrual fluid) is sufficient to invalidate tests for albuminuria. Therefore an elevated urine albumin should be repeated at least 1–3 months later to confirm the presence of diabetic kidney disease.

Patients with confirmed albuminuria are referred to as having incipient kidney disease and are at a higher risk for developing progressive kidney disease. Without specific interventions, ~80% of subjects with type 1 diabetes who develop sustained albuminuria have their urinary albumin excretion increase at a rate of ~10–20% per year. This leads to overt kidney disease or clinical albuminuria (>300 mg/24 h or ~300 µg/mg creatinine) over 10–15 years, with hypertension also developing.

In addition to being the earliest manifestation of kidney disease, increased urine albumin excretion is a marker of greatly increased cardiovascular risk for patients with either type 1 or type 2 diabetes. Thus, the finding of albuminuria is an indication for screening for possible vascular disease and aggressive intervention to reduce all cardiovascular risk factors (e.g., lowering of LDL cholesterol, antihypertensive therapy, smoking cessation, increased physical activity). In addition, some preliminary evidence suggests that lowering cholesterol may also reduce the level of proteinuria.

Once overt kidney disease occurs, without specific interventions, the GFR gradually falls over several years at a rate that is highly variable from individual to individual (2–20 mL/min/year). Kidney failure develops in 50% of patients with type 1 diabetes with overt kidney disease within 10 years and in >75% by 20 years.

Although the GFR may still be elevated at the onset of proteinuria, it usually declines by ~50% within 3 years, and the serum creatinine and urea nitrogen concentrations become frankly elevated. Hypertension starts to manifest itself and becomes progressively more difficult to treat. The mean duration of type 1 diabetes when end-stage renal disease (ESRD) develops is 23 years. With progression of diabetic kidney disease to end-stage renal disease, the uremic symptoms, e.g., drowsiness, lethargy, and nausea, appear and become progressively more pronounced. Most patients receive treatment before reaching this stage, and cardiovascular disease is now the most common cause of death in patients with diabetic kidney disease.

Traditionally, it has been considered unusual in type 1 diabetes to observe diabetic kidney disease in the absence of retinopathy, neuropathy, and hypertension. However, the correlation is close only in advanced kidney disease. As kidney failure progresses, the incidence and severity of all three disorders increases markedly, generally in parallel with renal status.

PATHOGENESIS

Considerable evidence suggests that diabetic kidney disease in type 1 diabetes is related primarily to the hyperglycemia induced by the diabetic state. First, renal changes are absent initially in people with type 1 diabetes biopsied around the time of onset of diabetes. Second, typical changes of diabetic kidney disease occur in all types of diabetes. Third, diabetic kidney disease appears in various animal models regardless of whether the diabetes is induced or spontaneous, and the damage occurs in both original and transplanted kidneys. Fourth, in these diabetic animals, intensive insulin therapy or islet cell transplantation completely prevents renal histopathologic changes from occurring in the healthy kidney, or may reverse early changes that have already occurred. Finally, improved blood glucose control can substantially delay the initial appearance of persistent and clinical-grade albuminuria in type 1 diabetes.

Possible Mechanisms of Damage

The mechanisms by which diabetes damages the kidney are not completely understood. Podocyte injury and depletion appear to play a role in the pathogenesis of diabetic kidney disease, and there is a strong correlation between podocyte density, albuminuria, and renal function decline. Understanding of the regulatory and signaling pathways involved in glomerular injury, including VEGF, Notch signaling, and others, might lead to novel therapies for prevention and treatment in the future. How these pathways might be triggered by elevated glucose *per se* or by some metabolic event that occurs as a consequence of hyperglycemia remains unknown. However, a plausible hypothesis based upon the final common pathway of hyperglycemia leading to oxidant stress via activation of protein kinase C, increased advanced glycation end products (AGEs), the polyol pathway, and activation of the renin-angiotensin-aldosterone system (RAAS) has been put forth and is supported by multiple lines of experimental evidence.

A genetic propensity to diabetic kidney disease has been noted. Thus, it is possible that metabolic disturbances initiate the processes responsible for diabetic kidney disease, but that these processes operate on a genetic background that predisposes to diabetic glomerulosclerosis. Some studies suggest the genetic predisposition relates to an increased familial incidence of essential hypertension.

One explanation for renal damage may involve the typical increases in GFR and renal blood flow that occur early in the course of diabetes. In animals, these alterations in renal hemodynamics are associated with increased intraglomerular pressure. Although it has not been possible to measure intraglomerular pressure in humans, it has been suggested that glomerular hypertension is the ultimate mediator of kidney damage in diabetic kidney disease. Measures aimed at reversing the resulting hemodynamic changes have proved useful in slowing the progression of kidney disease in human diabetes.

TESTING FOR DIABETIC KIDNEY DISEASE

As of the 2015 publication of the Standards of Medical Care in Diabetes, the terms "microalbuminuria" (albumin levels 30–299 mg/24 h) and "macroalbuminuria" (albumin levels 300 mg/24 h) were eliminated because albuminuria occurs along a continuum. Albuminuria is defined as a urine albumin-to-creatinine ratio of ≥30 mg/g. Because increased albumin excretion rarely occurs with short duration of type 1 diabetes or before puberty, screening in individuals with type 1 diabetes should begin after the child has had diabetes for 5 years. Evidence suggests that the prepubertal duration of diabetes may be important in the development of microvascular complications, so clinical judgment should be used when applying this recommendation to individual patients.

Screening for albumin-to-creatinine ratio can be performed using the following three methods: *1*) measurement of the albumin-to-creatinine ratio in a random spot collection, *2*) 24-h collection, and *3*) timed (e.g., 4-h or overnight) collection. The first method is the easiest to carry out in an office setting and generally provides accurate information. First-void or other morning collections are preferred because of the known diurnal variation in albumin excretion, but if this timing cannot be used, uniformity of timing for different collections in the same individual should be employed. Specific assays are needed to detect albumin levels 30–299 mg/dL/24 h, because both standard dipsticks and standard hospital laboratory assays for urinary protein are not sufficiently sensitive to measure such levels.

In addition to annual assessment of urinary albumin, serum creatinine should be measured at least annually and used to estimate GFR and determine the stage of chronic kidney disease (CKD), if present (see Table 6.2). GFR can be estimated using formulae such as the Cockroft-Gault equation or a prediction formula using data from the Modification of Diet in Renal Disease Study. GFR calculators are

Table 6.2 Stages of CKD

Stage	Description	GFR (mL/min/1.73 m^2)
1	Kidney damage* with normal or increased eGFR	≥90
2	Kidney damage* with mildly decreased eGFR	60–89
3	Moderately decreased eGFR	30–59
4	Severely decreased eGFR	15–29
5	Kidney failure	<15 or dialysis

eGFR, estimated glomerular filtration rate.
*Kidney damage is defined as abnormalities on pathological, urine, blood, or imaging tests.
Source: American Diabetes Association. Standards of medical care in diabetes—2016. *Diabetes Care* 2016;39(Suppl. 1):S73.

available at www.nkdep.nih.gov. Many clinical laboratories now report estimated GFR (eGFR) in addition to serum creatinine. Although in the DCCT/EDIC albuminuria was a strong predictor of eGFR loss and risk of developing sustained eGFR <60 mL/min/1.73 m^2, it is estimated that albumin excretion rate alone would have missed 24% of cases of sustained impaired eGFR. Therefore, it is recommended that serum creatinine be measured annually in adults regardless of the degree of urine albumin excretion.

Assessment of the urinary albumin excretion should be performed at least annually to monitor for progression and improvement after initiation of therapy, since an increase in urine albumin-to-creatinine ratio (UACR) can signal problems with medication adherence or worsening of effectiveness of therapy.

In addition, patients with relatively short duration of type 1 diabetes (<10 years duration), no other microvascular complications, nephrotic range proteinuria without increased UACR, presence of red cell casts, or other signs of glomerulonephritis should prompt a search for nondiabetic causes for kidney disease.

MANAGEMENT OF DIABETIC KIDNEY DISEASE

Incipient Diabetic Kidney Disease

The use of an ACE inhibitor or an angiotensin II receptor blocker (ARB) is not recommended in the primary prevention of diabetic kidney disease in patients with diabetes who have normal blood pressure and normal urinary albumin excretion. However, confirmation of increased urinary albumin excretion should trigger increased attention to improved glycemic control and the institution of ACE-inhibitor or ARB therapy, both of which have been shown to decrease the progression of diabetic kidney disease. The DCCT demonstrated conclusively that intensive glycemic control reduces the development and progression of early kidney disease. In the DCCT/EDIC follow-up study at 22 years, there remained a 50% risk reduction in the intensive therapy group. However, there is no evidence that tight glycemic control through intensive insulin therapy can reverse or even slow the progression of severely advanced kidney disease.

Patients with type 1 diabetes often develop albuminuria prior to developing hypertension, so the dosage of the ACE inhibitor may need to be low to avoid symptomatic hypotension. ARBs have been shown to reduce the rate of progression of albuminuria. Combination therapy with an ACE inhibitor and an ARB should *not* be used since an increased risk of serious adverse events has been found.

Overt Diabetic Kidney Disease

Once overt proteinuria or decreased GFR are detected, renal function should be monitored at least two to three times per year. Hypertension should be aggressively treated with an ACE inhibitor or an ARB and usually with adjunctive medications, as discussed in Table 6.3. Other interventions in the management of advanced diabetic kidney disease include: *1)* minimizing factors that are known to accelerate the natural progression of kidney disease or that may otherwise jeopardize the kidney, *2)* assessing for anemia and secondary hyperparathyroidism, and *3)* appropriately responding to decreasing insulin needs (Tables 6.3 and 6.4). The development of renal insufficiency may initially be associated with insulin resistance, resulting in an increase in insulin requirements. However, because insulin is cleared by the kidney and since the kidneys account for approximately 20% of gluconeogenesis, as kidney disease becomes more advanced, it is common to see a decrease in the daily insulin dose and/or an increase in hypoglycemic episodes, particularly in patients with a GFR <20 mL/min. For this reason, self-monitoring of blood glucose and use of the results to adjust the insulin dose are critical.

REFERRAL TO A NEPHROLOGIST

If there is uncertainty regarding the etiology of kidney disease, challenging management issues, and/or rapidly progressing kidney disease, patients should be

---

Table 6.3 Treatment of Diabetic Kidney Disease

The following are factors influencing diabetic kidney disease that should be addressed:

- **Hypertension.** This is the most important factor shown to accelerate progression of renal failure. Goal blood pressure is <140/90 mmHg, but clinicians should consider lower targets of <130/80 mmHg in individuals with albuminuria. Angiotensin-converting enzyme (ACE) inhibitors and angiotensin II receptor blockers (ARBs) have specific effects to preserve renal function, as do diuretics. There are some data supporting use of nondihydropyridine calcium channel blockers.

- **Hyperglycemia.** Control of blood glucose is extremely important in preventing and stopping the progression of albuminuria and proteinuria. The recommended glycemic goals are as close to normal as possible (Tables 2.1 and 2.2). Note that uremia may be associated with insulin resistance and increased insulin requirements. With advanced uremia (GFR 15–20 mL/min), insulin requirements may fall because the kidneys are no longer able to clear insulin as well, and hepatic degradation of insulin is inhibited by uremia. Consideration should be given to lowering the insulin dose when GFR drops below 60 mL/min.

- **Hyperlipidemia.** Control of lipids is essential in preventing cardiovascular disease and may aid in slowing the progression of kidney disease. There is insufficient evidence for a specific LDL target, but clinicians should use the maximally tolerated statin dose. In ESRD, there is no benefit for initiating statin therapy.

- **Overweight or obesity.** Evidence shows that weight loss can help in patients who are overweight or obese.

- **Tobacco use.** Smoking cessation can help protect kidney function.

- **Proteinuria.** Reducing proteinuria with ACE inhibitors or ARBs and nondihydropyridine calcium antagonists will result in additive effects to preserve renal function.

- **Protein restriction.** A low-protein diet (<0.8 g/kg body weight/day) should not be recommended to slow progression of renal disease in patients with diabetes with advanced renal insufficiency because it has not been shown to improve glycemic measures or cardiovascular risk or slow the rate of decline in GFR. Daily protein intake of 0.8 g/kg body weight is generally recommended, while a high-protein diet (>1.3 g/kg body weight/day) should be avoided.

Table 6.4 Other Threats to Diabetic Kidneys

Several conditions can endanger the kidneys of individuals with diabetes, even if renal insufficiency has not yet come into play. Among them are the following:

- **Urinary tract infection.** Older individuals with diabetes generally have an increased incidence of urinary tract infection. Therefore, for these patients, it is important that a urinalysis be performed if clinically indicated. If leukocytes or bacteriuria are detected, a urine culture should be obtained. Positive cultures should be treated with an appropriate bactericidal antibiotic.

- **Neurogenic bladder.** The development of a neurogenic bladder is common in patients with diabetes, especially if other evidence of autonomic neuropathy is present, and may predispose to infection. If the patient is on any medications with anticholinergic properties that could contribute to neurogenic bladder, the need for these medication(s) should be reviewed and discontinued if not necessary. Symptoms of neurogenic bladder (e.g., frequent voiding, nocturia, incontinence, and recurrent urinary tract infections) may be minimal or may mimic those of prostatic hypertrophy. Once suspected, the diagnosis is easily established if a cystometrogram demonstrates a large atonic bladder with low-pressure recordings. If the presence of a neurogenic bladder is confirmed, the patient should receive instruction in Credé's manual voiding maneuver, which should be performed about every 8 h. Often this will be sufficient to prevent excessive post-void residuals and will decompress the upper urinary tract. If not, parasympathetic agents such as bethanechol chloride may be tried. In some people with diabetes, β-adrenergic–blocking agents, such as phenoxybenzamine, have proved useful. If pharmacologic therapy proves unsuccessful, intermittent straight catheterization should be performed 2–3 times daily.

- **Intravenous pyelography and other dye studies.** Patients with diabetes are at increased risk for acute renal failure after any radiocontrast (intravenous and retrograde pyelography, arteriography, cholangiography, computed tomography scanning) procedure. With the judicious use of echography, radionuclide studies, magnetic resonance imaging, and noncontrast computed tomography scanning, studies employing iodinated radiocontrast dye are rarely necessary. If contrast media must be used, a minimum amount of dye should be given, and adequate hydration with half-normal or normal saline should be ensured before the dye study. Potentially nephrotoxic medications, including nonsteroidal anti-inflammatory drugs (NSAIDs), metformin, and diuretics, should be held prior to contrast administration. Use of iso-osmolar, dimeric, and nonionic iodinated contrast agents such as iodixanol should be considered in high-risk patients with kidney disease or serum creatinine concentrations >1.5 mg/dL. General recommendations cannot yet be made regarding the routine administration of specific agents to prevent contrast-induced reductions in renal function, such as acetylcysteine or fenoldopam, as they are still under intensive investigation. Serum creatinine concentration should be checked daily for 2–3 days after the contrast study.

referred promptly to a physician experienced in the care of kidney disease. A long-term therapeutic strategy needs to be planned, and the possibility and implications of kidney failure need to be discussed with the patient. Furthermore, patients should be referred for evaluation for renal replacement treatment if they have an estimated GFR <30 mL/min/1.73 m². The patient should understand the two options available for renal replacement therapy, dialysis and kidney transplantation, and have adequate medical and psychological preparation for renal replacement therapy.

HYPERTENSION

In type 1 diabetes, hypertension typically is secondary to the onset of more advanced kidney disease; long-term survivors of diabetes without kidney disease rarely have hypertension. Hypertension is the single most important factor accelerating the progression of established diabetic kidney disease and contributes to other causes of diabetes-related morbidity and mortality, such as retinopathy and heart disease. Aggressive treatment of hypertension is the only therapeutic intervention definitively shown to slow the progression of established kidney disease.

The diagnosis of hypertension should be based on multiple blood pressure determinations before beginning treatment. Orthostatic hypotension is frequent in patients with diabetic kidney disease; therefore, both supine and standing blood pressure should be measured. Ambulatory blood pressure monitoring is used in some centers to monitor patients during treatment.

According to recent data from the Action to Control Cardiovascular Risk in Diabetes blood pressure (ACCORD BP) trial and other trials, the patient with diabetes should have blood pressure treated to <140/85 mmHg, and those with overt diabetic kidney disease should be treated to <130/80 mmHg. For patients (generally older) with isolated systolic hypertension with a systolic pressure of >180 mmHg, the initial goal of treatment is to reduce the systolic blood pressure in stages. If these initial goals are met and well tolerated, further lowering should be pursued. Caution should be used because of the increased risk of dizziness and falls with low diastolic blood pressure, especially in the setting of limited autonomic drive.

Antihypertensive Therapy

ACE inhibitors. Many studies have shown that in hypertensive patients with type 1 diabetes, ACE inhibitors reduce the level of albuminuria and reduce the rate of progression of kidney disease to a greater degree than other antihypertensive agents that lower blood pressure by an equal amount. ACE inhibitors are recommended as the primary treatment for all hypertensive type 1 diabetes patients with albumin levels 30–299 mg/dL/24 h or overt diabetic kidney disease.

ACE inhibitors have few adverse effects and may even have modest beneficial effects on lipid metabolism and insulin sensitivity. The major serious side effect of ACE inhibitors is hyperkalemia, which is of particular concern in patients with more advanced diabetic kidney disease, who may have the syndrome of hyporeninemic hypoaldosteronism. In the presence of low renin, circulating aldosterone levels are decreased and the renal tubular secretion of potassium is impaired. Any drug that further impairs aldosterone secretion or action may lead to clinically significant hyperkalemia. If this occurs, the ACE inhibitor should be discontinued and the serum chemistries repeated. A rechallenge can be considered, but the clinician may need to find an alternative therapy. Mild hyperkalemia can occur during ACE/ARB therapy for hypertension with elevated albumin excretion in the absence of advanced diabetic kidney disease. So monitoring of serum potassium is needed, particularly when initiating ACE/ARB therapy, for dose increases, and in situations that put patients at higher risk for renal dysfunction.

Some patients may experience a precipitous rise in serum creatinine when initiating therapy with ACE inhibitors, especially those with bilateral renal artery stenosis or advanced kidney disease. In patients with impaired kidney function or suspected renovascular hypertension, the physician should determine serum creatinine and potassium levels ~1 week after therapy begins. An excessive increase in either level warrants discontinuation of the drug. Cough may also occur. Finally, ACE inhibitors are contraindicated in pregnancy and therefore should be used with caution in women of childbearing potential.

Angiotensin II receptor blockers. ARBs also slow the progression of kidney disease; studies have shown a slowing of the rate of transition from less severe (albumin excretion of 30–299 mg/dL/24 h) to more severe urine albumin excretion in hypertensive type 2 diabetes patients. Furthermore, in type 2 diabetes with hypertension, albuminuria, and elevated creatinine levels, ARBs clearly slow the progression of diabetic kidney disease compared with other antihypertensive agents. If ACE inhibitors cannot be tolerated because of side effects such as cough, substitution of an ARB should be considered. The simultaneous use of ARBs with ACE inhibitors should be avoided because there is no evidence for added ASCVD benefit, but there is increased incidence of side effects (hyperkalemia, syncope, renal dysfunction).

Diuretics. Because hypertension in the patient with diabetic kidney disease is often volume sensitive, therapy with a low-sodium diet and addition of a diuretic, especially when edema is present, may be needed to reach blood pressure treatment goals. Because many hypertensive individuals with type 1 diabetes have some degree of renal insufficiency, a loop diuretic is usually necessary. Thiazide diuretics do not promote natriuresis once the serum creatinine level has risen to ~2 mg/dL. In patients with renal insufficiency, diuretics that inhibit potassium secretion (e.g., spironolactone, triamterene) should be used with caution because of concern for inducing hyperkalemia.

β-adrenergic–blocking agents. β-adrenergic–blocking agents have also proven successful in treating the hypertensive patient with diabetes. However, this class of drugs may mask many of the warning symptoms of hypoglycemia (although sweating is not affected). β-blocking agents also predispose patients to the development of hyperkalemia, by inhibiting renin synthesis and impairing potassium uptake by extrarenal tissues, and may aggravate hypertriglyceridemia. Specific β_1-antagonists are the preferred β-blocking agents in patients with diabetes because they are less likely to cause hypoglycemia and hyperkalemia.

Calcium antagonists. Studies have shown that nondihydropyridine calcium antagonists reduce albuminuria and proteinuria; however, they have not been shown to have specific renal-protective effects, so they should be used as adjunctive rather than primary agents. This class of drugs is relatively free of harmful side effects and does not cause significant alterations in glucose or lipid metabolism.

OTHER ASPECTS OF TREATMENT

Low-Protein Diet

Over the last several years, there has been renewed interest in the use of low-protein diets to prevent the progression of chronic kidney failure. Animal studies have shown that restriction of dietary protein intake reduces hyperfiltration and intraglomerular pressure and retards the progression of several models of kidney disease, including diabetic glomerulopathy. However, data in humans are mixed, and adhering to this can be difficult in an already restricted diet. The general consensus is to prescribe a protein intake of approximately the adult recommended dietary allowance of 0.8–1.0 g/kg/day in early stages of CKD and 0.8 g/kg/day (~10% of daily calories) in patients with overt kidney disease. Reducing dietary protein below usual intake is not recommended because it does not alter glycemic measures or course of GFR decline.

Low-Sodium Diet

A diet lower in sodium has been shown to potentiate the beneficial effects of ACE-inhibitor and ARB therapy and should be recommended.

DIALYSIS AND KIDNEY TRANSPLANTATION

Once kidney disease progresses to stage 5 (kidney failure), prolonging life requires dialysis or a functioning kidney transplant. The latter provides the uremic patient with diabetes a greater survival with greater rehabilitation than does either continuous ambulatory peritoneal dialysis (CAPD) or maintenance hemodialysis. Therapy should be individualized to the patient's specific medical and family circumstances. The pros and cons of these procedures should be discussed with patients and their families well in advance of kidney failure. The prospect of needing such measures should never be a surprise. The ultimate choice among alternatives requires input from the patient, the patient's family, a nephrologist, and the primary care physician. In patients with diabetes, the absolute indications for dialysis or transplantation occur earlier than with other causes of kidney failure (i.e., at serum creatinine >6 mg/dL or creatinine clearance ≤20 mL/min). Urgent uremic symptoms (e.g., seizures, uremic pericarditis, unresponsive hypertension, and muscle deterioration) also occur earlier in patients with diabetes. More subjective criteria include worsening lethargy, nausea or vomiting, and progressive retinopathy and neuropathy. It is important not to delay the start of dialysis in patients with diabetes. No matter which renal replacement therapy has been elected, optimal rehabilitation in patients with kidney failure requires that effort be devoted to recognition and management of comorbid conditions.

Renal Dialysis

Of the various forms of renal dialysis, hemodialysis is the most frequently used in patients with diabetes, although peritoneal dialysis is also used with success. Some patients using peritoneal dialysis have insulin included with the dialysate. This procedure may help with the problematic blood glucose control that may occur due to high concentrations of dextrose in the dialysate; peritoneal insulin delivery is more physiologic than subcutaneous delivery. Icodextrin in peritoneal dialysate may result in artifactual hyperglycemia in some glucose monitors. However, peritoneal dialysis affords a motivated patient the greatest mobility. Treatment of anemia with erythropoietin or its analogs improves the general well-being both of patients on dialysis and of patients before the initiation of dialysis therapy. Dialysis may be associated with wide swings of glycemia, suggesting a role for increasing the number of glucose measurements in the peridialysis period or using CGM. In addition, A1C levels may significantly underestimate glycemia because of shortened red cell survival, use of erythropoietin, anemia, and uremia, while glycated albumin may be a more valid reflection of glucose control.

Kidney Transplantation

When the success rate of kidney transplantation in patients with diabetes approached the excellent success rate achieved in patients without diabetes, this procedure became the treatment of choice in patients with diabetic kidney failure. Living-donor kidneys (from first-degree relatives or, increasingly, from living unrelated donors) have higher organ survival rates than cadaveric kidneys, although the gap continues to narrow. The decision of whether to opt for a transplant is still not one to be taken lightly, and a patient must be well briefed on the chances of failure, the risks of immunosuppression, and the possibility that the new kidney will develop diabetic kidney disease in the future. This risk means that the patient should be committed to a program of intensive glycemic control post-transplantation. Serious consideration should be devoted to a combined kidney and pancreas transplant to control hyperglycemia in type 1 diabetes patients. Combined transplantation increases short-term morbidity, but properly selected patients may have better long-term rehabilitation.

CONCLUSION

Diabetic kidney disease is a major cause of morbidity and mortality in patients with type 1 diabetes of >15 years duration. Vigilant monitoring of evolving proteinuria, in particular its early detection with testing for urine albumin-to-creatinine ratio, striving for excellent glycemic control as early as possible after diagnosis and within patient-acceptable goals, early institution of ACE-inhibitor or ARB therapy, aggressive therapy of hypertension, and anticipating the need for dialysis or transplantation form the cornerstones of management. The primary care provider is pivotal in integrating available resources, including referral to a nephrologist. The options available in the event of kidney failure offer greater possibilities for salvaging quality of life and increasing longevity than were available in the past. When possible, renal transplantation is advised, as the treatment is more likely to enhance both quality and quantity of life.

BIBLIOGRAPHY

Ahn SH, Susztak K. Getting a notch closer to understanding diabetic kidney disease. *Diabetes* 2010;59:1865–1867

American Diabetes Association. Standards of medical care in diabetes—2016. *Diabetes Care* 2016;39(Suppl. 1):S72–S80

Brownlee M. Biochemistry and molecular cell biology of diabetic complications. *Nature* 2001;414:813–820

Chiang JL, Kirkman MS, Laffel LM, Peters AL; on behalf of the Type 1 Diabetes Sourcebook Authors. Type 1 diabetes through the life span: a position statement of the American Diabetes Association. *Diabetes Care* 2014;37:2034–2054

DCCT/EDIC Research Group, de Boer IH, Sun W, Cleary PA, et al. Intensive diabetes therapy and glomerular filtration rate in type 1 diabetes. *N Engl J Med* 2011;365:2366–2376

DCCT Research Group. Retinopathy and nephropathy in patients with type 1 diabetes four years after a trial of intensive therapy. *N Engl J Med* 2000;342:381–389

DCCT Research Group. The effect of intensive treatment of diabetes on the development and progression of long-term complications in insulin-dependent diabetes mellitus. *N Engl J Med* 1993;329:977–986

Diabetes Control and Complications Trial/Epidemiology of Diabetes Interventions and Complications Research Group, Nathan DM, Zinman B, Cleary PA, et al. The modern-day clinical course of type 1 diabetes mellitus after 30 years' duration: the Diabetes Control and Complications Trial/Epidemiology of Diabetes Interventions and Complications and Pittsburgh Epidemiology of Diabetes Complications Experience (1983-2005). *Arch Intern Med* 2009;169:1307–1316

Gross JL, de Azevedo MJ, Silveiro SP, Canani LH, Caramori ML, Zelmanovitz T. Diabetic nephropathy: diagnosis, prevention, and treatment. *Diabetes Care* 2005;28:164–176

La Rocca E, Fiorina P, di Carlo V, Astorri E, Rossetti C, Lucignani G, Fazio F, Giudici D, Cristallo M, Bianchi G, Pozza G, Secchi A. Cardiovascular outcomes after kidney-pancreas and kidney-alone transplantation. *Kidney Int* 2001;60:1964–1971

Molitch ME, DeFronzo RA, Franz MJ, et al.; American Diabetes Association. Nephropathy in diabetes. *Diabetes Care* 2004;27(Suppl. 1):S79–S83

Molitch ME, Steffes M, Sun W, Rutledge B, Cleary P, de Boer IH, Zinman B, Lachin J; the EDIC Study Group. Development and progression of renal insufficiency with and without albuminuria in adults with type 1 diabetes and the Diabetes and Control and Complications Trial and the Epidemiology of Diabetes Interventions and Complications Study. *Diabetes Care* 2010;33:1536–1543

National Kidney Foundation. Collaborators: Nelson RG, Tuttle KR, Bilous RW, Gonzalez-Campoy JM, Mauer M, Molitch ME, Sharma K, Fradkin JE, Narva AS, Wilt TJ, Ishani A, Rector TS, Slinin Y, Fitzgerald P, Carlyle M, Rocco MV, Berns JS, Nally JV Jr, Kramer H, Choi MJ, Willis K, Howell E, Cheung M, Slifer S. KDOQI clinical practice guideline for diabetes and CKD: 2012 update. *Am J Kidney Dis* 2012;60:850–886

Peacock TP, Shihabi ZK, Bleyer AJ, Dolbare EL, Byers JR, Knovich MA, Calles-Escandon J, Russell GB, Freedman BI. Comparison of glycated albumin and hemoglobin A_{1c} levels in diabetic subjects on hemodialysis. *Kidney Int* 2008;73:1062–1068

Tuttle KR, Bakris GL, Bilous RW, Chiang JL, deBoer IH, Goldstein-Fuchs J, Hirsch IB, Kalantar-Zadeh K, Narva AS, Navaneethan SD, Neumiller JJ, Patel UD, Ratner RF, Whaley-Connell AT, Molitch ME. Diabetic kidney disease: a report from an ADA Consensus Conference. *Diabetes Care* 2014;37:2864–2883

Yusef S, Teo KK, Pogue J, et al.; ONTARGET Investigators. Telmisartan, ramipril, or both in patients at high risk for vascular events. *N Engl J Med* 2008;358;1547–1559

Neuropathy is one of the most common and troubling chronic complications of diabetes, potentially affecting virtually all regions of the body and causing significant impairment alone or in concert with other conditions. Most notably, neuropathic loss of sensation in the foot often coexists with infection and/or vascular insufficiency, which is more common in people with diabetes, and results in diabetes being the most common cause of nontraumatic lower-limb amputations in the U.S. The frequency of diabetic neuropathy parallels the duration and severity of hyperglycemia in both type 1 and type 2 diabetes. In patients with type 1 diabetes, it rarely occurs within the first 5 years after diagnosis. The prevalence of neuropathy in the DCCT cohort increased from 9% to 25% between baseline and 13–14 years post-DCCT closeout in the intensive arm and increased from 17% to 35% in the conventional group, which provided evidence for the durable effect of prior intensive treatment on neuropathy. The prevention of neuropathy with strict glycemic control and comprehensive foot care is a key strategy to minimize this potentially devastating complication of diabetes.

OVERVIEW OF NEUROPATHIES

Histological Findings and Pathophysiology

Histologically, with neuropathy, there is loss of both large and small myelinated nerve fibers, accompanied by varying degrees of paranodal and segmental demyelination, connective tissue proliferation, and thickening and reduplication of capillary basement membranes with capillary closure. Pathways by which hyperglycemia (perhaps aided by other metabolic derangements of diabetes) may cause such changes include overactivity of the polyol pathway, advanced glycation end-products (AGEs), and altered intracellular oxidation-reduction potential.

Treatment of Neuropathies

There is no known direct treatment for established neuropathy, and the most effective strategies are preventive. The DCCT demonstrated that intensive glycemic control reduced the development and progression of early neuropathy by 60%. Aldose reductase inhibitors block the rate-limiting enzyme in the polyol pathway, which is activated in hyperglycemic states, and have appeared promising in animal studies but have been disappointing in human clinical trials. Clinical trials with protein kinase C inhibitors are ongoing. Treatment strategies for established neuropathies are directed at the symptoms and the dysfunction that result.

Clinical Syndromes

Diabetic neuropathy is classified into a set of discrete clinical syndromes, each with a characteristic presentation and clinical course (Table 6.5). Because the syndromes overlap clinically and frequently occur simultaneously, rigid classification of individual cases is often difficult. Identical neurological syndromes occur in other diseases and other conditions, such as alcoholic neuropathy and inflammatory neuropathies. Diabetic neuropathy is a diagnosis of exclusion, so

Table 6.5   Syndromes of Diabetic Neuropathy

Diffuse neuropathies (common, insidious onset, usually progressive)

- Distal symmetric sensorimotor polyneuropathy
- Autonomic neuropathy

Focal neuropathies (sudden onset, usually improve over time)

- Cranial neuropathy
- Radiculopathy
- Plexopathy
- Mononeuropathy/mononeuropathy multiplex
- Other mononeuropathies

in all patients with diabetes and peripheral neuropathy, other potential etiologies must also be considered (Table 6.6). Other causes include, but are not limited to, toxins (alcohol), neurotoxic medications (chemotherapy), vitamin B12 deficiency, hypothyroidism, renal disease, malignancies (multiple myeloma, bronchogenic carcinoma), infections (HIV), chronic inflammatory demyelinating neuropathy, inherited neuropathies, and vasculitis.

DISTAL SYMMETRIC SENSORIMOTOR POLYNEUROPATHY

Distal symmetric polyneuropathy is the most common form of diabetic neuropathy. Sensory signs and symptoms generally predominate over motor involvement and vary depending on the classes of nerve fibers. Loss of large fibers produces diminished proprioception and light touch, resulting in ataxic gait, unsteadiness, and weakness of intrinsic muscles in the hands and feet. Involvement of small fibers causes diminished pain and temperature sensation, resulting in significant problems such as unrecognized trauma (especially to the feet) and accidental burn injuries of the hands.

Typical neuropathic paresthesia (spontaneous uncomfortable sensations) or dysesthesia (contact paresthesia) may accompany both large- and small-fiber involvement. Sensory deficits first appear in the most distal portions of the extremities and spread proximally with disease progression in a "stocking-glove" distribution. In the most advanced cases, vertical bands of sensory deficit may develop on the chest or abdomen when the tips of the shorter truncal nerves become involved (Figure 6.6).

Occasionally, patients complain of exquisite hypersensitivity to light touch, superficial burning or stabbing pain, or bone-deep aching or tearing pain, usually most troublesome at night. Sometimes, neuropathic pain may become the overriding and disabling feature, especially in small-fiber neuropathy. Both neuropathic pain and paresthesia are thought to reflect spontaneous depolarization of newly regenerating nerve fibers.

Table 6.6 Common Conditions Resembling Various Forms of Diabetic Neuropathy

Distal symmetrical neuropathy

- Inflammatory neuropathies (vasculitic, i.e., systemic lupus erythematosus, polyarteritis, and other connective tissue diseases; sarcoidosis; leprosy)
- Metabolic neuropathies (hypothyroidism, uremic; nutritional; acute intermittent porphyria)
- Toxic neuropathies (alcohol; drugs; heavy metals, e.g., lead, mercury, and arsenic; industrial hydrocarbons)
- Other neuropathies (paraneoplastic; dysproteinemic, amyloid, hereditary)

Autonomic neuropathy

- Pure autonomic failure (idiopathic orthostatic hypotension, Bradbury-Eggleston syndrome)
- Autoimmune autonomic neuropathy

Cranial neuropathy

- Carotid aneurysm
- Intracranial mass
- Elevated intracranial pressure

Radiculopathy

- Spinal cord/root compression
- Transverse myelitis
- Coagulopathies
- Shingles

Plexopathy

- Mass lesions
- Coagulopathies
- Cauda equina lesions (femoral neuropathy)

Mononeuropathy/mononeuropathy multiplex

- Compression neuropathies
- Inflammatory (vasculitic) neuropathies
- Hypothyroidism, acromegaly

Patients should be screened annually for distal polyneuropathy using the following tests: pinprick sensation, vibration perception using a 1,280-Hz tuning fork, 10-g monofilament pressure sensation at the distal plantar aspect of both great toes and metatarsal joints, and assessment of ankle reflexes. More than one abnormal finding has >87% sensitivity in detecting polyneuropathy. Loss of 10-g monofilament perception and reduced vibration perception predict foot ulcers. Dermal markers, such as skin intrinsic fluorescence, may be useful in the future to indicate the presence of diabetic neuropathy.

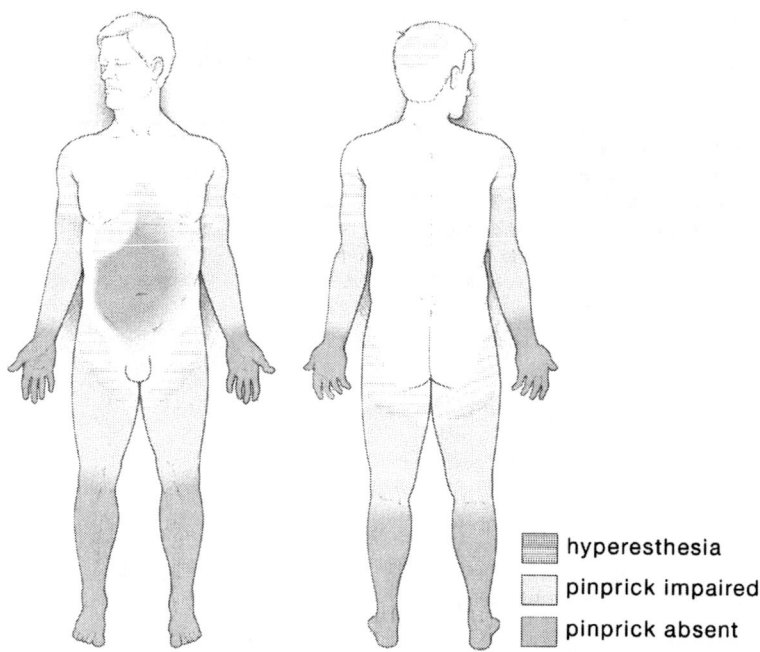

hyperesthesia

pinprick impaired

pinprick absent

Figure 6.6 Distribution of sensory loss in patient with severe chronic diabetic sensory polyneuropathy. Loss is maximal distally in limbs but also affects anterior trunk and vertex of head.

Asymptomatic Neuropathy

Many patients with distal symmetrical polyneuropathy remain free of troubling, subjective symptoms. In these cases, it may take careful questioning to learn of a patient's subtle feelings of numbness or cold or "dead" feet. Diminished or absent deep-tendon reflexes, especially the Achilles tendon reflex, or loss of ability to sense a 10-g monofilament, may be early indications of otherwise asymptomatic neuropathy. However, in the absence of pain or paresthesia, diabetic neuropathy may go unrecognized unless the physician routinely tests foot sensation during office visits.

LATE COMPLICATIONS OF POLYNEUROPATHY

Patients with chronic unrecognized neuropathy may present with late complications such as foot ulceration, foreign objects embedded in the foot, unrecognized trauma to the extremities, or neuroarthropathy (Charcot foot). All of these conditions are avoidable with proper early diagnosis of neuropathy and institution of appropriate foot care.

Foot Ulcerations and Infections

Acute foot ulcerations and resulting infections can occur when an individual cannot feel the pain caused by poorly fitting shoes (a source of blisters or penetrating abrasions), a retained foreign body, or accidental trauma (often unintentionally self-inflicted during nail trimming) because of neuropathy. Plantar ulcers, which form at the calloused sites of maximal walking pressure, can result from a combination of motor, sensory, and proprioceptive deficits. Patients with long-standing diabetes and neuropathy are also predisposed to vascular ulcers due to macrovascular and microvascular insufficiency and ischemic gangrene.

In a typical sequence of events, imbalance of extensor and flexor muscles in the feet resulting from impaired proprioception and atrophy of intrinsic extensor muscles leads to tendon shortening and chronic toe flexion (claw toe or hammer-toe deformity). This, in turn, shifts weight bearing from the padded ball of the foot to the unprotected metatarsal heads. With pain insensitivity, trauma to the overlying skin goes undetected, producing thick calluses that further concentrate weight bearing over the bony prominences. Splitting and fissuring of the thick callus or underlying pressure necrosis initiates ulcer formation, further aggravated by infection and vascular insufficiency.

Neuroarthropathy

Neuropathy impairs normal protective proprioceptive and nociceptive functions, which normally lead patients to recognize injury and protect the foot. Neuroarthropathy, or Charcot foot, refers to the joint erosions, unrecognized fractures, demineralization, and devitalization of bones in the foot resulting from unawareness of the minor injuries that occur during routine daily weight-bearing activities. The foot may be swollen and red but it is not painful. The problem may be misdiagnosed as cellulitis despite a normal leukocyte count and differential and the absence of fever. The patient may report relatively painless trauma, and initial radiographic examination may be unrevealing, whereas follow-up X-rays several days or weeks later may reveal clear traumatic changes. In more advanced cases, devitalization of bone may mimic osteomyelitis, and in the most advanced stages, the foot may look like a "bag of bones."

MANAGEMENT OF DISTAL SYMMETRIC POLYNEUROPATHY AND COMPLICATIONS

Treatment for diabetic distal symmetric polyneuropathy is symptomatic, palliative, and supportive, with primary emphasis on preventing the neuropathy and vasculopathy by near-normalization of glucose and lipids and smoking cessation. In most cases, the primary neuropathic symptoms consist of mild intermittent pain or paresthesia. Even severely painful symptoms generally remit spontaneously within a few months in most but not all patients.

Management of Pain

Persistent and severely painful neuropathy has been treated with various drugs, including standard analgesics and drugs normally used to treat pain in other conditions. Narcotics should generally be avoided. A recent evidence-based guideline on treatment of painful diabetic neuropathy recommended pregabalin as first-line therapy. Pregabalin, duloxetine, and tapentadol have all been approved for the treatment of diabetic peripheral neuropathy. Other drugs that may be effective in ameliorating, but not completely eliminating, symptoms include venlafaxine, amitriptyline, gabapentin, valproate, and opioids such as morphine sulfate, tramadol, and oxycodone controlled release. The antidepressant duloxetine, a serotonin and norepinephrine uptake inhibitor, is the only drug in this class to have a U.S. Food and Drug Administration (FDA) indication for treatment of painful diabetic neuropathy. It is a viable option for patients with anxiety and depression, fibromyalgia, and other chronic pain, but it is not recommended for patients with existing renal disease or hepatic impairment. A number of anticonvulsants have been used to treat painful neuropathy, but pregabalin has undergone the most rigorous testing and is the only anticonvulsant with an FDA indication for neuropathic pain. Topical capsaicin applied frequently to the hypersensitive areas may be useful in some cases, especially in those with more localized pain. Transcutaneous electrical nerve stimulation has also been used for refractory painful neuropathy.

Because early diagnosis of asymptomatic neuropathy is essential for preventing the late complications, every routine physician visit should include a thorough examination of the feet if the patient has preexisting risk factors or any foot symptoms. A list of neurologic and related symptoms to watch for is given in Table 6.7. In the absence of risk factors or symptoms, neuropathy screening is part of the annual comprehensive foot examination recommended for all patients with diabetes.

Callus Formation and Plantar Ulcers

Callus formation over weight-bearing areas indicates the need to consult an orthopedist and/or podiatrist for prescription of corrective footwear to redistribute weight bearing. Plantar ulcers should be managed by eliminating weight bearing either by special walking casts or by bed rest. Local debridement and application of growth factors may speed healing. Refractory and/or recurrent ulcers may be managed by surgical removal of the involved metatarsal. If there is evidence of impaired macrovascular circulation, vascular studies should be obtained and revascularization attempted when indicated. Neuroarthropathy is managed by reduced ambulation and weight bearing, as well as cushioned footwear.

Treatment of Infection

Infection must be treated aggressively with appropriate consultation from infectious disease specialists. Antibiotics effective against aerobic and anaerobic organisms should be included in the treatment regimen. Deep-wound cultures are necessary to direct antibiotic therapy properly. Vascular bypass surgery or percutaneous angioplasty should be considered if arterial insufficiency is a major contributing factor. Localized osteomyelitis may require a limited amputation.

AUTONOMIC NEUROPATHY

Neuropathy can affect virtually any autonomic function in patients with diabetes. Although autonomic neuropathy produces diffuse subclinical dysfunction, autonomic symptoms are usually confined to one or two organ systems, producing the discrete autonomic syndromes listed in Table 6.8.

Table 6.7　Warning Symptoms and Signs of Diabetic Foot Problems

SYMPTOMS

Vascular
- Cold feet
- Intermittent claudication involving calf or foot
- Pain at rest, especially nocturnal, relieved by dependency

Neurologic
- Sensory: burning, tingling, or crawling sensations; pain and hypersensitivity; complaints of cold or "dead" feet
- Motor weakness (drop foot)
- Autonomic: diminished sweating

Musculoskeletal
- Gradual change in foot shape
- Sudden painless change in foot shape, with swelling, without history of trauma

Dermatologic
- Exquisitely painful or painless wounds
- Slow-healing or nonhealing wounds, necrosis
- Skin color changes (cyanosis, redness)
- Chronic scaling, cracking, itching, or dry feet
- Recurrent infections (e.g., paronychia, athlete's foot)

SIGNS

- Absent pedal, popliteal, or femoral pulses
- Femoral bruits
- Dependent rubor, plantar pallor on elevation
- Prolonged capillary filling time (>3–4 sec)
- Decreased skin temperature
- Sensory: deficits (vibratory and proprioperceptive, then pain and temperature perception), hyperesthesia
- Motor: diminished to absent deep-tendon reflexes (Achilles then patellar), weakness
- Autonomic: diminished to absent sweating
- Cavus feet with claw toes
- Drop foot
- "Rocker-bottom" foot (Charcot foot)
- Neuropathic arthropathy

Skin
- Abnormal dryness
- Chronic tinea infections
- Keratotic lesions with or without hemorrhage (plantar or digital)
- Trophic ulcer

Hair
- Diminished to absent

Nails
- Trophic changes
- Onychomycosis
- Subungual ulceration or abscess
- Ingrown nails with paronychia

Source: Scardina RJ. Diabetic foot problems: assessment and prevention. *Clinical Diabetes* 1983;1(2):1–7.

Table 6.8 Syndromes of Autonomic Neuropathy

Cardiovascular Autonomic Neuropathy
- Resting sinus tachycardia without sinus arrhythmia (fixed heart rate)
- Exercise intolerance
- Painless myocardial infarction
- Orthostatic hypotension
- Sudden death

Gastrointestinal Autonomic Neuropathy
- Esophageal dysfunction
- Autonomic gastropathy and delayed gastric emptying (gastroparesis)
- Diabetic diarrhea
- Constipation
- Fecal incontinence
- Gallbladder atony

Genitourinary Autonomic Neuropathy
- Erectile dysfunction
- Retrograde ejaculation with infertility
- Bladder dysfunction

Sudomotor Neuropathy
- Distal hyperhidrosis or anhidrosis
- Facial sweating
- Heat intolerance
- "Gustatory" sweating

Hypoglycemia Unawareness

Cardiovascular Autonomic Neuropathy

The earliest clinical signs of cardiovascular autonomic neuropathy are absence of the normal sleep bradycardia and diminished variation of the pulse rate with inspiration-expiration or Valsalva (reduced sinus tachycardia), which are both due to early vagal involvement.

Later, sympathetic denervation interferes with normal cardiovascular reflexes thereby diminishing exercise tolerance, possibly hypersensitizing the heart to circulating catecholamines, and potentially causing tachyarrhythmias, and sudden death. It also predisposes to painless myocardial infarction.

Orthostatic hypotension. Orthostatic hypotension is managed by correcting hypovolemia with fluid replacement and improved glycemic control, elastic stockings, increased salt intake, mineralocorticoids, or vasoconstrictors. Midodrine, a specific β_1-agonist, has been shown to produce arteriolar constriction and a decrease in venous pooling via a constriction of venous capacitance vessels. It may exacerbate supine hypertension, which often coexists with orthostatic hypotension in patients with diabetes.

Gastrointestinal Autonomic Neuropathy

Nonspecific gastrointestinal (GI) symptoms in patients with diabetes often reflect diffuse but subtle GI autonomic dysfunction. Esophageal dysmotility can cause dysphagia, retrosternal discomfort, and heartburn. Delayed gastric emptying (gastroparesis) causes anorexia, nausea, vomiting, early satiety, and postprandial bloating and fullness. Delayed nutrient absorption can greatly complicate glycemic control, producing otherwise unexplained swings between severe hyperglycemia and hypoglycemia. Diagnosis of upper GI symptoms may be facilitated by liquid and solid-phase radionuclide gastric-emptying studies, although results do not correlate well with symptomatology nor with response to therapy. Management of esophageal dysmotility and delayed gastric emptying includes normalization of glucose, since hyperglycemia itself acutely decreases gastric emptying, and frequent small and/or primarily liquid feedings. High-fiber diets should be avoided, because they delay gastric emptying and may result in bezoar formation. The dopamine antagonist metoclopramide, or domperidone, may be helpful, but can cause acute or chronic dyskinesia. Irreversible tardive dyskinesia can occur after long-term use of metoclopramide, so the chronic use of metoclopramide should be avoided. Instead, metoclopramide should be reserved for patients with the most severe symptoms that are unresponsive to other therapies. The medication should be used at the lowest dose and for the shortest duration possible, generally not to exceed 3 months, and side effects should be closely monitored. Liquid erythromycin also sometimes improves symptoms. For patients suffering from constipation and lower GI motor issues, polyethylene glycol 3350 may be helpful. Newer therapeutic strategies for gastroparesis include drugs that target the underlying defects, prokinetic agents such as 5-hydroxytryptamine agonists that do not appear to have cardiac or vascular effects, and ghrelin agonists. Refractory cases may need gastric pacing or a feeding jejunostomy tube.

Diabetic diarrhea is classically painless, nocturnal, associated with fecal incontinence, and alternates with periods of constipation. Diagnostic studies of lower GI problems are necessary to define the multiple contributing factors that stem from widespread intestinal autonomic dysfunction in order to determine appropriate treatment. A therapeutic trial of broad-spectrum antibiotics may also be helpful, whereas evidence of bile salt malabsorption would argue in favor of bile salt–sequestering agents, both of which are effective in properly selected patients. Hypermotility is managed with diphenoxylate hydrochloride.

Fecal incontinence, which is also usually nocturnal, reflects impaired sensation of rectal distention, and in one small series of patients, it was effectively managed with biofeedback techniques. Clonidine may also be useful.

Sexual Dysfunction

Erectile dysfunction. Erectile dysfunction in men with diabetes is usually neuropathic. In 2003, an ancillary study to the DCCT/EDIC was conducted to assess erectile dysfunction in 571 men in both the primary and secondary cohorts. The prevalence of reported erectile dysfunction was 23%; it was significantly lower in the intensive compared to the conventional treatment groups in the secondary cohort (12.8% vs. 30.8%) but not in the primary cohort (17.0% vs. 20.3%). The risk of erectile dysfunction in the primary and secondary cohorts was directly associated with mean A1C during both the DCCT and EDIC trials combined; age, peripheral neuropathy, and lower urinary tract symptoms were additional risk factors for erectile dysfunction. In addition to neuropathy, erectile dysfunction can be psychogenic, endocrine, vascular, or drug or stress related. A normal erection on awakening or impotence only with a certain partner suggests a psychogenic cause. A band-type turgidity gauge or nocturnal penile tumescence monitoring at a sleep research facility can help clarify ambiguous situations.

Sex steroid imbalances, hypogonadism, and hyperprolactinemia should be excluded by appropriate endocrine studies. Proximal vascular insufficiency is usually evident on examination of the femoral pulses, although localized obstruction of the penile artery has been reported and can be excluded only by measurement of the brachial-penile blood pressure ratio with Doppler-flow studies. Proximal or localized vascular obstruction has been managed surgically, but the success rate is low.

Drugs known to produce erectile dysfunction include various antihypertensives, anticholinergics, antipsychotics, antidepressants, narcotics, barbiturates, alcohol, and amphetamines. Drug-induced impotence is managed by altering the treatment regimen when possible. Neuropathic impotence is generally, but not always, accompanied by other manifestations of diabetic neuropathy.

The main therapy for erectile dysfunction of neuropathic etiology consists of oral inhibitors of the phosphodiesterase type 5 enzyme (the predominant isoenzyme in human corpus cavernosum) which increase nitric oxide (sildenafil, vardenafil, tadalafil). Unfortunately, these medications are only effective in approximately 60% of men. The intracorporeal injection of vasoactive substances such as papaverine and prostaglandins is also effective in treating nonvascular erectile dysfunction. Patients who do not respond to pharmacologic therapy may opt for implantation of a penile prosthesis, but this is associated with risks of infection.

Retrograde ejaculation. Retrograde ejaculation, which may or may not occur in conjunction with erectile dysfunction, reflects loss of the coordinated closure of the internal and relaxation of the external vesicle sphincter during ejaculation. Patients usually present with infertility, and the diagnosis is confirmed by documenting azoospermia in ejaculate, and the presence of motile sperm in postcoital urine. Such sperm have been successfully used for artificial insemination.

Female sexual dysfunction. A recent review and meta-analysis found that female sexual dysfunction occurs more frequently in women with diabetes (particularly in type 1 versus type 2 diabetes) than in women without diabetes. Unfortunately, it is not well understood and has not been well studied. More studies are necessary to understand the risk factors for female sexual dysfunction, and potential treatment.

Other Autonomic Syndromes

Cystopathy initially diminishes sensation of bladder fullness, reducing urinary frequency. Later, efferent involvement produces incomplete urination, poor stream, dribbling, and overflow incontinence. Patients with cystopathy are predisposed to urinary tract infections. Conservative management involves scheduled voluntary urination with or without Credé's maneuver. Cholinergic-stimulating drugs, sphincter relaxants, periodic catheterization, and bladder-neck resection of the internal sphincter may be used in more advanced cases.

Hypoglycemia unawareness. Hypoglycemia unawareness may be related to autonomic neuropathy, which can blunt the usual adrenergic response to hypoglycemia. The condition predisposes to future episodes, and is worsened by antecedent episodes of severe hypoglycemia. Hypoglycemia awareness can be improved by strict avoidance of hypoglycemia. Relaxation of glycemic targets is imperative for patients who have one or more episodes of severe hypoglycemia or who have hypoglycemia unawareness. Insulin pump therapy and the use of CGM as well as the use of the low glucose suspend feature can help minimize or even prevent recurrent episodes of severe hypoglycemia.

Autonomic sudomotor dysfunction. Autonomic sudomotor dysfunction produces both asymptomatic anhydrosis of the extremities and central hyperhidrosis; the latter may be triggered by eating (gustatory sweating). Sudomotor dysfunction diminishes thermoregulatory reserve and predisposes to heat stroke and hyperthermia. Management includes avoidance of heat stress. Topical glycopyrrolate, an antimuscarinic compound, results in a marked reduction in sweating while eating a meal.

FOCAL NEUROPATHIES

Neural deficits corresponding to the distribution of single or multiple peripheral nerves (mononeuropathy and mononeuropathy multiplex), cranial nerves, areas of the brachial or lumbosacral plexuses (plexopathy), or the nerve roots (radiculopathy) are of sudden onset and are generally but not always self-limiting in patients with diabetes.

The third cranial nerve may be affected, presenting with unilateral pain, diplopia, and ptosis but with pupillary sparing. Differential diagnosis includes an aneurysm of the internal carotid artery and myasthenia gravis. Spontaneous remission usually occurs within a few months.

Radiculopathy presents as band-like thoracic or abdominal pain, often misdiagnosed as an acute intrathoracic or intra-abdominal emergency.

Femoral neuropathy in patients with diabetes often involves motor and sensory deficits at the level of the sacral plexus as well as the femoral nerve, with the relative excess of motor versus sensory involvement differentiating diabetic femoral neuropathy from that seen in other conditions. When bilateral, this is sometimes termed amyotrophy. Management of focal neuropathies includes exclusion of other causes, e.g., nerve entrapment or compression, and symptomatic palliation pending spontaneous resolution, which occurs generally but not always over periods of months to years.

CONCLUSION

Diabetic neuropathy is an extremely common complication of diabetes that becomes more prevalent with increasing duration and severity of hyperglycemia. Manifestations include diffuse and focal, painful and painless neurological deficits in the peripheral nervous system and widespread autonomic dysfunction. Prompt and proper diagnosis is essential to effective management and avoidance of serious secondary musculoskeletal and visceral complications.

BIBLIOGRAPHY

Albers AW, Herman WH, Pop-Busui R, Feldman EL, Martin CL, Cleary PA, Waberski BH, Lachin JM; for the DCCT/EDIC Research Group. Effect of prior intensive insulin treatment during the Diabetes Control and Complications Trial on peripheral neuropathy in type 1 diabetes during the Epidemiology of Diabetes Interventions and Complications Study. *Diabetes Care* 2010;33:1090–1096

Bril V, England J, Franklin GM, Backonja M, Cohen J, Del Toro D, Feldman E, Iverson DJ, Perkins B, Russell JW, Zochodne D, et al. Evidence-based guideline: treatment of painful diabetic neuropathy. *Neurology* 2011;76:1758–1765

Camilleri M, Bharucha AE, Farrigia G. Epidemiology, mechanisms and management of diabetic gastroparesis. *Clin Gastroenterol Hepatol* 2011;9:5–12

Conway BN, Aroda VR, Maynard JD, Matter N, Fernandez S, Ratner RE, Orchard TJ. Skin intrinsic fluorescence correlates with autonomic and distal symmetrical polyneuropathy in individuals with type 1 diabetes. *Diabetes Care* 2011;34:1000–1005

DCCT Research Group. The effect of intensive treatment of diabetes on the development and progression of long-term complications in insulin-dependent diabetes mellitus. *N Engl J Med* 1993;329:977–986

Gries FA, Cameron NE, Low PA, Ziegler D (Eds.). *Textbook of Diabetic Neuropathy*. New York, Thieme, 2003

Gruden G, Bruno G, Chaturvedi N, Burt D, Schalkwijk C, Pinach S, Stehouwer CD, Witte DR, Fuller JH, Perin PC; the EURODIAB Prospective Complications Study Group. Serum heat shock protein 27 and diabetes complications in the EURODIAB prospective complications study: a novel circulating marker for diabetic neuropathy. *Diabetes* 2008;57:1966–1970

Maser RE, Mitchell BD, Vinik AI, Freeman R. The association between cardiovascular autonomic neuropathy and mortality in individuals with diabetes: a meta-analysis. *Diabetes Care* 2003;26:1895–1901

Mayfield JA, Reiber GE, Sanders LJ, Janisse D, Pogach LM; American Diabetes Association. Preventive foot care in people with diabetes (Position Statement). *Diabetes Care* 2004;27(Suppl. 1):S63–S64

Ormseth MJ, Scholz BA, Boomershine CS. Duloxetine in the management of diabetic peripheral neuropathic pain. *Patient Prefer Adherence* 2011;5:343–356

Pontiroli AE, Cortelazzi D, Morabito A. Female sexual dysfunction and diabetes: a systematic review and meta-analysis. *J Sex Med* 2013;10:1044–1051

Scardina RJ. Diabetic foot problems: assessment and prevention. *Clinical Diabetes* 1983;1(2):1–7

Shaw JE, Abbott CA, Tindle K, Hollis S, Boulton AJ. A randomized controlled trial of topical glycopyrrolate, the first specific treatment for diabetic gustatory sweating. *Diabetologia* 1997;40:299–301

Vinik AI, Maser RE, Mitchell BD, Freeman R. Diabetic autonomic neuropathy. *Diabetes Care* 2003;26:1553–1579

Wessells H, Penson DF, Cleary P, Rutledge BN, Lachin JM, McVary KT, Schade DS, Sarma AV; and the DCCT/EDIC Research Groups. Effect of intensive glycemic therapy on erectile function in men with type 1 diabetes. *J Urology* 2011;185:1828–1834

MACROVASCULAR DISEASE

Coronary heart disease, peripheral arterial disease, and cerebrovascular disease all occur more commonly, at an earlier age, with a more diffuse distribution, and with greater severity and mortality in people with diabetes compared to patients without diabetes. Current recommendations for macrovascular disease prevention in individuals with type 1 diabetes have largely been extrapolated from populations with type 2 diabetes. In general, the American Diabetes Association recommends applying the same preventive and treatment strategies to patients with type 1 and type 2 diabetes, who have high lifetime cardiovascular risk. There is evidence that levels of risk factors for cardiovascular disease have improved in U.S. adults with diabetes in the past decade, but there is still room for considerable improvement.

PREVALENCE AND RISK FACTORS

Although cardiovascular deaths are less common in patients with type 1 diabetes than in generally older patients with type 2 diabetes, mortality rates among individuals with type 1 diabetes are excessive. Patients with type 1 diabetes have at least a 10-fold increase in mortality compared to individuals of the same age without diabetes. Overall, atherosclerotic cardiovascular disease (ASCVD) accounts for ~25% of the deaths among patients with the onset of diabetes before age 20 years. Premature coronary heart disease (CHD) and stroke cause 27% and 6%, respectively, of deaths among patients with diabetes age <45 years. Many of these deaths occur in patients with diabetic kidney disease, and a large percentage of them result from the unfavorable and avoidable interactions of diabetes, hypertension, and cigarette smoking.

Diabetes is an independent risk factor for ASCVD, increasing risk two- to threefold in men and even more in women. Women with diabetes are at equivalent CHD risk to men with diabetes. They lose the normally assumed "protection" of the female gender, and their cardiovascular disease rates parallel those of men with diabetes, even before menopause. In general, A1C and mean glucose levels are associated with ASCVD risk factors; it is controversial as to the strength of the relationship between ASCVD risk factors and postprandial glycemia and glucose variability.

The prevalence of lipid abnormalities varies significantly, depending on the characteristics of the study population such as age, gender, type of diabetes, severity of obesity, glycemic control, nondiabetes drugs, and thyroid and renal status. In patients with type 1 diabetes and good glycemic control, lipid levels are no different from an age- and sex-matched control population. In fact, with excellent glycemic control, the lipid profile may show lower total cholesterol and higher HDL cholesterol levels than in control subjects. Levels of cholesterol, ratios of total cholesterol to HDL cholesterol, and triglyceride levels are generally higher in patients with type 1 diabetes during periods of poor glycemic control and then become powerful risk factors for cardiovascular disease. Diabetic ketoacidosis may be associated with a profound temporary hypertriglyceridemia. Although improved glycemic control corrects elevated triglyceride levels and may help to raise HDL cholesterol slightly, a lower A1C will usually not improve LDL cholesterol levels. Separate treatment for LDL cholesterol will be required.

Even minimal urine excretion of albumin becomes a potent risk factor for CHD and stroke events. When proteinuria reaches the level of early diabetic kidney disease (300–1,000 mg/24 h), lipid levels may begin to reveal a more atherogenic pattern: decreased HDL cholesterol, increased triglyceride levels, and a shift toward larger numbers of smaller, more dense LDL particles without necessarily raising LDL cholesterol levels. The most extreme example is with nephrotic syndrome. Even when the lipid levels are acceptable by standard lipid profile measures, glycation of lipoproteins and other lipoprotein compositional abnormalities, including oxidation of the LDL particles induced by diabetes and/or hyperglycemia, may make those lipid levels more atherogenic. The precise role of advanced lipid testing for patients with diabetes remains under investigation.

Hypertension and cigarette smoking are major cardiovascular risk factors. In health surveys of people age 20–44 years, 29% of those with diabetes (compared with only 8% of those without diabetes) report having hypertension. Hypertension is especially seen in men, those with microangiopathy, those who are overweight or obese, those who are older, and those with longer diabetes duration. Hypertension also increases in prevalence with the degree of renal impairment. Fortunately, the percentage of smokers is decreasing, but young patients with diabetes should always be reminded not to begin this habit and reminded of effects of tobacco on the many complications of diabetes.

In the DCCT, subjects with intensively treated type 1 diabetes and lower A1C levels had trends toward lower levels of LDL cholesterol and fewer myocardial infarctions and peripheral vascular events. Long-term follow-up of the intensively treated group revealed a significant reduction in ASCVD events and mortality in this group. Thirty-year data from the DCCT/EDIC and the Pittsburgh Epidemiology of Diabetes Complications Experience (EDC) studies, encompassing the years 1983–2005, showed the differential risk by conventional and intensive treatment groups for the DCCT/EDIC compared to the EDC cohort. After 30 years of diabetes, the cumulative incidences of cardiovascular disease were 14% in the DCCT conventional treatment group, 14% in the EDC cohort, and 9% in the DCCT intensive therapy group.

ASSESSMENT AND TREATMENT

Because of the high prevalence of cardiovascular risk factors in patients with diabetes and the ability of hyperglycemia to magnify the impact of these risk factors, physicians should consider all patients with type 1 diabetes to be at risk for developing macrovascular disease. They should systematically assess patients for risk factors for ASCVD (those mentioned above plus a family history of ASCVD), question them about symptoms of ASCVD, and be alert for signs of atherosclerosis. Lifestyle and pharmacologic treatments for modifying specific risk factors should be started. All patients with type 1 diabetes need to understand the critical importance of following a healthy lifestyle from childhood onward.

Although assessment of ASCVD can be done with noninvasive tests, for example with computed tomography angiography, and novel blood markers, such as inflammatory cytokines, it has not been determined how these tests add to risk stratification.

Dyslipidemia

Dyslipidemia in a patient with diabetes may result from poor metabolic control; use of certain drugs, including high-dose β-blockers (other than carvedilol), high-dose diuretics, systemic corticosteroids or other immunosuppressants, protease inhibitor antiviral agents, androgens, progestins (other than micronized progesterone or drospirenone), or estrogens; obesity; associated conditions such as hypothyroidism (the frequency of which is increased in type 1 diabetes); or inherited dyslipidemia. Each cause must be considered in assessing patients with diabetes and abnormal blood lipid levels.

Adults. The American Diabetes Association recommends that adult patients with diabetes undergo a screening lipid profile at the time of first diagnosis and/ or at age 40 years, and then every 1–2 years thereafter.

If dyslipidemia is present, the patient should be assessed for factors that aggravate dyslipidemia. Insulin treatment should be intensified in poorly controlled patients, but retesting will be necessary to be sure that additional therapy will be provided if abnormalities persist. Any drugs that might exacerbate hyperlipidemia should be discontinued or reduced where possible. The patient should be evaluated for renal disease and alcohol abuse. Genetic hyperlipidemia, separate from diabetes, is often the cause of moderate to marked hypercholesterolemia, and the treatment should be based on the etiology of the disorder and not limited to intensified insulin therapy.

The physician should be cognizant of the American College of Cardiology/ American Heart Association (ACC/AHA) 2013 cholesterol guidelines and the recently updated American Diabetes Association guidelines regarding dyslipidemia. Lifestyle factors, including medical nutrition therapy (MNT) and exercise, are a crucial component of cholesterol treatment for individuals with diabetes. In addition, the ACC/AHA guidelines recommend moderate or high-intensity statin treatment for all individuals with diabetes aged 40–75. The 2016 American Diabetes Association guidelines are generally in concordance with these recommendations (see Table 6.9). This approach is a departure from previous guidelines, and represents a shift away from older, more target-oriented guidelines.

Children. In children ≥10 years of age, a fasting lipid profile should be done soon after the diagnosis of diabetes once glucose control has been established. If lipids are abnormal then annual monitoring would be reasonable. If the LDL cholesterol values are within the accepted range (<100 mg/dL [2.6 mmol/L]) the lipid profile can be repeated every 3–5 years. For children with a significant family history of ASCVD, the National Heart, Lung, and Blood Institute recommends obtaining a fasting lipid panel beginning at 2 years of age. Initial therapy should involve glucose control and MNT. After the age of 10 years, the addition of a statin could be considered in children with LDL cholesterol >160 mg/dL or LDL cholesterol >130 mg/dL and one or more cardiovascular risk factors. The goal of therapy is an LDL cholesterol value <100 mg/dL. Statins are not approved for use in patients under 10 years of age, and are contraindicated in pregnancy. The SEARCH for Diabetes in Youth study has shown that mean

Table 6.9 American Diabetes Association Recommendations for Statin Treatment in People with Diabetes

Age	Risk Factors	Recommended Statin Dose*	Monitoring with Lipid Panel
<40 years	None	None	Annually or as needed to monitor for adherence
	ASCVD risk factor(s)**	Moderate or high	
	Overt ASCVD***	High	
40–75 years	None	Moderate	As needed to monitor adherence
	ASCVD risk factors	High	
	Overt ASCVD	High	
	ACS and LDL cholesterol >50 mg/dL in patients who cannot tolerate high-dose statins	Moderate plus ezetimibe	
>75 years	None	Moderate	As needed to monitor adherence
	ASCVD risk factors	Moderate or high	
	Overt ASCVD	High	
	ACS and LDL cholesterol >50 mg/dL in patients who cannot tolerate high-dose statins	Moderate plus ezetimibe	

* In addition to lifestyle therapy.

**ASCVD risk factors include LDL cholesterol $\geq$100 mg/dL (2.6 mmol/L), high blood pressure, smoking, and being overweight or obese.

***Overt ASCVD includes those with previous cardiovascular events or acute coronary syndromes (ACS).

Source: Adapted from American Diabetes Association. Standards of medical care in diabetes—2016. *Diabetes Care* 2016;39:S60–S71.

LDL-C is 100 mg/dL, HDL-C 55 mg/dL, and triglycerides 64 mg/dL in the cohort, and that 18% of youth with type 1 diabetes have high triglycerides, 10% have low HDL-C, 15% have a high LDL-C, and 21% have the metabolic syndrome.

Hypertension

Blood pressure should be measured in all patients with type 1 diabetes, including children and adolescents, at each physical examination. If hypertension develops, treatment should be initiated to reduce the risk of macrovascular and microvascular disease. Adults with blood pressure >120/80 mmHg should receive counseling about lifestyle modification. Adults with hypertension and diabetes should receive pharmacologic treatment with a goal blood pressure of <140/90 mmHg. In children, lifestyle intervention should be started in individuals with diabetes with high-normal blood pressure ($\geq$90th percentile for age, sex, and height). Children with hypertension (blood pressure $\geq$95th percentile for age, sex, and height) should be started on pharmacologic treatment, with a goal blood pressure <90th percentile for age, sex, and height.

When prescribing pharmacologic therapy, the clinician should consider the adverse effects of various antihypertensive drugs on hyperglycemia and hypoglycemia, electrolyte balance, renal function, lipid metabolism, ASCVD status, and neuropathic symptoms including orthostatic hypotension and impotence (Table 6.10). Overall, first-line therapy should include an ACE inhibitor or an ARB, with the addition of a second agent if blood pressure targets are not reached. The Eighth Joint National Committee (JNC 8) no longer singles out ACE inhibitors or ARBs for treatment of hypertension in individuals with diabetes, and now recommends either thiazide-type diuretics, calcium channel blockers, ACE inhibitors, or ARBs for first-line treatment. This is due largely to the lack of consistent evidence in populations with diabetes showing the superiority of ACE inhibitors and ARBs on ASCVD outcomes. However, due in part to the clear benefits of ACE inhibitors and ARBs in individuals with albuminuria or renal insufficiency, the American Diabetes Association continues to recommend ACE inhibitors or ARBs as first-line therapy in individuals with diabetes and hypertension. Kidney function and potassium should be monitored if blockers of the renin-angiotensin system are used. Studies have shown that renal protection ensues even if creatinine levels rise on a drug in this class. Women of childbearing potential should be counseled regarding the potential teratogenic effects of ACE inhibitors and ARBs. Ultimately, lowering of blood pressure may require multiple agents including ACE inhibitors, ARBs, β-blockers, diuretics, and calcium-channel blockers.

Cigarette Smoking

Each patient's smoking history should also be determined. Nonsmokers, particularly children and adolescents, should be encouraged not to begin, and

Table 6.10   Potential Interactions of Antihypertensive Medications in Type 1 Diabetes

Medication	Impact on Glycemia	Advantages/Disadvantages*
Diuretics	None (unlike type 2 diabetes, where hypokalemia reduces β-cell function)	None
Calcium-channel	None	Edema, increased blockers GI symptoms in patients with neuropathy
β-Blockers	May increase	Decreased hypoglycemic awareness
ACE inhibitors	None	Proven to reduce risk of diabetic kidney disease
ARBs	None	ARBs, like ACE inhibitors, can slow the progression of diabetic kidney disease
α-Blockers	None	Increased risk of orthostasis in patients with neuropathy

*Advantages and disadvantages are meant to be specific to type 1 diabetes and not to focus on generally appreciated attributes of the drugs.

smokers should be strongly urged to stop. The physician's advice not to smoke has an impact and represents time well spent. Advice should be reinforced with educational materials, medications, and referral to a smoking-cessation program.

SYMPTOMS AND SIGNS OF ATHEROSCLEROSIS

The physician should be particularly alert to the symptoms and signs of atherosclerosis in all patients with diabetes.

Cerebrovascular Disease

Symptoms of cerebrovascular disease include intermittent dizziness, transient loss of vision, slurring of speech, and paresthesia or weakness of one arm or leg. Vascular bruits may be heard over the carotid arteries. Noninvasive procedures, including Doppler and carotid ultrasound studies, may be helpful to confirm the diagnosis or detect earlier disease that can still be associated with symptoms.

Aspirin at a dose of 325 mg/day may prevent a recurrence of symptoms, and use of anticoagulant medications after a transient ischemic attack may help some patients. For many patients, 75–162 mg aspirin/day appear to provide comparable benefit with reduced risk of bleeding. Clopidogrel may be considered in aspirin-intolerant patients or patients who fail to respond to aspirin. Use of aspirin has not been studied in people with diabetes age <30 years.

Coronary Heart Disease

As in people without diabetes, CHD may be associated with chest pain, arm pain, or nausea. However, in people with diabetes, ischemia may occur in the absence of chest pain, particularly in women and those with cardiac autonomic neuropathy. Atypical symptoms such as fatigue, unexplained onset of congestive heart failure, and deterioration of glycemic control to the point of diabetic ketoacidosis may indicate silent myocardial ischemia. Myocardial infarction should be considered in the differential diagnosis of these conditions. Noninvasive procedures, including exercise tolerance tests, exercise thallium studies, and gated blood pool scans, may help establish the diagnosis of silent ischemia and/or myocardial perfusion defects. The utility, frequency, and cost-benefit ratios of these studies in older, asymptomatic patients to screen for CHD have not been determined. However, a plan to substantially increase physical activity in a previously inactive patient with long-standing type 1 diabetes should include consideration of stress test evaluation.

Therapy for CHD may be medical or surgical. Medical treatments include aspirin, nitrates, calcium-channel blockers, and cardioselective β-adrenergic blockers and agents that modify the renin-angiotensin system. Coronary angiography is necessary if bypass surgery or angioplasty is being considered. Bypass surgery is recommended for left main coronary artery disease and is generally indicated for triple-vessel disease, particularly in the presence of left ventricular dysfunction. Aggressive treatment of ASCVD risk factors, such as hypertension and dyslipidemia, is warranted in all patients with diabetes and CHD, and has been shown to have equal efficacy to aggressive risk factor treatment plus percutaneous procedures in patients with stable angina (including those with diabetes).

Peripheral Arterial Disease

Peripheral arterial disease (PAD) should be suspected in patients who complain of buttock, calf, or thigh pain that occurs during exercise and is relieved with rest (intermittent claudication) and/or who exhibit decreased pulses in the lower extremities. The diagnosis can be confirmed with noninvasive Doppler studies. Simple office screens for an abnormal ankle-brachial index (<0.9) can help to detect early disease.

The American Diabetes Association recommends that a screening ankle-brachial index be performed in patients over 50 years of age and be considered in patients under 50 years of age who have other risk factors for PAD such as smoking, hypertension, hyperlipidemia, or duration of diabetes >10 years. Sclerotic vessels can lead to falsely elevated systolic blood pressure and invalid results. Otherwise, a decreased index not only indicates a patient with peripheral arterial disease but is also a strong indicator of possible coronary artery disease and future cardiac mortality.

Aspirin, exercise, and smoking cessation are critical components of treatment. If pain is incapacitating or persists at rest, or if a foot infection results from impaired blood flow through the major leg arteries, angioplasty or surgery to bypass the diseased vessels may be indicated. Treatment with either cilostazol or pentoxifylline may improve symptoms. But aspirin and exercise are important adjuncts to treatment.

Aspirin Therapy in Type 1 Diabetes

Aspirin therapy (75–162 mg/day) should be used as a secondary prevention strategy in those with diabetes and a history of atherosclerotic cardiovascular disease. Aspirin therapy (75–162 mg/day) should be considered for primary ASCVD prevention in type 1 diabetes in patients with an increased risk of ASCVD, defined as a 10-year risk >10%. This includes most men >50 years of age and women >60 years of age who have at least one additional major risk factor including family history of ASCVD, hypertension, smoking, dyslipidemia, or albuminuria. Aspirin is not recommended for primary ASCVD prevention for adults with diabetes at low risk of ASCVD, defined as a 10-year risk <5%, such as men <50 years of age and women <60 years of age with no major additional ASCVD risk factors. Clinical judgment is required for adults with diabetes with intermediate risk.

CONCLUSION

Patients with type 1 diabetes should be aware of their increased risk of ASCVD and advised of the importance of modifying risk factors such as hypertension, hyperlipidemia, and cigarette smoking. Clinicians should systematically assess patients for risk factors for ASCVD and attempt to modify them. They should question patients about symptoms of ASCVD, examine them for signs of atherosclerosis, and seek the expertise of appropriate specialists when needed.

BIBLIOGRAPHY

Ali MK, Bullard KM, Saaddine JB, Cowie CC, Imperatore G, Gregg EW. Achievement of goals in U.S. diabetes care, 1999–2010. *N Eng J Med* 2013;368:1613–1624

American Diabetes Association. Standards of medical care in diabetes—2016. *Diabetes Care* 2016;39(Suppl. 1):S1–S112

American Diabetes Association. Peripheral arterial disease in people with diabetes. *Diabetes Care* 2003;26:3333–3341

Bax JJ, Young LH, Frye RL, Bonow RO, Steinberg HO, Barrett EJ; American Diabetes Association. Screening for coronary artery disease in patients with diabetes (Consensus Statement). *Diabetes Care* 2007;30:2729–2736

Borg R, Kuenen JC, Cartensen B, Zheng H, Nathan DM, Heine RJ, Nerup J, Borch-Johnsen K, Witte DR; on behalf of the ADAG Study Group. HbA1C and mean blood glucose show stronger associations with cardiovascular disease risk factors than do postprandial glycaemia or glucose variability in persons with diabetes: the A1C-Derived Average Glucose (ADAG) study. *Diabetologia* 2011;54:69–72

Campos H, Moye LA, Glasser SP, Stampfer MJ, Sacks FM. Low-density lipoprotein size, pravastatin treatment, and coronary events. *JAMA* 2001;286:1468–1474

DCCT Research Group. The effect of intensive treatment of diabetes on the development and progression of long-term complications on insulin-dependent diabetes mellitus. *N Engl J Med* 1993;329:977–986

De Ferranti SD, de Boer IH, Fonseca V, Fox CS, Golden SH, Lavie CJ, Magge SN, Marx N, McGuire DK, Orchard TJ, Zinman B, Eckel RH. Type 1 diabetes mellitus and cardiovascular disease: a scientific statement from the American Heart Association and American Diabetes Association. *Diabetes Care* 2014;37:2843–2863

Diabetes Control and Complications Trial/Epidemiology of Diabetes Interventions and Complications Research Group, Nathan DM, Zinman B, Cleary PA, et al. The modern-day clinical course of type 1 diabetes mellitus after 30 years' duration: the Diabetes Control and Complications Trial/Epidemiology of Diabetes Interventions and Complications and Pittsburgh Epidemiology of Diabetes Complications Experience (1983-2005). *Arch Intern Med* 2009;169:1307–1316

Eeg-Olofsson K, Cederholm J, Nilsson PM, Zethelius B, Svensson AM, Gudbjornsdottir S, Eliasson B. Glycemic control and cardiovascular disease in 7454 patients with type 1 diabetes: an observational study for the Swedish National Diabetes Register. *Diabetes Care* 2010;33:1640–1646

James PA, Oparil S, Carter BL, Cushman WC, Dennison-Himmelfarb C, Handler J, Lackland DT, LeFevre ML, MacKenzie TD, Ogedegbe O, Smith SC Jr,

Svetkey LP, Taker SJ, Townsend RR, Wright JT Jr, Narva AS, Ortiz E. 2014 evidence-based guideline for the management of high blood pressure in adults: report from the panel members appointed to the Eighth Joint National Committee (JNC 8). *JAMA* 2014;311:507–520

Kavey RE, Allada V, Daniels SR, Hayman LL, McCrindle BW, Newburger JW, Parekh RS, Steinberger J, et al. Cardiovascular risk reduction in high-risk pediatric patients: a scientific statement from the American Heart Association Expert Panel on Population and Prevention Science; the Councils on Cardiovascular Disease in the Young, Epidemiology and Prevention, Nutrition, Physical Activity and Metabolism, High Blood Pressure Research, Cardiovascular Nursing, and the Kidney in Heart Disease; and the Interdisciplinary Working Group on Quality of Care and Outcomes Research. Endorsed by the American Academy of Pediatrics. *Circulation* 2006;114:2710–2738

Lachin JM, Orchard TJ, Nathan DM; for the DCCT/EDIC Research Group. Update on cardiovascular outcomes at 30 years of the Diabetes Control and Complications Trial/Epidemiology of Diabetes Interventions and Complications Study. *Diabetes Care* 2014;37:39–43

Maahs DM, Daniels SR, de Ferranti SD, Dichek HL, Flynn J, Goldstein BI, Kelley AS, Nadeau KJ, Nartyn-Nemeth P, Osganian SK, Quinn L, Shah AS, Urbina E, et al. Cardiovascular disease risk factors in youth with diabetes mellitus: a scientific statement from the American Heart Association. *Circulation* 2014;130:1532–1558

Nathan DM, Cleary PA, Backlund JY, Genuth SM, Lachin JM, Orchard TJ, Raskin P, Zinman B; DCCT/EDIC Study Research Group. Intensive diabetes treatment and cardiovascular disease in patients with type 1 diabetes. *N Engl J Med* 2005;353:2643–2653

Polak JF, Backlund JY, Cleary PA, Harrington AP, O'Leary DH, Lachin JM, Nathan DM; for the DCCT/EDIC Research Group. Progression of carotid artery intima-media thickness during 12 years in the Diabetes Control and Complications Trial/Epidemiology of Diabetes Interventions and Complications (DCCT/EDIC) Study. *Diabetes* 2011;60:607–613

Rodriguez BL, Fujimoto WY, Mayer-David EJ, Imperatore G, Williams DE, Bell RA, Wadwa RP, Palla SL, Liu LL, Kershnar A, Daniels SR, Linder B; for the SEARCH for Diabetes in Youth Study Group. Prevalence of cardiovascular disease risk factors in U.S. children and adolescents with diabetes. *Diabetes Care* 2006;29:1891–1896

Stone NJ, Robinson JG, Lichtenstein AH, Bairey Merz CN, Blum CB, Eckel RH, Goldberg AC, Gordon D, Levy D, Lloyd-Jones DM, McBride P, Schwartz JS, Shero ST, Smith SC Jr, Watson K, Wilson PW; American College of Cardiology/American Heart Association Task Force on Practice Guidelines. 2013 ACC/AHA guideline on the treatment of blood cholesterol to reduce atherosclerotic cardiovascular risk in adults: a report of the American College of Cardiology/American Heart Association Task Force on Practice Guidelines. *J Am Coll Cardiol* 2014;63(25 Pt B):2889–2934

MUSCULOSKELETAL COMPLICATIONS

Diabetes is associated with complications in multiple organ systems, and the musculoskeletal system must be not be forgotten among the systems involved. Patients with type 1 diabetes are at increased risk for fragility fractures and limited joint mobility. These complications are discussed in this section.

OSTEOPOROSIS

Type 1 diabetes is associated with low bone density, particularly in the radius in children and adolescents, which is postulated to be due to low peak bone mass from impaired peak bone formation. Adults with type 1 diabetes tend to have lower bone density at the femur but similar bone mineral density (BMD) at the lumbar spine when compared with individuals without diabetes, although this also depends on the specific population examined. However, patients with diabetes are at higher risk for fractures at all sites despite similar BMD, so dual energy X-ray absorptiometry (DEXA) scores may not accurately represent bone strength and risk for fractures in this population. A large meta-analysis including data from more than 1 million patients showed an odds ratio (OR) of 6.3–6.9 for hip fracture in patients with type 1 diabetes (Merlotti D 2010), and the Women's Health Study reported an OR of 12.3 for hip fracture in postmenopausal women with type 1 diabetes as compared with an OR of 1.7 in patients with type 2 diabetes.

The mechanisms underlying this increased risk are poorly understood, although *in vitro* and *in vivo* studies support the presence of impaired bone formation but not to excessive bone resorption. There have been suggestions that insulin itself may have osteometabolic effects, although this has been difficult to separate from the effects of glycemic control and other complications that affect BMD. In addition, β-cells produce osteotropic factors such as amylin, which is a member of the calcitonin gene–related peptide family and appears to play a role in bone mass and strength. Osteocalcin is another factor that may play an important role.

Risk factors for fragility fractures appear to include degree of glycemic control and presence and severity of vascular complications (particularly neurologic and renal), although in some studies, age and body mass index appear to play a role while A1C, duration of diabetes, and vascular complications do not. The presence of diabetic kidney disease increases the risk of hip fracture 12-fold. In addition, patients lose whole body calcium via hypercalciuria during periods of glycosuria associated with poor glycemic control. Periods of poor glycemic control may also be associated with higher risk for falls (because of dehydration), slower-to-heal fractures, and higher risk for infection.

It is important to identify at-risk patients prior to development of fractures. Relevant history includes a history of falls, gait disturbances, visual impairment, polyneuropathy, and hypoglycemic episodes. Medication review must include a specific focus on those that may increase the risk of falls, such as medications for insomnia and other medications that may cause drowsiness such as antidepressants. Physical exam should include an assessment of body weight (risk factors would include low body weight or evidence of malnutrition), hypogonadism, and muscle atrophy. Laboratory studies for suspected osteoporosis include a complete blood count (CBC), complete chemistries for renal and liver function, calcium, phosphate, 25-hydroxyvitamin D level, thyroid-stimulating hormone, and depending on suspicion of hypogonadism, reproductive hormones. In older adults with suspected osteoporosis, evaluation of serum protein electrophoresis/urine protein electrophoresis (SPEP/UPEP) may be appropriate. Other testing may be required depending on comorbidities and findings in history or exam. There are no standard recommendations regarding screening for osteoporosis with DEXA scan for BMD. Bone turnover markers are of limited value.

The online fracture risk assessment (FRAX) tool (www.shef.ac.uk/FRAX/) for calculation of an individual's 10-year risk of major osteoporotic fracture and hip fracture considers patients with type 1 diabetes to have secondary osteoporosis, and fracture risk thresholds of ≥3% for hip fracture and ≥20% for major osteoporotic fracture are used to help guide the need for specific osteoporosis therapy.

Treatment should include good glycemic control with prevention of and screening for vascular complications, assessing risk for and prevention of falls, adequate calcium and vitamin D supplementation if needed, and if indicated, osteoporosis-specific therapy. However the latter are usually not indicated in children and adolescents, and in women of childbearing age, clinicians must take into consideration the prolonged half-life in bone of bisphosphonates, which may have unintended long-term consequences. Other therapies including anabolic therapies should be reserved for patients with clear evidence of osteoporosis and/or osteoporotic fractures.

LIMITED JOINT MOBILITY (CHEIROARTHROPATHY)

Limited joint mobility, or what is now termed cheiroarthropathy, was formerly one of the earliest and most common clinical complications seen in type 1 diabetes. Since the Diabetes Control and Complications Trial, it was believed that there was a marked decrease in prevalence of cheiroarthropathy in both children and adults. Unfortunately, this long-term complication of diabetes has received little attention, has not been well studied in clinical research studies, and likely is not well recognized in clinical care. However, if cheiroarthropathy is present, it is a potentially important clinical marker for diabetes complications such as retinopathy, diabetic kidney disease, neuropathy, and abnormalities in growth stature.

Risk Factors

Cheiroarthropathy is strongly associated with duration of diabetes, particularly individuals with a ~30 year history of type 1 diabetes or longer. Accumulation of advanced glycation end products associated with chronic hyperglycemia may be responsible for cheiroarthropathy. Other risk factors include advanced age and the presence of microvascular complications.

Definition

Diabetic cheiroarthropathy is characterized by thickened skin and limited mobility of joints in the hands and fingers leading to flexion contractures. In a recent analysis by the DCCT/EDIC investigators, it was defined as the presence of any one of the following findings: adhesive capsulitis, carpal tunnel syndrome, flexor tenosynovitis, Dupuytren's contracture, or positive prayer sign.

Detection and Evaluation

Cheiroarthropathy may occur in children or adults, is painless, and may cause little disability at first. Thus, it is unlikely to be brought to the attention of family members or health-care professionals. The best way to detect early cheiroarthropathy is to examine hands and joints as part of routine physical examinations.

To evaluate for cheiroarthropathy, the following should be included: 1) observe and shake both hands of the patient, noting any scleroderma-like stiffness of the skin, and 2) ask the patient to place the hands in a clapping or "prayer" position with forearms as parallel to the floor as possible (Figure 6.7). Any inability to oppose the joints of the fingers and any limitation of flexion or extension of wrist, elbow, neck, or spine should be documented.

If pain or neuromuscular findings (e.g., atrophy, paresthesia) are present, other disorders, such as tenosynovitis or carpal tunnel syndrome, should be considered. In adults, another possibility is Dupuytren's contracture, which is painless and characterized by palmar nodules and involvement of the third and fourth fingers.

Because there is a relationship between the severity of cheiroarthropathy and the microvascular complications of diabetes, patients found to have cheiroarthropathy at an office visit should be carefully examined for clinical evidence of retinopathy via ophthalmoscopy; for diabetic kidney disease by a quantitative determination of urinary albumin excretion; and for hypertension, hepatomegaly, and neuropathy by careful clinical examination.

Although the prevalence of cheiroarthropathy has markedly decreased in children and adults due to improved glycemic control, a recent analysis by the DCCT/EDIC Research Group demonstrated that the prevalence was 66% among study

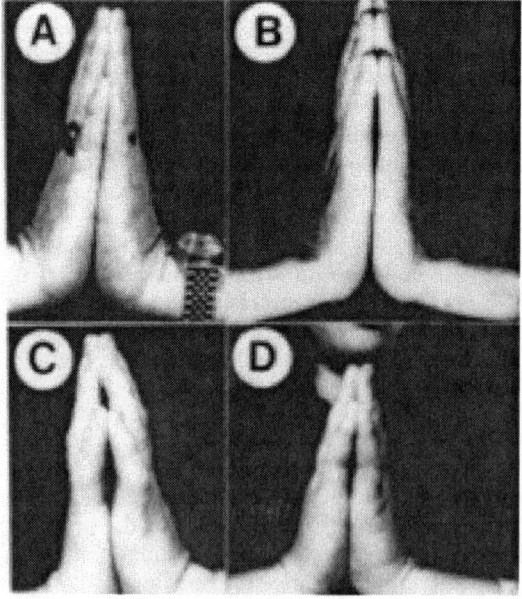

Figure 6.7 LJM of increasing severity.
A: Normal joint mobility.
B: Bilateral contracture of 5th fingers.
C: Bilateral contracture of more than fifth fingers.
D: Bilateral wrist involvement.

participants after a mean duration of diabetes of 30 years, with adhesive capsulitis of the shoulder being the most frequent disorder (31%), followed closely by carpal tunnel syndrome (30%), and flexor tenosynovitis (28%). The presence of cheiroarthropathy remains an important clinical marker of coexistent microvascular disease. In addition, the presence of this disorder may cause significant morbidity with decreased function and quality of life. Surveillance for cheiroarthropathy should be included in the routine screening for complications in patients with type 1 diabetes.

BIBLIOGRAPHY

Aljahlan M, Lee KC, Toth E. Limited joint mobility in diabetes. *Postgrad Med* 1999;105:99–101, 105–106

Duffin AC, Conaghue KC, Potter M, McInnes A, Chan AK, King J, Howard NJ, Silink M. Limited joint mobility in the hands and feet of adolescents with type 1 diabetes mellitus. *Diabet Med* 1999;16:125–130

Frost D, Beischer W. Limited joint mobility in type 1 diabetic patients: associations with microangiopathy and subclinical macroangiopathy are different in men and women. *Diabetes Care* 2001;24:95–99

Hamann C, Kirschner S, Klaus-Peter G, Hofbauer LC. Bone, sweet bone—osteoporotic fractures in diabetes mellitus. *Nat Rev Endocrinol* 2012;8:297–305

Hofbauer LC, Brueck CC, Singh SK, Dobnig H. Osteoporosis in patients with diabetes mellitus. *J Bone Min Res* 2007;22:1317–1328

Larkin ME, Barnie A, Braffett BH, Cleary PA, Diminick L, Harth J, Gatcomb P, Golden E, Lipps J, Lorenzi G, Mahony C, Nathan DM; and the Diabetes Control and Complications Trial/Epidemiology of Diabetes Interventions and Complications Research Group. Musculoskeletal complications in type 1 diabetes. *Diabetes Care* 2014;37:1863–1869

Leidig-Bruckner G, Grobholz S, Bruckner T, Scheidt-Nave C, Nawroth P, Schneider JG. Prevalence and determinants of osteoporosis in patients with type 1 and type 2 diabetes mellitus. *BMC Endocrine Disord* 2014;14:33

Lindsay JR, Kennedy L, Atkinson AB, Bell PM, Carson DJ, McCance DR, Hunter SJ. Reduced prevalence of limited joint mobility in type 1 diabetes in a U.K. clinic population over a 20-year period. *Diabetes Care* 2005;28:658–661

Merlotti D, Gennari L, Dotta F, Lauro D, Nuti R. Mechanisms of impaired bone strength in type 1 and type 2 diabetes. *Nutr Metab Cardiovasc Dis* 2010;20:683–690

Nicodemus KK, Folsom AR; Iowa Women's Health Study. Type 1 and type 2 diabetes and incident hip fractures in postmenopausal women. *Diabetes Care* 2001;24:1192–1197

Vestergaard P, Renjmark L, Mosekilde L. Relative fracture risk in patients with diabetes mellitus, and the impact of insulin and oral antidiabetic medication on relative fracture risk. *Diabetologia* 2005;48:1292–1299

ABNORMAL LINEAR GROWTH

Abnormalities of height (absolute short stature as well as decreased growth velocity) are known consequences of insulin deficiency. Although the classic example occurs in the extreme and relatively rare Mauriac syndrome (diabetic dwarfism), subtle abnormalities of growth and development are not uncommon among young people with type 1 diabetes. Patients with poorly controlled diabetes have decreased insulin-like growth factor-1 levels and paradoxical increments in growth hormone levels during the night and in response to provocative stimuli. These abnormalities can be prevented or corrected with better glycemic control.

SUBTLE GROWTH ABNORMALITIES

Growth abnormalities become apparent when large patient populations are studied and subtle growth changes are sought, including a lag in height or weight or a deviation from previously established growth curves (Figures 6.8 and 6.9). Defined in this fashion, 5–10% of young people with type 1 diabetes will not grow well. Children most likely to be affected are those with the earliest onset of diabetes and those who have the worst day-to-day glycemic control and the highest A1C levels. Boys are two or three times more likely to have a growth abnormality than girls.

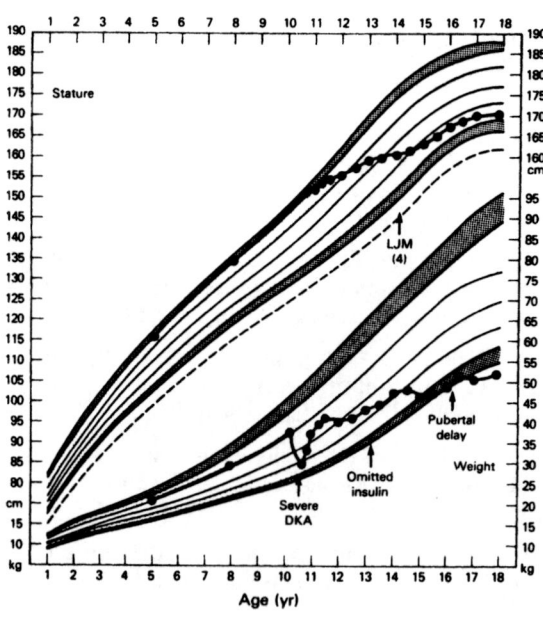

Figure 6.8 Inadequate diabetes control and growth abnormalities. Growth deceleration solely from uncontrolled diabetes. Patient refused to take two shots of insulin each day. Most of the time, patient omitted morning insulin and refused to follow any type of meal plan. The family refused psychiatric consultation.

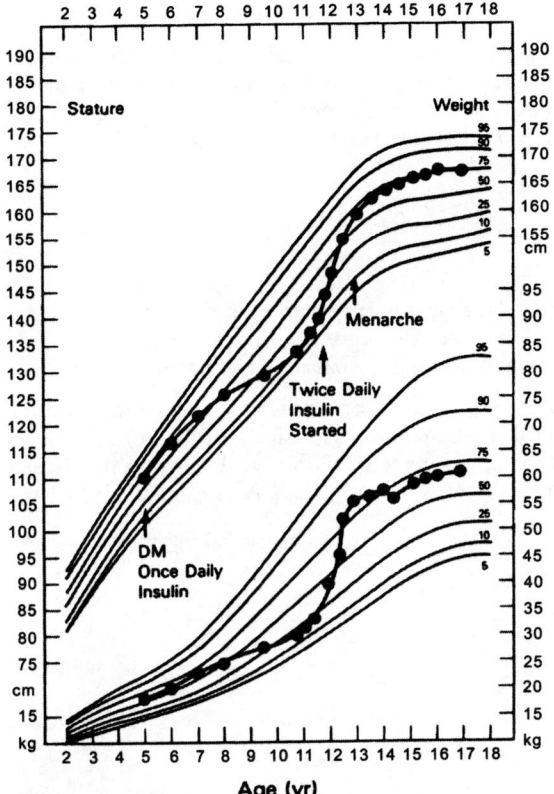

Figure 6.9 Catch-up growth phenomenon with adequate insulin. Growth data from child with type 1 diabetes treated with one shot of morning insulin, showing growth deceleration and catch-up growth phenomenon after twice-daily insulin was started.

DETERMINING GROWTH RATE

The only way to determine whether growth is adequate is to measure height and weight at each office visit and to plot data on standardized growth charts. Ideally, data should be recorded at least every 3–4 months; at minimum, height and weight should be measured and recorded annually. Growth data obtained from other family members may be extremely valuable in placing an individual patient's growth in perspective. Bone age determination (single radiograph of left wrist and hand compared with standard radiographs) coupled with other hormonal measurements may help assess the need for further evaluation. If growth abnormalities are found, the child should be evaluated for the presence of hypothyroidism and celiac disease. If no comorbidity is found, metabolic status should be carefully evaluated and appropriate recommendations for improvement made, such as changing to an intensified insulin treatment program.

CONCLUSION

Although mild growth retardation may not be totally preventable, evidence strongly indicates that major alterations in growth rate can be avoided by better blood glucose control in children. Therefore, the definition of adequate diabetes control must include the attainment and maintenance of normal growth and development.

BIBLIOGRAPHY

Chiang JL, Kirkman MS, Laffel LM, Peters AL; on behalf of the Type 1 Diabetes Sourcebook Authors. Type 1 diabetes through the life span: a position statement of the American Diabetes Association. *Diabetes Care* 2014;37:2034–2054

Silverstein J, Klingensmith G, Copeland K, Plotnick L, Kaufman FR, Laffel L, Deeb L, Grey M, Anderson B, Holzmeister LA,Clark N; American Diabetes Association. Care of children and adolescents with type 1 diabetes mellitus: a statement of the American Diabetes Association. *Diabetes Care* 2005;28:186–212

Index

Note: Page numbers followed by *t* refer to tables. Page numbers followed by *f* refer to figures. Page numbers in **bold** indicate an in-depth discussion on the topic.

A

α-1 antitrypsin, 24
A1C. *See* glycated hemoglobin (A1C)
abatacept (CTLA-4 Ig), 24
ABCC8, 10*t*, 11*t*, 12, 99
abdominal pain, 56*t*, 170, 179
α-blockers, 291*t*
abnormal linear growth, 300–301
Academy of Nutrition and Dietetics, 144
ACE inhibitor, 188
acesulfame potassium, 133
acetoacetic acid, 17, 169
acetone, 119
acetylcysteine, 268*t*
acidosis, 169, 172, 173*t*, 174–175, 179
Action to Control Cardiovascular Risk in Diabetes blood pressure (ACCORD BP) trial, 269
Addison's disease, 22
adequate intake (AI), 133
adherence, 94–95, 225–226, 232
adiponectin, 9
adipose tissue, 17*t*, 151*t*, 152
adjunctive therapy, 104, 105*t*, 106–110
adolescent
  A1C values, 41–42
  caloric requirement, 127
  continuous glucose monitoring, 234
  developmental considerations, 229*t*, 231–236

diabetes management team factor, 233–234
diabetic ketoacidosis, 170*t*
disordered eating, 140
education, 233
Estimated Energy Requirement, 128
exercise, 150
family, 229*t*, 233
glucagon-like peptide-1 (GLP-1), 107
growth years, 137
hormonal change, 232
hypertension, 290
idiopathic type 1 diabetes, 9
long-term therapy, 78
management priorities, 229*t*
metformin, 108
monitoring, 234–236
nocturnal hypoglycemia, 118
patient factor, 233
peer influence, 232
psychosocial issue, 54
self-care regimen, 231
self-monitoring of blood glucose, 234–236
treatment regimen, 226
type 2 diabetes, 8
adrenergic counterregulatory response, 109, 152
adult, 236
adult-onset diabetes. *See* type 2 diabetes

CPSIA information can be obtained
at www.ICGtesting.com
Printed in the USA
FFOW05n0357010317